GERIATRICS *At Your* FINGERTIPS®

2019, 21st EDITION

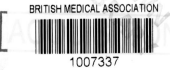

GERIATRICS *At Your* FINGERTIPS®

2019, 21st EDITION

AUTHORS

David B. Reuben, MD

Keela A. Herr, PhD, RN

James T. Pacala, MD, MS

Bruce G. Pollock, MD, PhD

Jane F. Potter, MD

Todd P. Semla, MS, PharmD

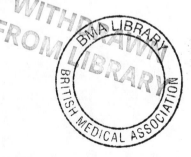

Geriatrics At Your Fingertips® is published by the American Geriatrics Society as a service to healthcare providers involved in the care of older adults.

Although *Geriatrics At Your Fingertips*® is distributed by various companies in the healthcare field, it is independently prepared and published. All decisions regarding its content are solely the responsibility of the authors. Their decisions are not subject to any form of approval by other interests or organizations.

Some recommendations in this publication suggest the use of agents for purposes or in dosages other than those recommended in product labeling. Such recommendations are based on reports in peer-reviewed publications and are not based on or influenced by any material or advice from pharmaceutical or healthcare product manufacturers.

No responsibility is assumed by the authors or the American Geriatrics Society for any injury or damage to persons or property, as a matter of product liability, negligence, warranty, or otherwise, arising out of the use or application of any methods, products, instructions, or ideas contained herein. No guarantee, endorsement, or warranty of any kind, express or implied (including specifically no warrant of merchantability or of fitness for a particular purpose) is given by the Society in connection with any information contained herein. Independent verification of any diagnosis, treatment, or drug use or dosage should be obtained. No test or procedure should be performed unless, in the judgment of an independent, qualified physician, it is justified in the light of the risk involved.

Citation: Reuben DB, Herr KA, Pacala JT, et al. *Geriatrics At Your Fingertips: 2019, 21st Edition*. New York: The American Geriatrics Society; 2019.

Copyright © 2019 by the American Geriatrics Society.

ISSN 1553-152X
ISBN 978-1-886775-62-6

TABLE OF CONTENTS

AUTHORS

David B. Reuben, MD
Director, Multicampus Program in Geriatric Medicine and Gerontology
Chief, Division of Geriatrics
Archstone Foundation Chair
Professor of Medicine
David Geffen School of Medicine at UCLA, Los Angeles, CA

Keela A. Herr, PhD, RN
Kelting Professor in Nursing and Associate Dean for Faculty
Co-Director, Csomay Center for Gerontological Excellence
College of Nursing
The University of Iowa, Iowa City, IA

James T. Pacala, MD, MS
Professor and Head
Department of Family Medicine and Community Health
University of Minnesota Medical School, Minneapolis, MN

Bruce G. Pollock, MD, PhD, FRCPC, DFAPA
Peter and Shelagh Godsoe Chair in Late-Life Mental Health
Vice President, Research
Director, Campbell Family Mental Health Research Institute
Centre for Addiction and Mental Health
Professor of Psychiatry and Pharmacology
University of Toronto, Toronto, Ontario, Canada

Jane F. Potter, MD
Professor, Internal Medicine, Geriatrics
Director, Home Instead Center for Successful Aging
University of Nebraska Medical Center, Omaha, NE

Todd P. Semla, MS, PharmD
Associate Professor, Clinical
Departments of Medicine and Psychiatry & Behavioral Sciences
The Feinberg School of Medicine
Northwestern University, Chicago, IL

1,25(OH)2D	1,25-dihydroxyvitamin D
25(OH)D	25-hydroxyvitamin D
A_{1c}	glycosylated hemoglobin
AAA	abdominal aortic aneurysm
AAOS	American Academy of Orthopaedic Surgeons
AASM	American Academy of Sleep Medicine
ABG	arterial blood gas
ABI	ankle-brachial index
ACC	American College of Cardiology
ACEI	angiotensin-converting enzyme inhibitor
ACI	anemia of chronic inflammation
ACIP	Advisory Committee on Immunization Practices
ACOG	American College of Obstetrics and Gynecology
ACP	advance care planning
ACR	American College of Rheumatology
ACS	acute coronary syndrome
ACTH	adrenocorticotropic hormone
AD	Alzheimer disease
ADA	American Diabetes Association
ADLs	activities of daily living
ADT	androgen deprivation therapy
AE	adverse event
AF	atrial fibrillation
AGS	American Geriatrics Society
AHA	American Heart Association
AHI	Apnea-Hypopnea Index
AHRQ	Agency for Healthcare Research and Quality
AIDS	acquired immune deficiency syndrome
AIMS	Abnormal Involuntary Movement Scale
ALS	amyotrophic lateral sclerosis
ALT	alanine aminotransferase
AMD	age-related macular degeneration
APAP	acetaminophen
APRN	advanced practice nurse
ARB	angiotensin receptor blocker
AS	aortic stenosis
ASA	acetylsalicylic acid or aspirin
ASA Class	American Society of Anesthesiologists grading scale for surgical patients
AST	aspartate aminotransferase
ATA	American Thyroid Association
ATS	American Thoracic Society
AUA	American Urological Association
BC	Beers Criteria
BMD	bone mineral density
BMI	body mass index
BP	blood pressure
BPH	benign prostatic hyperplasia
bpm	beats per minute

BUN	blood urea nitrogen
C&S	culture and sensitivity
CABG	coronary artery bypass graft
CAD	coronary artery disease
CAM	Confusion Assessment Method
CBC	complete blood cell count
CBD	cannabidiol
CBT	cognitive-behavioral therapy
CCB	calcium-channel blocker
CCP	cyclic citrullinated peptide (antibody test)
CDC	US Centers for Disease Control and Prevention
CDR	Clinical Dementia Rating Scale
cfu	colony-forming unit
$CHADS_2$	Congestive heart failure, Hypertension, Age ≥75, Diabetes, Stroke (doubled) (score)
CHA_2DS_2- VASc	Congestive heart failure, Hypertension, Age ≥75 (doubled), Diabetes, Stroke (doubled), Vascular disease, Age 65–74, and Sex (female) (score)
CHD	coronary heart disease
CKD	chronic kidney disease
CMS	Centers for Medicare and Medicaid Services
CNS	central nervous system
COPD	chronic obstructive pulmonary disease
CPAP	continuous positive airway pressure
Cr	creatinine
CrCl	creatinine clearance
CRP	C-reactive protein
CSF	cerebrospinal fluid
CT	computed tomography
CVD	cardiovascular disease
cw	Choosing Wisely recommendation
CXR	chest x-ray
CYP	cytochrome P-450
D&C	dilation and curettage
D5W	dextrose 5% in water
DASH	Dietary Approaches to Stop Hypertension
DBP	diastolic blood pressure
D/C	discontinue
DHIC	detrusor hyperactivity with impaired contractility
DM	diabetes mellitus
DMARD	disease-modifying antirheumatoid drug
DOAC	direct oral anticoagulant
DPI	dry powder inhaler
DPP-4	dipeptidyl peptidase 4
DSM-5	Diagnostic and Statistical Manual of Mental Disorders, 5th ed. (Arlington, VA: American Psychiatric Association; 2013)
DVT	deep-vein thrombosis
EBRT	external beam radiation therapy
ECF	extracellular fluid
ECG	electrocardiogram, electrocardiography
ED	erectile dysfunction
EEG	electroencephalogram
EF	ejection fraction
eGFR	estimated glomerular filtration rate

EHR	electronic health record
EPS	extrapyramidal symptoms
ESA	erythropoietin-stimulating agents
ESRD	end-stage renal disease
ESR	erythrocyte sedimentation rate
EULAR	European League Against Rheumatism
FAST	Reisberg Functional Assessment Staging Scale
FDA	Food and Drug Administration
FEV_1	forced expiratory volume in 1 sec
FI	fecal incontinence
FOBT	fecal occult blood test
FRAX	WHO Fracture Risk Assessment Tool
FTD	frontotemporal dementia
FVC	forced vital capacity
GAD	generalized anxiety disorder
GDS	Geriatric Depression Scale
GERD	gastroesophageal reflux disease
GFR	glomerular filtration rate
GI	gastrointestinal
GLP–1	glucagon-like peptide–1
GnRH	gonadotropin-releasing hormone
GU	genitourinary
Hb	hemoglobin
HCTZ	hydrochlorothiazide
HDL	high-density lipoprotein
HF	heart failure
HR	heart rate
HT	hormone therapy
HTN	hypertension
hx	history
IADLs	instrumental activities of daily living
IBS	irritable bowel syndrome
IBS-C	irritable bowel syndrome with constipation
IBW	ideal body weight
ICD	implantable cardiac defibrillator
ICU	intensive care unit
Ig	immunoglobulin (eg, IgE, IgM)
IL	interleukin (eg, IL-1, IL-6)
INH	isoniazid
INR	international normalized ratio
IOP	intraocular pressure
iPTH	intact parathyroid hormone
JNC 8	Eighth Joint National Committee on Prevention, Detection, Evaluation, and Treatment of High Blood Pressure
K^+	potassium ion
LBD	Lewy body dementia
LBW	lean body weight
LDL	low-density lipoprotein
L-dopa	levodopa
LFT	liver function test
LMWH	low-molecular-weight heparin
LVEF	left ventricular ejection fraction

LVH	left ventricular hypertrophy
MAOI	monoamine oxidase inhibitor
MCI	mild cognitive impairment
MCV	mean corpuscular volume
MDI	metered-dose inhaler
MDRD	Modification of Diet in Renal Disease
MDS	myelodysplastic syndromes
MI	myocardial infarction
MMA	methylmalonic acid
MMSE	Mini-Mental State Examination (Folstein's)
MoCA	Montreal Cognitive Assessment
MRA	magnetic resonance angiography
MRI	magnetic resonance imaging
MRSA	methicillin-resistant *Staphylococcus aureus*
MSE	mental status examination
NICE	National Institute for Health and Clinical Excellence (for the United Kingdom)
NIH	National Institutes of Health
NIHSS	National Institutes of Health Stroke Scale
NNRTI	non-nucleoside reverse transcriptase inhibitor
NPH	neutral protamine Hagedorn (insulin)
NSAID	nonsteroidal anti-inflammatory drug
NYHA	New York Heart Association
OA	osteoarthritis
OGTT	oral glucose tolerance test
OIC	opioid-induced constipation
ORT	Opioid Risk Tool
OSA	obstructive sleep apnea
OT	occupational therapy
PAD	peripheral arterial disease
PAH	pulmonary arterial hypertension
PCA	patient-controlled analgesia
PCSK9	proprotein convertase subtilisin/kexin type 9
PDE5	phosphodiesterase type 5
PE	pulmonary embolism
PET	positron-emission tomography
POLST	Physician Orders for Life-Sustaining Treatment
PONV	postoperative nausea and vomiting
PPD	purified protein derivative (of tuberculin)
PPI	proton-pump inhibitor
PSA	prostate-specific antigen
PT	prothrombin time *or* physical therapy
PTH	parathyroid hormone
PTT	partial thromboplastin time
PUVA	psoralen plus ultraviolet light of A wavelength
QTc	QT (cardiac output) corrected for heart rate
RA	rheumatoid arthritis
RBC	red blood cells *or* ranitidine bismuth citrate
RCT	randomized controlled trial
RF	rheumatoid factor
RLD	restrictive lung disease
RLS	restless legs syndrome
RR	respiratory rate

sats	saturations
SBP	systolic blood pressure
SD	standard deviation
SGLT2	sodium glucose co-transporter 2
SIADH	syndrome of inappropriate secretion of antidiuretic hormone
SLUMS	St Louis University Mental Status (examination)
SMI	soft mist inhalers
SNRI	serotonin norepinephrine-reuptake inhibitor
SPEP	serum protein electrophoresis
SSRI	selective serotonin-reuptake inhibitor
TBW	total body weight
TCA	tricyclic antidepressant
TD	tardive dyskinesia
TG	triglycerides
THC	tetrahydrocannabinol
TIA	transient ischemic attack
TIBC	total iron-binding capacity
TNF	tumor necrosis factor
TSH	thyroid-stimulating hormone
TURP	transurethral resection of the prostate
tx	treatment(s), therapy (-ies)
U	unit(s)
UA	urinalysis
UFH	unfractionated heparin
UI	urinary incontinence
USPSTF	US Preventive Services Task Force
UTI	urinary tract infection
UV	ultraviolet
VEGF	vascular endothelial growth factor
VF	ventricular fibrillation
VIN	vulvar intraepithelial neoplasia
VT	ventricular tachycardia
VTE	venous thromboembolism
WBC	white blood cell(s)
WHO	World Health Organization

Drug Prescribing and Elimination

Drugs are listed by generic names; trade names are in *italics*. An asterisk (*) indicates that the drug is available OTC. Check marks (✓) indicate drugs preferred for treating older adults. A triangle (▲) after the drug name indicates that the drug is available as a generic formulation. A triangle after a combination medication indicates that the combination is available as a generic, not the individual drugs (ie, even though individual drugs in a combination medication are available as generics, the combination may not be).

Formulations in text are bracketed and expressed in milligrams (mg) unless otherwise specified. Information in parentheses after dose ranges indicate the number of doses into which the daily dose can be split. Abbreviations for dosing, formulations, and route of elimination are defined below.

ac	before meals	OU	both eyes
C	capsule, caplet	pc	after meals
ChT	chewable tablet	pch	patch
conc	concentrate	pk	pack, packet
CR	controlled release	po	by mouth
crm	cream	pr	per rectum
d	day(s)	prn	as needed
ER	extended release	pwd	powder
F	fecal elimination	qam	every morning
fl	fluid	qhs	each bedtime
g	gram(s)	S	liquid (includes concentrate,
gran	granules		elixir, solution, suspension,
gtt	drop(s)		syrup, tincture)
h	hour(s)	SC	subcutaneous(ly)
hs	at bedtime	sec	second(s)
IM	intramuscular(ly)	shp	shampoo
inj	injectable(s)	sl	sublingual
IR	immediate release	sol	solution
IT	intrathecal(ly)	Sp	suppository
IV	intravenous(ly)	spr	spray(s)
K	renal elimination	SR	sustained release
L	hepatic elimination	sus	suspension
lot	lotion	syr	syrup
max	maximum	T	tablet
mcg	microgram(s)	tab(s)	tablet(s)
min	minute(s)	tbsp	tablespoon(s)
mo	month(s)	tinc	tincture
npo	nothing by mouth	TR	timed release
NS	normal saline	tsp	teaspoon(s)
ODT	oral disintegrating tablet	wk	week(s)
oint	ointment	XR	extended release
OL	off-label use	y	year(s)
OTC	over-the-counter		

INTRODUCTION

Providing high-quality healthcare for older adults requires special knowledge and skills. *Geriatrics At Your Fingertips® (GAYF)* is an annually updated, pocket-sized reference that provides quick, easy access to the specific information clinicians need to make decisions about the care of older adults. Since its initial publication in 1998, GAYF's up-to-date content and portable format quickly made it the American Geriatrics Society's (AGS) best-selling publication.

In response to the increased use of electronic media in clinical settings, the AGS has also developed GAYF for the Web and for mobile devices. Schools can acquire licenses to provide mobile device access for all their faculty and trainees. More information on these formats can be found at www.geriatricscareonline.org.

In this updated 21st edition, we have made several changes regarding medications and brand-name products. First, we have listed trade names only for drugs that are not available generically. Second, we have not listed the trade names of combination drugs. The rationale for these decisions is the proliferation of drug names and combinations, which would add considerable length to the book. This information is also readily available from other sources and in electronic health records at the time of prescribing. Similarly, for skin and wound care, we have eliminated any product listing other than the category and its use and contraindications.

We have added sections on endovascular thrombectomy for strokes, and reversal of direct-acting oral anticoagulants, and blepharitis. New guidelines for dual and triple therapy for diabetes mellitus and clostridia difficile treatment are included. The text and tables contain updated and newly recommended diagnostic tests and management strategies. Among the many updates included in this edition are recommendations about tests and procedures that follow the American Board of Internal Medicine Foundation's Choosing Wisely® Campaign (indicated by a ᶜᵂ). Medication tables were updated shortly before publication and include specific caveats and cautions to facilitate appropriate prescribing in older adults.

Given its portable size, GAYF does not explain in detail the rationale underlying the strategies presented. Many of these strategies have been derived from guidelines published by medical societies and professional organizations. When no such guidelines exist, the strategies recommended represent the best opinions of the authors and reviewers, based on clinical experience and the most recent medical and health literature. References are provided sparingly, but many others are available from the AGS Geriatrics Review Syllabus.

The authors welcome comments about GAYF, which should be addressed to the AGS at info.amger@americangeriatrics.org or 40 Fulton Street, 18th Floor, New York, NY 10038. The authors are particularly grateful to the following organizations and individuals: the John A. Hartford Foundation, for generously supporting the initial development and distribution of GAYF and its PDA version; AGS staff, Nancy Lundebjerg, Carol Goodwin, and Elvy Ickowicz, who have served a vital role in GAYF's development and its continued distribution and expansion; and the following experts who reviewed portions of this edition:

Daniel Blumberger, MD
Ab Brody, PhD, RN
Catherine E. DuBeau, MD
Sherry Greenberg, PhD, RN
Gail Greendale, MD
Peter Hollmann, MD

Jason M. Johanning, MD
Jerry C. Johnson, MD
James Judge, MD
Andrew Lee, MD
Jeffrey Levine, MD
Debra Weiner, MD

FORMULAS AND REFERENCE INFORMATION

Table 1. Conversions		
Temperature	**Liquid**	**Weight**
F = (1.8)C + 32	1 fl oz = 30 mL	1 lb = 0.453 kg
C = (F − 32) / (1.8)	1 tsp = 5 mL	1 kg = 2.2 lb
	1 tbsp = 15 mL	1 oz = 30 g

Alveolar-Arterial Oxygen Gradient

$A - a = 148 - 1.2(PaCO_2) - PaO_2$ [normal = 10–20 mmHg, breathing room air at sea level]

Calculated Osmolality

$Osm = 2Na + glucose / 18 + BUN / 2.8$ [normal = 280–295]

Golden Rules of Arterial Blood Gases

• $PaCO_2$ change of 10 corresponds to a pH change of 0.08.
• pH change of 0.15 corresponds to base excess change of 10 mEq/L.

Creatinine Clearance

See Appropriate Prescribing, p 19.

For renally eliminated drugs, dosage adjustments may be necessary if CrCl <60 mL/min/1.73 m^2.

Cockcroft-Gault formula:

$$\frac{IBW(140 - age) (0.85 \text{ if female})}{(72) \text{ (stable serum Cr)}}$$

Many laboratories report an estimate of GFR (eGFR) using the Chronic Kidney Disease Epidemiology Collaboration (CKD-EPI) equation. This measure is used for staging CKD. eGFR should not be equated with CrCl or eCrCl. The use of eGFR to adjust drug dosages overestimates kidney function in many older adults, placing them at risk for ADEs. The Cockcroft-Gault is the least biased estimate of kidney function compared to measures of eGFR. FDA-labeled dosing is based on the Cockcroft-Gault formula.

The validity of the Cockcroft-Gault estimate of CrCl in obese patients has been questioned because total body weight (TBW) tends to overestimate CrCl in obese patients, while lean body weight (LBW) tends to underestimate CrCl. In obese patients, use of adjusted body weight (ABW) with correction of 0.3 [ABW(0.3)=(TWB − IBW)0.3 + IBW] or 0.4 [ABW(0.4)=(TBW − IBW)0.4 + IBW] and actual serum Cr in Cockcroft-Gault formula is recommended.

Ideal Body Weight

• Men = 50 kg + (2.3 kg) (each inch of height >5 feet)
• Women = 45.5 kg + (2.3 kg) (each inch of height >5 feet)

Body Mass Index

$$\frac{\text{weight in kg}}{(\text{height in meters})^2} \quad or \quad \frac{\text{weight in lb}}{(\text{height in inches})^2} \quad \times \quad 704.5$$

Age-adjusted Erythrocyte Sedimentation Rate

Westergren:
women = (age + 10) / 2
men = age / 2

Partial Pressure of Oxygen, Arterial (PaO$_2$) While Breathing Room Air

100 − (age/3) estimates decline

Table 2. Motor Function by Nerve Roots			
Level	**Motor Function**	**Level**	**Motor Function**
C4	Spontaneous breathing	L1–L2	Hip flexion
C5	Shoulder shrug	L3	Hip adduction
C6	Elbow flexion	L4	Hip abduction
C7	Elbow extension	L5	Great toe dorsiflexion
C8/T1	Finger flexion	S1–S2	Foot plantar flexion
T1–T12	Intercostal abdominal muscles	S2–S4	Rectal tone

Table 3. Lumbosacral Nerve Root Compression			
Root	**Motor**	**Sensory**	**Reflex**
L4	Quadriceps	Medial foot	Knee jerk
	Dorsiflexors	Dorsum of foot	Medial hamstring
L5	Great toe dorsiflexors	Dorsum of foot	Medial hamstring
S1	Plantar flexors	Lateral foot	Ankle jerk

Figure 1. Dermatomes

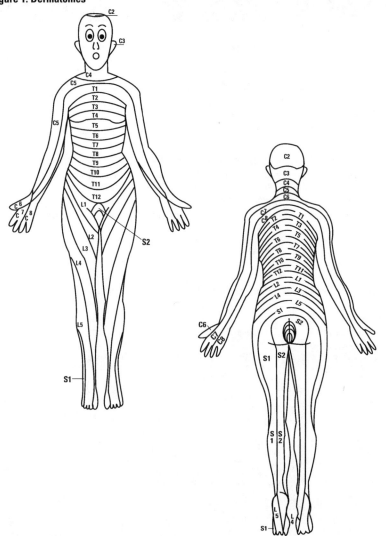

Source: Hamilton RJ, ed. *The Tarascon Pocket Pharmacopoeia*, 2014 classic shirt-pocket edition. Jones and Bartlett Learning, 2014:143. Sudbury, MA. jblearning.com. Reprinted with permission.

ASSESSMENT

Table 4. Assessing Older Adults

Assessment Domain	Screening Methods	Further Assessments (if screen is positive)	See Page(s)
Medical			
Medical illnesses[1,2]	Hx, screening physical examination	Additional targeted physical examination, laboratory and imaging tests	—
Medications[1,2]	Medications review/reconciliation	Pharmacy referral	19
Nutrition[1,2]	Inquire about weight loss (>10 lb in past 6 mo), calculate BMI	Dietary hx, malnutrition evaluation	203
Dentition	Oral examination	Dentistry referral	—
Hearing[1]	Handheld audioscope, Brief Hearing Loss Screener, whisper test	Ear examination, audiology referral	146
Vision[1]	Inquire about vision changes, Snellen chart testing	Eye examination, ophthalmology referral	114
Pain	Inquire about pain	Pain inventory	252
Urinary incontinence	Inquire if patient has lost urine >5 × in past year	UI evaluation	161
Mental			
Cognitive status[1,2]	3-item recall, Mini-Cog	MSE, dementia evaluation	5
Emotional status[1] Depression	PHQ-2: "Over the past month, have you often had little interest or pleasure in doing things? Over the past month, have you often been bothered by feeling down, depressed, or hopeless?"	PHQ-9 or other depression screen, in-depth interview	—
Anxiety	GAD-2: "Over the last 2 weeks, how often have you been bothered by the following problems: Feeling nervous, anxious, or on edge? Not being able to stop or control worrying?" (Scoring for each item: not at all = 0, several days = 1, more than half the days = 2, nearly every day = 3; total score of 3 or more is a positive screen)	GAD-7	41
Spiritual status	Spiritual hx	In-depth interview, chaplain or spiritual advisor referral	—

(cont.)

Table 4. Assessing Older Adults* (cont.)			
Assessment Domain	**Screening Methods**	**Further Assessments (if screen is positive)**	**See Page(s)**
Physical			
Functional status[1]	ADLs, IADLs	PT/OT referral	—
Balance and gait[1]	Observe patient getting up and walking, orthostatic BP and HR, Romberg test, semitandem stand	Formal gait evaluation, measurement of gait speed, 6-min walk test	
Falls	Inquire if patient has had ≥2 falls in past y or is afraid of falling due to balance and/or walking problem	Falls evaluation	123
Environmental			
Social, financial status[1]	Social hx, assess risk factors for mistreatment	In-depth interview, social work referral	11–13
Environmental hazards[1]	Inquire about living situation, home safety checklist	Home evaluation	128
Care Preferences			
Life-sustaining tx[1,2]	Inquire about preferences; complete POLST form		11

[1]Required elements of the Medicare Initial Annual Wellness Visit

[2]Required elements of Medicare Subsequent Annual Wellness Visits

MINI-COG™ SCREEN FOR DEMENTIA

Step 1: Three Word Registration

Look directly at person and say, "Please listen carefully. I am going to say 3 words that I want you to repeat back to me now and try to remember. The words are [select a list of words from the versions below]. Please say them with me now." If the person is unable to repeat the words after 3 attempts, move on to Step 2 (clock drawing).

The following and other word lists have been used in one or more clinical studies. For repeated administrations, use of an alternative word list is recommended.

Version 1	**Version 2**	**Version 3**	**Version 4**	**Version 5**	**Version 6**
Banana	Leader	Village	River	Captain	Daughter
Sunrise	Season	Kitchen	Nation	Garden	Heaven
Chair	Table	Baby	Finger	Picture	Mountain

Step 2: Clock Drawing

Say: "Next, I want you to draw a clock for me. First, put in all the numbers where they go." When that is completed, say, "Now, set the hands to 10 past 11."

Use preprinted circle (see mini-cog.com) for this exercise. Repeat instructions as needed as this is not a memory test. Move to Step 3 if the clock is not complete within 3 minutes.

Step 3: Three Word Recall

Ask the person to recall the 3 words you stated in Step 1. Say: "What were the 3 words I asked you to remember?" Record the word list version number and the person's answer.

Scoring

Word Recall: 0–3 points	1 point for each word spontaneously recalled without cueing.
Clock Draw: 0 or 2 points	Normal clock = 2 points. A normal clock has all numbers placed in the correct sequence and approximately correct position (eg, 12, 3, 6, and 9 are in anchor positions) with no missing or duplicate numbers. Hands are pointing to the 11 and 2 (11:10). Hand length is not scored. Inability or refusal to draw a clock (abnormal) = 0 points.
Total Score: 0–5 points	Total score = Word Recall score + Clock Draw score. A cut point of <3 on the Mini-Cog has been validated for dementia screening, but many individuals with clinically meaningful cognitive impairment will score higher. When greater sensitivity is desired, a cut point of <4 is recommended as it may indicate a need for further evaluation of cognitive status.

Medicare Annual Wellness Visit (AWV)

- Can be performed by a physician, physician assistant, nurse practitioner, clinical nurse specialist, or a health professional (eg, health educator, dietitian) under the direct supervision of a physician.
- Initial and subsequent AWVs must include documentation of elements indicated in **Table 4**, plus the following items that are to be established at the initial AWV and updated at subsequent AWVs:
  - A family hx
  - A list of current providers caring for the patient
  - A written 5- to 10-y schedule of screening activities based on USPSTF/CDC recommendations (Prevention, p 289)
  - A list of risk factors and conditions for which primary, secondary, and tertiary preventive interventions are being applied
- If face-to-face discussions of advance directives are performed as part of the AWV, providers may bill for it separately using the Advance Care Planning (ACP) CPT billing code of 99497 for initial ACP and 99498 for additional add-on of 30 min of face-to-face discussion.

INTERPROFESSIONAL GERIATRIC TEAM CARE

- Most effective for care of frail older adults with multiple comorbidities
- Also appropriate for management of complex geriatric syndromes (eg, falls, confusion, dementia, depression, incontinence, weight loss, persistent pain, immobility)
- Common features of team care include:
  - Proactive assessment of multiple domains (**Table 4**)
  - Care coordination, usually performed by an advanced practice nurse or social worker
  - Care planning performed by team members (**Table 5**), also p 9

Table 5. Interprofessional Team Members[1]

Profession	Degree	Training	Team Role
Advance practice nurse	APRN	2–4 y PB	Disease management, care coordination, patient education, primary care, skin and pain assessment
Nurse	RN/LPN (LVN)	2–4 y B/1–2 y B	Care coordination, patient education, skin and pain assessment, ADL/IADL screening, symptom management
Occupational therapist	OTR	2–4 y PB	ADL/IADL assessment and improvement (including driving and home safety assessments)
Pharmacist	PharmD	4-6 y PD ± 1–2 y PG	Medication review/reconciliation, patient education, drug monitoring, drug-related problems
Physician assistant	PA	3 y PB	Disease management, primary care
Physical therapist	PT, DPT	3 y PB	Mobility, strength, extremity assessment and improvement
Physician	MD, DO	4 y PB + ≥3 y PG	Diagnosis and management of medical problems, primary care
Social worker	MSW, DSW, LMHP	2–4 y PB	Complete psychosocial assessment and improvement, individual and family counseling
Speech therapist	SLP	2 y PB	Communication and swallowing disorders

B = baccalaureate (post–high school), PB = postbaccalaureate, PD = professional degree,
PG = postgraduate (ie, residency training)

[1] This is not an exhaustive list. Other common team members include audiologists, dentists, dietitians, speech therapists, and spiritual care professionals.

SITES OF CARE FOR OLDER ADULTS

Table 6. Sites of Care[1]

Site	Patient Needs and Services	Principal Funding Source
Home	ADL or IADL assistance	PP for caregiving services
	Skilled nursing and/or rehabilitation services when patient can only occasionally leave the home at great effort	Medicare Part A for nonphysician homecare services (eg, nursing, OT, PT); Part B for outpatient PT/ST/OT services independent of a home care agency[2]
Senior citizen housing	Housing	PP[3]
Assisted living, residential care, board-and-care facilities	IADL assistance, primarily with meals, housekeeping, and medication management	PP, Medicaid for some facilities
Hospital		
Acute care	Acute hospital care	Medicare Part A

(cont.)

Table 6. Sites of Care[1] (cont.)

Site	Patient Needs and Services	Principal Funding Source
Chronic care/ long-term acute care (LTAC facility)	Chronic skilled care (eg, chronic ventilator)	Medicare Part A, PP, Medicaid
Inpatient rehabilitation	Intensive multidisciplinary team rehabilitation	Medicare Part A
Skilled nursing facility		
Transitional care unit	Skilled nursing care and/or intensive multidisciplinary team rehabilitation	Medicare Part A[4]
Short stay/ Rehabilitation	Skilled nursing care and/or straight-forward rehabilitation	Medicare Part A[4]
Long-term care	ADL assistance and/or skilled nursing care	PP, Medicaid
Continuing care retirement communities	Variety of living arrangements ranging from independent to skilled	PP
Hospice (home- or facility-based)	Palliative/comfort care for life expectancy <6 mo	Medicare Part A

PP = private pay (may include long-term care insurance).

[1] For useful information about sites of care for patients and families, see payingforseniorcare.com.

[2] A yearly cap of $2040 for these services can be exceeded if the therapist documents a "medically reasonable and necessary" exception.

[3] May be subsidized for older adults spending over one-third of income for rent. Some facilities may have access to a social worker or caregiving services for hire.

[4] Medicare Part A pays for 20 d after a hospital stay of ≥3 d, patient or co-insurance pays $170.50/d (in 2019) for days 21–100 with Part A covering the rest; patient or co-insurance pays 100% after day 100.

HOSPITAL CARE

Common Problems to Monitor

- Delirium (p 72)
- Intra- and postoperative coronary events: postoperative ECG to check
- Malnutrition (p 203)
- Pain (p 252)
- Polypharmacy: review medications daily
- Pulmonary complications: minimized by incentive spirometry, coughing, early ambulation after surgery
- Rehabilitation: encourage early mobility
- Skin breakdown (p 331)

Discharge Planning

- Ideally, all team members should participate in discharge planning, beginning early in the hospitalization.
- Site of care after discharge should be determined by patient's needs (**Table 6**).
- Evidence-based procedures for preventing hospital readmissions include:
  ○ A discharge coordinator (usually a specially trained nurse) who oversees appropriate patient and caregiver education regarding diagnoses and self-care, arrangement of posthospital care, reconciliation of medications, and follow-up with the patient within 72 h of discharge
  ○ Clearly written discharge plans geared toward the patient, caregivers, and healthcare team members

- Medication reconciliation at the time of discharge and within 1 wk of discharge by a clinical pharmacist
- Tools for achieving effective transitions of care out of the hospital are available through the RED: Re-Engineered Discharge project (ahrq.gov/professionals/systems/hospital/red/toolkit), the Transitional Care Model (transitionalcare.info), and the Care Transitions Program (caretransitions.org/tools-and-resources).
- For a safe and effective transfer from the hospital to the nursing home, the following should be completed by the time the patient arrives at the nursing home:
  - Interfacility transfer form (the medication administration record is inadequate) that includes a discharge medication list noting new and discontinued medications, discontinuation dates for short-term medications, and any dosage changes in all medications
  - Discharge summary (performed by physician) that includes the patient's baseline functional status, "red flags" for rare but potentially serious complications of conditions or tx, orders including medications, important tests for which results are pending, and needed next steps
  - Verbal provider-to-provider sign-out

SCHEDULED NURSING-HOME VISIT CHECKLIST

1. Evaluate patient for interval functional change
2. Check vital signs, weight, laboratory tests, consultant reports since last visit
3. Review medications (correlate to active diagnoses)
4. Sign orders
5. Address nursing staff concerns
6. Write a SOAP note (subjective data, objective data, assessment, plan)
7. Revise problem list as needed
8. Update advance directives at least yearly
9. Update resident; update family member(s) as needed

PATIENT-CENTERED CARE AND MEDICAL DECISION MAKING

Goal-Oriented Care

- Goals of care should be established for individual patients
- Goals of care should be based on:
  - Disease-specific care processes and outcomes (eg, A1c and retinopathy for patients with DM)—useful for healthier patients with isolated conditions.
  - Goal-oriented outcomes (an individual's goals potentially encompassing a variety of dimensions, including symptoms, functional status, social engagement, etc)—useful for patients with multiple conditions or who are frail.

Care Planning — a healthcare team process with patient and caregivers

- Elucidate patient's goal-oriented outcomes; operationalize goals to be specific, measurable, and time bound
- Identify chronic conditions and other stressors that threaten the achievement of goal-oriented outcomes
- Propose interventions and discuss possible risks and benefits of each for attaining goals
- Negotiate and implement the plan, which can address the following elements (all of which are required for chronic care management codes [see CODES section]):
  - Physical, mental, cognitive, psychosocial, and functional assessments

- ◦ Preventive care services
- ◦ Medication reconciliation
- ◦ Therapeutic and psychosocial support services
- ◦ Defined roster of healthcare team members and responsibilities of each
- ◦ Timeline for follow-up and reassessment of goal attainment
- Formal care planning is a requirement for Chronic Care Management coding (99490, 99487, 99489) and for the Cognition Assessment and Care Plan Code (99483).

Life Expectancy
- Many medical decisions are predicated on estimated life expectancy of the patient. **Table 7** shows life expectancy by age and sex.
- Life expectancy is associated with a number of factors in addition to age and sex, including health behaviors, presence of disease, nutritional status, race/ethnicity, and educational and financial status.
- Conditions commonly leading to death are frailty, cancer, organ failure (heart, lung, kidney, liver), and advanced dementia.
- Active life expectancy reflects the remaining years of disability-free existence. At age 65, active life expectancy is about 90% of total life expectancy; this percentage decreases with further aging.
- Estimated life expectancy can aid individualized medical decision making, particularly when considering preventive tests. A clinician can judge the patient's health status as being above (75th percentile), at (50th percentile), or below average (25th percentile) for age and sex, and then roughly determine life expectancy using **Table 7**. Another way to estimate individual life expectancy is by comorbidity; no comorbidity will add 3–4 y to average life expectancy (the 50th percentile in **Table 7**) while high comorbidity will decrease life expectancy by 3–4 y.

Table 7. Life Expectancy (y) by Age (United States)[1]						
	25th percentile		50th percentile		75th percentile	
Age	Men	Women	Men	Women	Men	Women
65	12	14	18	21	24	27
70	8	11	14	17	20	22
75	6	8	11	13	16	18
80	4	5	8	10	11	14
85	3	3	6	7	9	10
90	2	2	4	5	6	7
95	1	1	3	3	4	5

[1] Figures indicate the number of years in which a percentage of the corresponding age and sex cohort will die. For example, in a cohort of men aged 65, 25% will be dead in 11 y (by age 76), 50% in 18 y, and 75% in 24 y.

Source: Arias E et al. United States Life Tables, 2012. *National Vital Statistics Reports*. 2016;65(8).

- After individual life expectancy is estimated, the period of time needed for the tx to result in a positive clinical outcome is estimated and compared with the life expectancy of the patient.
- ◦ If estimated life expectancy is longer than the time needed to achieve a positive outcome, the tx is encouraged.
- ◦ If estimated life expectancy is shorter than the time needed to achieve a positive outcome, the tx is discouraged.

- If estimated life expectancy is about the same as the time needed to achieve a positive outcome, the potential risks and benefits of the tx should be discussed neutrally with the patient.

For example, the benefit of many cancer screening tests is not realized for ~10 y after detection of asymptomatic malignancies. If a patient's life expectancy is significantly less than 10 y based only on age and sex, and the patient has poor overall health status compared with age-matched peers, cancer screening would be discouraged because the likelihood of benefit from having the test is low.

INFORMED DECISION MAKING AND PATIENT PREFERENCES FOR LIFE-SUSTAINING CARE

Healthcare providers have no ethical obligation to offer care that is judged to be futile.

Three elements are needed for a patient's choices to be legally and ethically valid:

- A capable decision maker: Capacity is for the decision being made; patient may be capable of making some but not all decisions. If a person is sufficiently impaired, a surrogate decision maker must be involved (**Figure 2**).
- Patient's voluntary participation in the decision-making process.
- Sufficient information: Patient must be sufficiently informed; items to disclose in informed consent include:
  - Diagnosis
  - Nature, risks, costs, and benefits of possible interventions
  - Alternative tx; relative benefits, risks, and costs
  - Likely results of no tx
  - Likelihood of success
  - Advice or recommendation of the clinician

Ideally, patient preferences for life-sustaining care should be established before the patient is critically ill.

- Preferences should be established for use of the following interventions and the conditions under which they would be used: cardiopulmonary resuscitation, hospitalization, IV hydration, antibiotics, artificially administered nutrition, other life-extending medical tx, and palliative/comfort care (Palliative Care, p 272).
- Patients should be encouraged to complete a living will and/or to establish a durable power of attorney for healthcare decision making.
- Use of a POLST form can be very useful in formalizing patient preferences (polst.org).
- Providers may bill for discussions of patient preferences using the ACP CPT billing code of 99497 for initial ACP and 99498 for additional add-on of 30 min of face-to-face discussion.

MISTREATMENT OF OLDER ADULTS

Risk Factors for Inadequate or Abusive Caregiving

- Cognitive impairment in patient, caregiver, or both
- Dependency (financial, psychological, etc) of caregiver on elderly patient, or vice versa
- Family conflict
- Family hx of abusive behavior, alcohol or drug problems, mental illness, or developmental disability
- Financial stress
- Isolation of patient or caregiver, or both
- Depression or malnutrition in the patient
- Living arrangements inadequate for needs of the patient
- Stressful events in the family, such as death of a loved one or loss of employment

Figure 2. Informed Decision Making

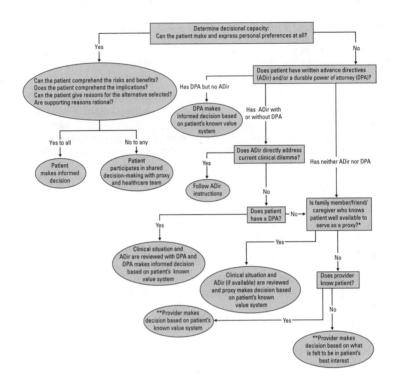

* Most states have laws specifying who should serve as proxy when no ADir or DPA exists. For most of these states, the specified hierarchy of decision makers is (in order): legal guardian, spouse or domestic partner, adult children, parents, adult siblings, closest living relative, close friend.

** Or court-appointed decision maker; laws vary by state.

Assessment and Management

• Interview patient and caregiver separately.

• Ask patient some general screening questions, such as, "Are there any problems with family or household members that you would like to tell me about?" Follow-up a positive response with more direct questions such as those suggested in **Table 8**.

• On physical examination, look for any unusual marks, signs of injury, or conditions listed in **Table 8**.

• If mistreatment is suspected, report case to Adult Protective Services (most states have mandatory reporting laws).

• If patient is in immediate danger of harm, create and implement plan to remove patient from danger (hospital admission, court protective order, placement in safe environment, etc).

Table 8. Determining Suspicion and Clinical Signs of Possible Mistreatment of Older Adults

Abandonment

Question to Ask Patient: Is there anyone you can call to come and take care of you?

Clinical Signs:
- Evidence that patient is left alone unsafely
- Evidence of sudden withdrawal of care by caregiver
- Statements by patient about abandonment

Physical Abuse

Question to Ask Patient: Has anyone at home ever hit you or hurt you?

Clinical Signs:
- Anxiety, nervousness, especially toward caregiver
- Bruising, in various healing stages, especially bilateral or on inner arms or thighs
- Fractures, especially in various healing stages
- Lacerations
- Repeated emergency department visits
- Repeated falls
- Signs of sexual abuse
- Statements by patient about physical abuse

Exploitation

Question to Ask Patient: Has anyone taken your things?

Clinical Signs:
- Evidence of misuse of patient's assets
- Inability of patient to account for money and property or to pay for essential care
- Reports of demands for money or goods in exchange for caregiving or services
- Unexplained loss of Social Security or pension checks
- Statements by patient about exploitation
- Requests for more frequent medication refills (possible indicator of diversion of patient's medications to others)

Neglect

Question to Ask Patient: Are you receiving enough care at home?

Clinical Signs:

- Contractures
- Dehydration
- Depression
- Diarrhea
- Fecal impaction
- Malnutrition
- Failure to respond to warning of obvious disease
- Inappropriate use of medications
- Poor hygiene
- Pressure ulcers
- Repeated falls
- Repeated hospital admissions
- Urine burns
- Statements by patient about neglect

Psychological Abuse

Questions to Ask Patient: Has anyone ever scolded or threatened you? Has anyone made fun of you?

Clinical Signs:
- Observed impatience, irritability, or demeaning behavior toward patient by caregiver
- Anxiety, fearfulness, ambivalence, or anger shown by patient about caregiver
- Statements by patient about psychological abuse

CROSS-CULTURAL GERIATRICS

Clinicians should remember that:
- Individuals within every ethnic group can differ widely.
- Familiarity with a patient's background is useful only if his or her preferences are linked to the cultural heritage.
- Ethnic groups differ widely in:
  ○ approach to decision making (eg, involvement of family and friends)
  ○ disclosure of medical information (eg, cancer diagnosis)
  ○ end-of-life care (eg, advance directives and resuscitation preferences)

In caring for older adults of any ethnicity:
- Use the patient's preferred terminology for his or her cultural identity in conversation and in health records.
- Determine whether interpretation services are needed; if possible, use professional interpreter rather than family member. When interpreters are not available, online translation services (eg, babelfish.com or translate.google.com) or telephone translation services can be useful.
- Recognize that the patient may not conceive of illness in Western terms.
- Determine whether the patient is a refugee or survivor of violence or genocide.
- Explore early on the patient's preferences for disclosure of serious clinical findings, and reconfirm at intervals.
- Ask if the patient prefers to involve or defer to others in the decision-making process.
- Follow the patient's preferences regarding gender roles.

For further information, see *Doorway Thoughts: Cross Cultural Health Care for Older Adults Series* (geriatricscareonline.org/ProductAbstract/doorway-thoughts-cross-cultural-health-care-for-older-adults/B016).

LESBIAN, GAY, BISEXUAL, AND TRANSGENDER (LGBT) HEALTH

Background
- At least 1–2 million LGBT older adults reside in the US and grew up in a time when their behavior was criminalized and considered pathological.
- Because of discrimination many hid their sexual orientation/gender identity. Many continue to do so and may distrust healthcare providers.
- To inquire about sexual identity, ask patients about past and present relationships, living situation, and sources of support to learn this information.
  ○ "What is your preferred name?"
  ○ "How do you refer to your loved ones?"
  ○ "Who lives with you at home?"
  ○ "What is your relationship status (are you single, partnered, married, open)?"
  ○ "Are your sexual partners women, men, or both?"
- Of LGBT people aged 65–75, about 50% are sexually active, as are 25% aged 75–85.

Medical Issues

- Provide the same basic geriatric care: syndromes, health maintenance, etc.
- Medical concerns with increased risk and or prevalence in LGBT patients:
  - *CVD:* especially in bisexual men but also lesbians; related to smoking, high BP, drug use; plus obesity in women; and the use of sex hormones in transgender people
  - *Anal cancer:* human papilloma virus, especially in men who have sex with men; if also HIV positive, consider screening with cytology using a PAP smear technique (*Dacron* or polyester swab moistened with water and inserted 2–3 inches into the anus, rotate 360°, fix to glass slide or place in preservative vial).
  - *Prostate cancer:* surgical and radiation tx has additional negative consequences on anal intercourse.
  - *Breast and cervical cancer:* lower prior screening rates increase risk.
  - *HIV/AIDS and other sexually transmitted infections:* less likely to use condoms and to be screened than younger persons; counsel on safe sex; evaluate for pre-exposure prophylaxis and renal function.
  - *Palliative care:* complicated by stigma; estrangement from family; partnerships not recognized.
  - *Advance care planning:* may need to name family of "choice" rather than biology.
  - Genital cancers in transgender people need screening based on biological sex if organs (prostate, uterus) are not removed.

Mental Health Issues

- LGBT persons have higher lifetime risk of depression and anxiety disorders; highest rates in transgender older adults.
- High suicide rates in young LGBT persons may not persist into late life.
- Important to assess for intimate partner violence.
- Better mental health results by more people (including healthcare professionals) being aware of the individual's sexual orientation.

Social and Economic Issues

- Older LGBT residents of long-term care facilities report higher frequency of verbal or physical harassment from other residents and staff, refused admission, or attempted discharge.
- LGBT older adults (especially lesbians) are more likely to live in poverty compared to heterosexual peers.
- Same-sex marriage is legal in all 50 states in 2015 and since 2013 recognition of federal benefits including Social Security spousal and survivor benefits, VA spousal benefits, and tax treatment of health insurance and retirement savings. However, there continues to be variability in state laws concerning private-sector job discrimination, adoption, transgender insurance coverage, and other relationship recognition (domestic partnerships).
  - SAGE, Services and Advocacy for LGBT Elders: www.sageusa.com
  - National Resource Center on LGBT Aging: lgbtagingcenter.org

COMPLETING A DEATH CERTIFICATE

- The **Cause of Death** statement in Section 32 of a Death Certificate indicates the provider's opinion, with reasonable probability, of the immediate, intermediate, and underlying causes of death and other significant contributing conditions. See below for details on completing this section.
- The **Manner of Death** statement in Section 37 indicates the provider's opinion of whether the death was natural or unnatural. Unnatural deaths will be reviewed by the coroner or medical examiner; the specific criteria for triggering a review vary by county and state.
- If a patient is on hospice care, the hospice provider will usually complete the death certificate.

Immediate Cause of Death Statement (Section 32.Part I.a)

- Indicates the final disease, injury, or complication causing death (eg, aspiration pneumonia, pulmonary embolism, aortic rupture)
- The approximate interval between the onset of the immediate cause and death is estimated (eg, 4 wk, minutes, 1 h for the above examples).
- If the cause of death is not apparent (eg, a very elderly man without clinically apparent major illnesses is found by his daughter to have died in his sleep), some states allow the clinician to indicate "Undetermined natural causes".
- Mechanistic terminal events such as asystole, electromechanical dissociation, cardiac arrest, and respiratory arrest should not be listed in this or any other cause-of-death section.

Intermediate/Underlying Causes of Death "Due to/Consequence of" Statement (Section 32.Part I.b–d)

- Indicates conditions and their sequence leading to the immediate cause of death, listed in reverse chronologic order.
- The last of these conditions listed is the **underlying** cause—the disease or injury that initiated the events leading to the patient's death.
- Examples:
  - A patient with osteoporosis fractures her hip, develops a DVT in the hospital, and dies of a pulmonary embolus. Pulmonary embolus would be cited as the immediate cause in Section 32.I.a, DVT would be cited as an intermediate ("due to/consequence of") cause in Section 32.I.b, hip fracture would be cited as another intermediate cause in Section 32.I.c, and osteoporosis would be entered in Section 32.I.d as the underlying cause.
  - A patient with late-state Alzheimer disease (AD) dies from apparent aspiration pneumonia. Aspiration pneumonia would be listed as the immediate cause in Section 32.I.a, and AD would be entered as the intermediate/underlying cause in Section 32.I.b.
- The approximate intervals between the onset of the intermediate/underlying causes and death is estimated.

Other Significant Conditions Leading to Death Statement (Section 32.Part II)

- Indicates conditions that likely contributed to death but did not result in underlying causes.
- Risk factors for underlying causes are often listed in this section, eg, hypertension for cerebrovascular disease (the underlying condition) leading to a massive hemorrhagic stroke (the immediate cause of death).

FRAILTY

- General definition: increased vulnerability to adverse outcomes (eg, falls, disability, delirium, failure to return to functional baseline) after exposure to a stressful event
- Frailty models are organized around different domains:
  - Phenotypic models (eg, the phenotype Cardiovascular Health Study [CHS] scale) characterize frailty around the presence of 5 indicators:
    - weight loss (>4–5 kg or >5%/y)
    - exhaustion/fatigue (inability to walk several hundred yards or >3–4 d/wk feeling exhausted)
    - low activity (<383 kcal/wk in men or <270 kcal/wk in women)
    - weakness (low grip strength)
    - slowness (slow gait speed)
  - Cumulative deficit models (eg, the Frailty Index) classify frailty by the presence of 25 or more functional deficits, conditions, symptoms, and/or laboratory values, scored as the proportion of total indicators present in the patient.
  - Other models (eg, FRAIL scale) combine elements of functional and biologic indicators.
- Frailty indicators can be measured clinically through direct observation or self-report.
- Frailty prevalence varies widely according to scale used; ~10% of older adults are frail using either the CHS scale or the FRAIL.
- Frailty is associated with numerous adverse outcomes, including geriatric syndromes (falls, delirium, immobility, incontinence, dementia), poor surgical outcomes, hospitalization, and death.
- It is unknown if frailty can be arrested or reversed. Frail individuals should be strongly considered for interprofessional geriatric team care (p 6).

MULTIMORBIDITY

- More than 50% of older adults have ≥3 chronic conditions.
- Management of patients with multimorbidity involves balancing issues of patient preferences and tx goals, prognosis, the evidence of outcomes for tx strategies of individual conditions, interactions among conditions and tx, and feasibility of tx (**Figure 3**).

Figure 3. Approach to the Evaluation and Management of the Older Adult with Multimorbidity

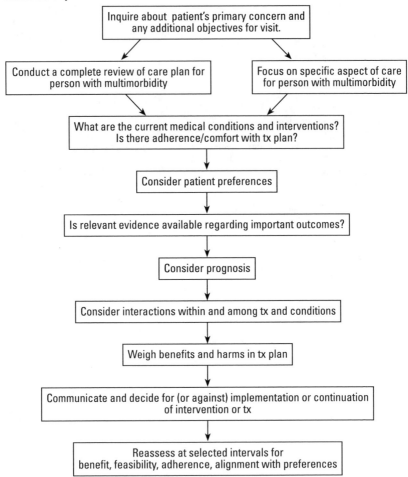

Source: AGS Expert Panel on the Care of Older Adults with Multimorbidity. *J Am Geriatr Soc* 2012;60(10):1957–1968.

APPROPRIATE PRESCRIBING, DRUG INTERACTIONS, AND ADVERSE EVENTS

HOW TO PRESCRIBE APPROPRIATELY AND REDUCE MEDICATION ERRORS

- **Obtain a complete medication history.** Ask about allergies, OTC drugs, nutritional supplements, alternative medications, alcohol, tobacco, caffeine, recreational drugs, and other prescribers.
- **Use e-prescribing to reduce risk of transcription and medication errors and to check insurance coverage.**
- **Avoid prescribing before a diagnosis is made except in severe acute pain.** Consider nondrug tx.
- **Review medications regularly and before prescribing a new medication.** D/C medications that are no longer needed, ineffective, or do not have a corresponding diagnosis.
- **Know the actions, AEs, drug interactions, monitoring requirements, and toxicity profiles of prescribed medications.** Avoid duplicative effects.
- **Consider the following for new medications:** Is the dosing regimen practical? Is the new medication affordable?
- **Start long-term medications at a low dose and titrate dose on the basis of tolerability and response.** Use drug concentration monitoring when available.
- **Attempt to reach a therapeutic dose before switching to or adding another medication.** Use combinations cautiously: titrate each medication to a therapeutic dose before switching to a combination product.
- **Avoid using one medication to treat the AEs caused by another.**
- **Attempt to use one medication to treat 2 or more conditions.**
- **Communicate with other prescribers.** Don't assume patients do—they assume you do!
- **Avoid using drugs from the same class or with similar actions** (eg, multiple opioids).
- **Avoid confusion and know the difference between products:** Brand name products can contain different ingredients depending on their indication, eg, *Mylanta Ultimate Strength* liquid contains aluminum and magnesium hydroxide, *Mylanta* maximum and regular strength liquid contains aluminum and magnesium hydroxide plus simethicone, while *Mylanta Supreme* contain calcium carbonate and magnesium hydroxide; *Lotrimin Ultra* crm contains butenafine, while *Lotrimin AF for Her* and *Gyne-Lotrimin* crm contain clotrimazole, and *Lotrimin AF* deodorant powder contains miconazole.
- **Write legibly** to avoid misreading of the drug name (eg, *Lamictal* vs *Lamisil*).
- **Write out the directions:**
    (1) Strength, route, quantity, and number of refills.
    (2) Avoid using abbreviations, especially easily confused ones (qd and qid).
    (3) Always precede a decimal expression of <1 with a zero (0); never use a zero after a decimal.
    (4) Do not use ambiguous directions (eg, as directed [ud] or as needed [prn]).
    (5) Include the medication's purpose in the directions (eg, for high blood pressure).
    (6) Write dosages for thyroid replacement tx in mcg, not mg.
    (7) Always reread what you've written.

Medication errors associated with e-prescribing:

  (1) Prescribing the wrong drug; look-alike errors (eg, metoprolol succinate instead of tartrate)
  (2) Choosing wrong dosage form (eg, tsp instead of tab)
  (3) Choosing wrong strength (1 mg for 10 mg)
  (4) Choosing wrong directions, quantity, or days of tx
  (5) To avoid delays and server errors, send e-prescriptions after seeing each patient instead of in batches.

• **Educate patient and/or caregiver about each medication.** Include the regimen, therapeutic goal, cost, and potential AEs or drug interactions. Provide written instructions. Assess health literacy using the Rapid Estimate of Adult Literacy in Medicine - Short Form (REALM-SF) tool. See ahrq.gov/professionals/quality-patient-safety/quality-resources/tools/literacy/index.html

• **Create a pill card for patients** or encourage them to create their own. See AHRQ's software program online at ahrq.gov/patients-consumers/diagnosis-treatment/treatments/pillcard/index.html. For more information, see www.fda.gov/drugs/drugsafety/medicationerrors or ismp.org/tools/abbreviations/

Medications listed as AVOID or Use with Caution in the 2019 AGS Beers Criteria are indicated in GAYF by [BC]. Some recommendations state to AVOID the drug without exceptions or USE WITH CAUTION, and others apply only to patients with a specific disease or syndrome, or for a specific duration of use, or a specific dose below a level of kidney function (CrCl), or in combination with other drugs (drug-drug interactions [DDI]). A detailed description of the 2019 AGS Beers Criteria including evidence tables, useful clinical tools, and patient education materials are available at the AGS website: GeriatricsCareOnline.org.

DEPRESCRIBING: WHEN AND HOW TO DISCONTINUE MEDICATIONS

• Recognize opportunities to stop a medication:
  ○ Care transitions (ie, medication reconciliation)
  ○ Annual/semiannual medication review (eg, annual wellness visit)
  ○ Review existing medications before starting a new medication
  ○ Presentation or identification of a new problem or complaint
  ○ Palliative care or end of life
• D/C medication if:
  ○ Harms outweigh benefits
  ○ Minimal or no effectiveness
  ○ No indication
  ○ Not being taken, and adherence is not critical
• Plan, communicate, and coordinate:
  ○ Include patient, caregiver, and other healthcare providers
    ▪ Prescribers: cancel discontinued medications in the EHR (eg, CancelRx or other available process) or by contacting the dispensing pharmacy.
    ▪ Patients and caregivers: remove discontinued medications from the home.
  ○ Use motivational interviewing to link reasons to discontinue (harms) with outcomes to get patient buy-in
  ○ What to expect/intent
  ○ Instructions, eg, how to taper (if indicated)

- Monitor and follow-up:
  - Withdrawal reactions
  - Exacerbation of underlying conditions

Examples of medications eligible for deprescribing: ASA, bisphosphonates, antiallergy (seasonal), antidiabetic agents, PPIs (taper off) and H_2 antagonists, cholinesterase inhibitors, memantine, iron, antipsychotics, antidepressants, and beta-blockers 1–3 y post MI.

Useful resources on deprescribing at www.deprescribingnetwork.ca:

- Algorithms for deprescribing antipsychotics, antidiabetic agents, benzodiazepines, and PPIs, brochures, and other materials to help prescribers and patients decide if and how to stop a medication.

CMS GUIDANCE ON UNNECESSARY DRUGS IN THE NURSING HOME

See Appendix PP of the CMS State Operations Manual. Updated survey guidelines for antipsychotic drugs in dementia are at https://www.cms.gov/Regulations-and-Guidance/Guidance/Manuals/downloads/som107ap_pp_guidelines_ltcf.pdf

CDC GUIDANCE ON USE OF OPIOIDS FOR CHRONIC PAIN

- See complete guidance at cdc.gov/drugoverdose/prescribing/guideline.html.
- Tx should be individualized.

MEDICATIONS THAT SHOULD NOT BE CRUSHED

Medications that have enteric-coated (EC), sustained-release (SR), extended-release (ER), sustained-action (SA), and other long-acting oral dosage forms should not be crushed. Crushing may result in the immediate release of the entire dose and toxicity. Immediate-release (IR) tablets can be crushed and IR capsules can usually be opened for easier administration. For more information, see ismp.org/tools/donotcrush.pdf or a drug's FDA label.

PHARMACOTHERAPY AND AGE-ASSOCIATED CHANGES

Table 9. Age-associated Changes in Pharmacokinetics and Pharmacodynamics			
Parameter	**Age Effect**	**Disease, Factor Effect**	**Prescribing Implications**
Absorption	Rate and extent are usually unaffected	Achlorhydria, concurrent medications, tube feedings	Drug-drug and drug-food interactions are more likely to alter absorption
Distribution	Increase in fat:water ratio; decreased plasma protein, particularly albumin	HF, ascites, and other conditions increase body water	Fat-soluble drugs have a larger volume of distribution; highly protein-bound drugs have a greater (active) free concentration
Metabolism	Decreases in liver mass and liver blood flow decrease drug clearance; may be age-related changes in CYP2C19, while CYP3A4 and CYP2D6 are not affected	Smoking, genotype, concurrent drug tx, alcohol and caffeine intake may have more effect than aging	Lower dosages may be therapeutic
Elimination	Primarily renal; age-related decrease in GFR	Kidney impairment with acute and chronic diseases; decreased muscle mass results in less Cr production	Serum Cr not a reliable measure of kidney function; best to estimate CrCl using formula (see p 1)

(cont.)

Parameter	Age Effect	Disease, Factor Effect	Prescribing Implications
Pharmaco-dynamics	Less predictable and often altered drug response at usual or lower concentrations	Drug-drug and drug-disease interactions may alter responses	Prolonged pain relief with opioids at lower dosages; increased sedation and postural instability to benzodiazepines; altered sensitivity to β-blockers

Table 9. Age-associated Changes in Pharmacokinetics and Pharmacodynamics (cont.)

COMPLICATING FACTORS

Drug-Food or -Nutrient Interactions

Physical Interactions: Mg++, Ca++, Fe++, Al++, or zinc can lower oral absorption of levothyroxine and some quinolone antibiotics. Tube feedings decrease absorption of oral phenytoin and levothyroxine.

Decreased Drug Effect: Warfarin and vitamin K-containing foods

Decreased Oral Intake or Appetite: Medications can alter the taste of food (dysgeusia) or decrease saliva production (xerostomia), making mastication and swallowing difficult. Medications associated with dysgeusia include captopril and clarithromycin. Medications that can cause xerostomia include antihistamines, antidepressants, antipsychotics, clonidine, and diuretics.

Drug-Drug Interactions

A drug's effect can be altered, displacement from protein-binding sites, inhibition or induction of metabolic enzymes, or because 2 or more drugs have a similar pharmacologic effect. For more information, consult a drug-drug interaction text, software, or Internet resource (eg, fda.gov/Drugs/DevelopmentApprovalProcess/DevelopmentResources/DrugInteractionsLabeling/ucm080499.htm and medicine.iupui.edu/clinpharm/ddis/), and **Table 10**.

Pharmacogenomics Resources

Pharmacogenomics Knowledge Base (Pharm GKB; www.pharmgkb.org) provides comprehensive knowledge to clinicians and researchers about how genetic variations impact drug response.

Clinical Pharmacogenetics Implementation Consortium (CPIC; https://cpicpgx.org) is a useful aid for clinicians when interpreting pharmacogenetic tests. CPIC guidelines are also available at guidelines.gov.

Drug-induced Changes in Cardiac Conduction (Table 11)

- Intrinsic changes associated with aging in cardiac pacemaker cells and conduction system
- Increased sensitivity to drug-induced conduction disorders, eg, bradycardia and tachyarrhythmias
- Acute lowering of serum calcium, potassium, and magnesium
- Other causes: genetic mutations (usually younger persons); medical conditions including hypothyroidism, DM, HF, and sepsis
- QTc prolongation exacerbated by drugs alone, drug interactions, and altered pharmacokinetics (eg, reduced kidney function)

- A comprehensive list of drugs associated with QTc prolongation, increase the risk of Torsades de Pointes, or should be avoided by patients with congenital long QT syndrome is available at crediblemeds.org.
- If possible, do not prescribe QT-prolonging drugs to anyone with a QTc >440 millisec (women) or >420 millisec (men). Each 10 millisec increase in QTc is estimated to increase the risk of torsades de pointes (TdP) by 5–7%.
- Do not allow the QTc to exceed 500 millisec during titration with these drugs as the risk of TdP is markedly increased and intervention considered necessary.

Table 10. Potentially Clinically Important Drug-Drug Interactions That Should Be Avoided in Older Adults

Object Drug/Class	Interacting Drug/Class	Rationale	Recommendation
Renin-angiotensin system (RAS) inhibitor (ACEIs, ARBs, aliskiren) or potassium-sparing diuretics (amiloride, triamterene)	Another RAS inhibitor or potassium-sparing diuretic	Increased risk of hyperkalemia	Avoid routine use in those with CKD Stage 3a or higher.
Opioids	Benzodiazepines	Increased risk of overdose	Avoid.
Opioids	Gabapentin, pregabalin	Increased risk of severe sedative AEs, including respiratory depression and death	Avoid. Exceptions are when transitioning from opioid tx to gabapentin or pregabalin, or when using gabapentinoids to reduce opioid dose, although caution should be used in all circumstances.
Anticholinergic	Other anticholinergic	Cognitive decline	Avoid, minimize the number of anticholinergic drugs (**Table 35**).
Antidepressants (TCAs, SSRIs, and SNRIs) Antipsychotics Antiepileptics Benzodiazepines and nonbenzodiazepines, benzodiazepine receptor agonists (ie, Z-drugs) Opioids	Any combination of ≥3 of these CNS-active drugs[1]	Increased risk of falls (all) and of fracture (benzodiazepines, nonbenzodiazepines, benzodiazepine receptor agonist hypnotics)	Avoid total of ≥3 CNS-active drugs[1]; minimize number of CNS-active drugs.
Corticosteroids, oral or parenteral	NSAIDs	Peptic ulcer disease and GI bleeding	Avoid; if not possible, provide GI protection.
Lithium	ACEIs	Lithium toxicity	Avoid, monitor lithium concentrations.
Lithium	Loop diuretics	Lithium toxicity	Avoid, monitor lithium concentrations.

(cont.)

Object Drug/Class	Interacting Drug/Class	Rationale	Recommendation
Lithium	NSAIDs (including ASA)	Lithium toxicity	Avoid, monitor lithium concentrations. Extent of effect varies by NSAID.
Peripheral α-1 blockers	Loop diuretics	Urinary incontinence in older women	Avoid in older women, unless conditions warrant both drugs.
Phenytoin	Trimethoprim-sulfamethoxazole	Increased risk of phenytoin toxicity	Avoid.
Theophylline	Cimetidine	Theophylline toxicity	Avoid.
Theophylline	Ciprofloxacin	Increased risk of theophylline toxicity	Avoid.
Warfarin	Amiodarone	Bleeding	Avoid when possible, monitor INR closely.
Warfarin	Ciprofloxacin	Increased risk of bleeding	Avoid when possible; if used together, monitor INR closely.
Warfarin	Macrolides (excluding azithromycin)	Increased risk of bleeding	Avoid when possible; if used together, monitor INR closely.
Warfarin	Trimethoprim-sulfamethoxazole	Increased risk of bleeding	Avoid when possible; if used together, monitor INR closely.
Warfarin	NSAIDs	Bleeding	Avoid when possible, monitor INR closely.

[1]CNS-active drugs: antiepileptics, antipsychotics, benzodiazepines, nonbenzodiazepines, benzodiazepine receptor agonist hypnotics, TCAs, SSRIs, SNRIs, and opioids.

Table 11. Examples of Medications With Known Risk to Prolong the QTc Interval Alone*†

Analgesics
Methadone
Antidepressants
Citalopram
Escitalopram
Antiemetics
Ondansetron

Anti-infectives
Azithromycin
Ciprofloxacin
Clarithromycin
Erythromycin
Fluconazole
Levofloxacin
Moxifloxacin
Antipsychotics
Haloperidol
Chlorpormazine
Pimozide
Thioridazine

Cardiovascular
Amiodarone
Cilostazol
Dispyramide
Dofetilide
Dronederone
Flecainide
Ibutilide
Procainamide
Quinidine
Soltaolol
Cholinesterase Inhibitors
Donepezil

*Level of risk depends on dosage, baseline QTc (mild risk if <450 millisec), other patient characteristics, and comorbidity.

†For a comprehensive list, see crediblemeds.org.

COMMONLY USED HERBAL AND ALTERNATIVE MEDICATIONS

Note: Herbal and dietary supplements are not subject to the same regulatory process by the FDA as prescription and OTC medications. Product and lot-to-lot variations can occur in composition and concentration of active ingredient(s), or be tainted with heavy metals or prescription medications (eg, sildenafil). Consumers are advised to purchase products by reputable manufacturers who follow good manufacturing procedures that contain the United States Pharmacopeia (USP) seal. For additional information on herbal and alternative medications, see NIH National Center for Complementary and Integrative Health (nccih.nih.gov).

Chondroitin/Glucosamine

Common Uses: Osteoarthritis, RA

Adverse Events: Chondroitin: nausea, dyspepsia, changes in IOP; Glucosamine: anorexia, insomnia, painful and itchy skin, peripheral edema, tachycardia

Comments: Meta-analyses have reached mixed conclusions of chondroitin's effectiveness in osteoarthritis of the knee. Neither the AAOS (2010) nor the ACR (2012) recommend chondroitin/glucosamine for knee arthritis. In one trial, knee pain did not respond better to chondroitin alone or in combination with glucosamine compared with placebo in >1500 patients with osteoarthritis. If patients choose a trial of chondroitin plus glucosamine, it should be glucosamine sulfate.

Cinnamon

Common Uses: DM, AD, heart disease, analgesia, and anti-inflammatory

Adverse Events: Allergy to cinnamon or Peru balsam; cassia cinnamon contains coumarin and may increase risk of bleeding; contact dermatitis and vasomotor symptoms with large doses

Comments: May lower A1c and blood pressure; clinical trials have concluded cinnamon does not affect factors related to DM or heart disease

Coenzyme Q_{10}

Common Uses: CVD (angina, HF, HTN), musculoskeletal disorders, periodontal diseases, DM, obesity, AD, Parkinson disease; may lessen toxic effects of doxorubicin and daunorubicin; reversal of statin myopathy

Adverse Events: Abdominal discomfort, headache, nausea, vomiting

Comments: May increase risk of bleeding; use with caution in patients with hepatic impairment, may decrease response to warfarin; may further decrease BP if taking antihypertensives or other medications that decrease BP; ubiquinol is a reduced form of coenzyme Q_{10}

Echinacea

Common Uses: Immune stimulant

Adverse Events: Hepatotoxicity, allergic reactions, GI upset, rash

Drug Interactions: Immunosuppressants; reportedly inhibits CYP1A2, −3A4; induces CYP3A4

Comments: D/C ≥2 wk before surgery; cross-sensitivity with chrysanthemum, ragweed, daisy, and aster allergies; kidney disease; immunosuppression; mixed results regarding effectiveness to shorten duration, reduce severity, or prevent colds; should not be taken for >10 d because of concern about immunosuppression

Feverfew

Common Uses: Anti-inflammatory, migraine prophylaxis

Adverse Events: Platelet inhibition, bleeding, GI upset, swelling of the lips, tongue, and oral mucosa; allergic contact dermatitis from handling fresh leaves

Drug Interactions: NSAIDs, antiplatelet agents, anticoagulants

Comments: D/C 7 d before surgery, active bleeding; cross-sensitivity with chrysanthemum and daisy; evidence lacking for either indication; minimum of 1-mo trial for migraine prophylaxis suggested

Fish oil (omega-3 fatty acids, *Lovaza*)

Common Uses: Decrease risk of CAD and CHD, hypertriglyceridemia, symptomatic tx of RA, inflammatory bowel disease, asthma, bipolar disorder, schizophrenia, and in cases of immunosuppression

Adverse Events: GI upset, dyspepsia, diarrhea, nausea, bleeding, increased ALT and LDL-C

Drug Interactions: Anticoagulants, antiplatelet agents

Comments: Use with caution if allergic to seafood; monitor LFTS, TG, and LDL-C at baseline, then periodically; a 2-mo trial is adequate for hypertriglyceridemia; not proven effective for primary or secondary prevention

Flaxseed and flaxseed oil

Common Uses: RA, asthma, constipation, DM, hyperlipidemia, menopausal symptoms, prevention of stroke and CHD, BPH, laxative

Adverse Events: Bleeding, hypoglycemia, hypotension, allergy; Flaxseed only: abdominal pain and bloating, flatulence, diarrhea

Drug Interactions: NSAIDs, antiplatelet agents, anticoagulants, insulin and hypoglycemic agents, lithium (mania)

Garlic

Common Uses: HTN, hypercholesterolemia, platelet inhibitor

Adverse Events: Bleeding, GI upset, hypoglycemia

Drug Interactions: NSAIDs, antiplatelet agents, anticoagulants, INH, NNRTIs, protease inhibitors

Comments: D/C 7 d before surgery; effect on lipid lowering modest and of questionable clinical value

Ginger

Common Uses: Antiemetic, anti-inflammatory, dyspepsia

Adverse Events: GI upset, heartburn, diarrhea, irritation of the mouth and throat

Drug Interactions: NSAIDs, antiplatelet agents, anticoagulants

Comments: D/C 7 d before surgery

Ginkgo biloba

Common Uses: AD, memory, migraine, CVD and stroke prophylaxis

Adverse Events: Bleeding, nausea, headache, GI upset, diarrhea, dizziness, heart palpitations

Drug Interactions: MAOIs (increased effect and toxicity), antiplatelet agents, anticoagulants, NSAIDs, midazolam

Comments: D/C 36 h before surgery; mixed results in dementia trials; recent trials tend to have negative results

Ginseng

Common Uses: Physical and mental performance enhancer, digestive, diuretic, immunomodulator, antineoplastic, cardiovascular, CNS, and endocrine effects

Adverse Events: HTN, tachycardia, insomnia, diarrhea, confusion, depression

Drug Interactions: Antiplatelet agents, anticoagulants, NSAIDs, imatinib

Comments: D/C 7 d before surgery, kidney failure

Glucosamine (see Chondroitin)

Kava kava

Common Uses: Anxiety, sedative

Adverse Events: Sedation, hepatotoxicity, GI upset, headache, dizziness, EPS, scaly skin rash, urinary retention, exacerbation of PD, rhabdomyolysis

Drug Interactions: Anticonvulsants (increased effect), benzodiazepines, CNS depressants, L-dopa

Comments: D/C 24 h before surgery; compared with placebo, kava kava has demonstrated antianxiety efficacy, but effect small and not robust

Melatonin

Common Uses: Sleep disorders, insomnia, jet lag

Adverse Events: Daytime drowsiness, headache, dizziness, enuresis, nausea, transient depression

Drug Interactions: Warfarin, ASA, clopidogrel, ticlopidine, dipyridamole (loss of hemostasis), antidiabetic agents (decreased glucose tolerance and insulin sensitivity), CNS depressants

Methyl sulfonylmethane (MSM)

Common Uses: Anti-inflammatory, analgesia, osteoarthritis, chronic pain, GI upset

Adverse Events: Nausea, diarrhea, fatigue, bloating, insomnia, headache

Comments: A derivative of dimethyl sulfoxide (DMSO) that produces less odor

Red yeast rice (*Monascus purpureus*, Xue Zhi Kang, natural source of mevinolin, the active ingredient of lovastatin)

Common Uses: CHD, DM, hypercholesterolemia

Adverse Events: Nausea, vomiting, GI upset, hepatic disorders, myopathy, rhabdomyolysis

Drug Interactions (theoretical): Cyclosporine, CYP3A4 substrates, digoxin, statins, niacin

Comments: Use with caution in patients taking other lipid-lowering agents

Rhodiola rosea (*Arctic Root*, golden root)

Common Uses: Energy, stamina, strength, enhanced cognitive capacity, stress, improved sexual function, mood and anxiety

Adverse Events: Dizziness, dry mouth

Drug Interactions: Antidiabetic drugs (hypoglycemia), antihypertensives (hypotension), moderate CYP3A4 inhibitor, immunosuppressants (may be an immunostimulant)

SAMe (S-adenosyl-methionine)

Common Uses: Depression, fibromyalgia, insomnia, osteoarthritis, RA

Adverse Events: GI distress, insomnia, dizziness, dry mouth, headache, restlessness

Drug Interactions: Antidepressants, St. John's wort, NSAIDs, antiplatelet agents, anticoagulants, other drugs affecting serotonin (serotonin syndrome)

Comments: Not effective for bipolar depression, hyperhomocysteinemia (theoretical), D/C ≥14 d before surgery

Saw palmetto

Common Uses: BPH

Adverse Events: Headache, nausea, GI distress, erectile dysfunction, dizziness

Drug Interactions: Finasteride, α_1-adrenergic agonist properties in vitro may decrease efficacy; may prolong bleeding time, so use with caution with antiplatelet agents, anticoagulants, NSAIDs

Comments: Efficacy in BPH did not differ from placebo in an adequately powered, randomized clinical trial

St. John's wort (*Hypericum perforatum*)

Common Uses: Depression, anxiety

Adverse Events: Photosensitivity, hypomania, insomnia, GI upset, dry mouth, itching, fatigue, dizziness, headache

Drug Interactions: Potent CYP3A4 inducer, finasteride (decreased finasteride concentration and possible effectiveness)

Comments: Wear sunscreen with UVA and UVB coverage; avoid in fair-skinned patients; D/C 5 d before surgery; not effective in severe depression; effects reported to vary from those of conventional antidepressants, yet no more effective than placebo; evaluation of effectiveness may be complicated by product, extraction process, and composition

Valerian

Common Uses: Anxiety, insomnia

Adverse Events: Sedation, benzodiazepine-like withdrawal, headache, GI upset, insomnia

Drug Interactions: Benzodiazepines, CNS depressants

Comments: Taper dose several weeks before surgery

NON-VTE INDICATIONS FOR ANTITHROMBOTIC MEDICATIONS

Table 12. Antithrombotic Medications for Selected Conditions

Indication	Antiplatelet (Table 17)	Anticoagulant (Table 18)						
		VK Antagonist	Heparin	LMWH	Factor Xa Inhibitor	Direct Thrombin Inhibitor	Glycoprotein IIb/IIIa Inhibitor
Atrial fibrillation	ASA	**Warfarin**	—	—	**Apixaban**[1] Rivaroxaban[2,4] **Edoxaban**[3,4]	Dabigatran[2]	—
Valvular disease	ASA	**Warfarin**	—	—	—	—	—
Acute coronary syndrome	**ASA Clopidogrel** Prasugrel[BC] **Ticagrelor**	—	**UFH**	Enoxaparin[2] Dalteparin	**Fondaparinux**[2]	**Bivalirudin**	**Abciximab Eptifibatide Tirofiban**
Cardio-vascular disease prevention	**ASA**	—	—	—	—	—	—
Prior TIA/ Stroke	**ASA** Clopidogrel Dipiridamole/ ASA	—	—	—	—	—	—
Peripheral arterial disease	**ASA Clopidogrel**	—	—	—	—	—	—
Heparin-induced thrombo-cytopenia	—	—	—	—	—	**Argatroban**	—

First choice in bold text; Secondary or alternate choice in regular text; LMWH = low-molecular-weight heparin; UFH = unfractionated heparin; VK = vitamin K. CrCl unit = mL/min/1.73 m²

[1] Avoid in patients with CrCl <25.[BC]
[2] Avoid in patients with CrCl <30.[BC]
[3] Avoid in patients with CrCl <30 or >95. [BC]
[4] Reduce dose if CrCl = 30–50. [BC]

VTE PROPHYLAXIS, DIAGNOSIS, AND MANAGEMENT

Prophylaxis

- Prophylaxis of medical and surgical inpatients is based on patient risk factors and type of surgery.
- See **Tables 13** and **14** for choice of antithrombotic strategy.
- See **Tables 17** and **18** for dosages of antithrombotic medications.

Table 13. DVT/PE Prophylaxis Strategies for Older Medical and Surgical Inpatients

DVT/PE Risk	Surgery Type or Medical Condition	Thromboprophylactic Options
Low	Healthy and mobile patients undergoing minor surgery Brief (<45 min) laparoscopic procedures Transurethral or other low-risk urologic procedures Joint arthroscopy Spine surgery	Aggressive early ambulation after procedure +/– intermittent pneumatic compression
Medium	Immobile (>72 h) patients Inpatients at bed rest with active malignancy, prior VTE, or sepsis Most general surgeries Open abdominopelvic surgeries Thoracic surgery Vascular surgery	Antithrombotic **(Table 14** and **Table 18)** +/– intermittent pneumatic compression
High	Acute stroke Hip or knee arthroplasty Hip, pelvic, or leg fracture Acute spinal cord injury	**Table 14**

Table 14. Antithrombotic Medications for VTE Prophylaxis

		Anticoagulant (Table 18)				
Indication	Anti-platelet (Table 17)	VK Antagonist	Heparin	LMWH	Factor Xa Inhibitor	Direct Thrombin Inhibitor
Medical inpatients at moderate/high risk for VTE; patients with acute stroke or spinal cord injury	—	—	UFH	**Enoxaparin**[1] **Dalteparin**	**Fondaparinux**[1] **Betrixaban**	—
Knee or hip replacement	ASA	Warfarin	UFH	**Enoxaparin**[1] **Dalteparin**	Apixaban[2] Fondaparinux[1] Rivaroxaban[1,3]	Dabigatran[1] Desirudin
Hip fracture surgery	ASA	Warfarin	UFH	**Enoxaparin**[1] **Dalteparin**	Fondaparinux[1]	—
Non–orthopedic surgery patients at moderate/high risk of VTE	ASA	**Warfarin**	**UFH**	**Enoxaparin**[1] **Dalteparin**	Fondaparinux[1] Rivaroxaban[1,3]	—

First choice(s) in bold text; Secondary or alternate choice(s) in regular text; LMWH = low-molecular-weight heparin, UFH = unfractionated heparin, VK = vitamin K; VTE = venous thromboembolism (DVT/PE). CrCl unit = mL/min/1.73 m²

[1]Avoid in patients with CrCl <30. **BC** [2]Avoid in patients with CrCl <25. **BC** [3]Reduce dose if CrCl = 30–50. **BC**

DVT Diagnosis

DVT diagnosis is directed by risk score, D-dimer testing, and duplex ultrasound imaging.
- Determine risk score
  - 1 point for each of the following:
    - active cancer
    - paralysis, paresis, or plaster immobilization of lower limb
    - bedridden for 3 d or major surgery in past 12 wk
    - localized tenderness along distribution of deep venous system

- entire leg swelling
- calf swelling ≥3 cm over diameter of contralateral calf
- pitting edema confined to symptomatic leg
- collateral superficial veins
- prior DVT
  - −2 points for alternative diagnosis as likely as DVT
- Interpret risk score and further testing
  - ≤0 points = low risk: Obtain moderately or highly sensitive D-dimer test. If negative (D-dimer ≤ patient age × 10), DVT is excluded. If positive, obtain ultrasound of proximal veins for diagnosis. Don't obtain imaging studies as the initial diagnostic test in patients with low pretest probability (low risk) of VTE.[CW]
  - 1–2 points = moderate risk: Obtain highly sensitive D-dimer. If negative, (D-dimer ≤ patient age × 10), DVT is excluded. If positive, obtain ultrasound of either proximal veins or whole leg for diagnosis.
  - ≥3 points = high risk: Obtain ultrasound of either proximal veins or whole leg. If proximal leg ultrasound is negative, repeat proximal ultrasound in 1 wk, obtain immediate highly sensitive D-dimer test, or obtain whole leg ultrasound; negative results of any of these rules out DVT.

PE Diagnosis

- Consider PE with any of the following (classic triad of dyspnea, chest pain, and hemoptysis seen in only ≤20% of cases):
  - Chest pain
  - Hemoptysis
  - Hypotension
  - Hypoxia
  - Shortness of breath
  - Syncope
  - Tachycardia
- If patient presents with shock or hypotension, obtain CT pulmonary angiography, and if positive, anticoagulate immediately with UFH and prepare for thrombolytic tx.
- If shock and hypotension are absent, calculate clinical probability of PE using clinical decision rule (**Table 15**), then follow evaluation of PE algorithm (**Figure 4**). Clinical probability of PE unlikely: total ≤4 points; clinical probability of PE likely: total >4 points.

Table 15. Clinical Decision Rule for PE Probability

Variable	Points
Clinical signs and symptoms of DVT (minimal leg swelling and pain with palpation of the 3 deep veins)	3
Alternative diagnosis less likely than PE	3
Heart rate >100/min	1.5
Immobilization (>3 d) or surgery in the previous 4 wk	1.5
Previous PE or DVT	1.5
Hemoptysis	1
Malignancy (receiving tx, treated in last 6 mo, or palliative)	1
Total	

Source: Wells PS et al. *Thromb Haemost* 2000;83(3):416–420. Reprinted with permission.

Figure 4. Evaluation of Suspected Pulmonary Embolism

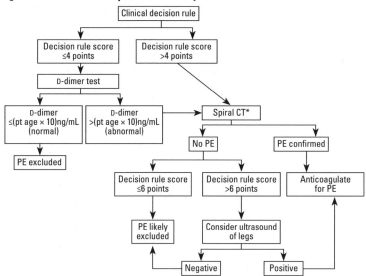

* Multidetector-row CT more sensitive than single-detector CT. Patient must be able to hold breath for 10 sec. Use ventilation perfusion scan when unable to use contrast (eg, renal dysfunction), or need to avoid ionizing radiation.

Management

Table 16. Antithrombotic Medications for VTE Management

			Anticoagulant (Table 18)				
Indication	Antiplatelet (Table 17)	VK Antagonist	Heparin	LMWH	Heparinoid	Factor Xa Inhibitor	Direct Thrombin Inhibitor
Acute VTE tx	—	—	UFH	**Enoxaparin**[1] Dalteparin **Tinzaparin**	—	**Apixaban**[2] **Fondaparinux**[1] **Rivaroxaban**[1,4]	—
Long-term VTE tx	—	**Warfarin**	—	Enoxaparin[1] Dalteparin Tinzaparin	—	Apixaban[2] Rivaroxaban[1,4] Edoxaban[3,4]	Dabigatran[1]

First choice(s) in bold text; Secondary or alternate choice(s) in regular text; LMWH = low-molecular-weight heparin; UFH = unfractionated heparin; VK = vitamin K; VTE = venous thromboembolism (DVT/PE). CrCl unit = mL/min/1.73 m^2

[1] Avoid in patients with CrCl <30.[BC]

[2] Avoid in patients with CrCl <25.[BC]

[3] Avoid in patients with CrCl <30 or >95.[BC]

[4] Reduce dose if CrCl = 30–50.[BC]

- For acute VTE, LMWH or fondaparinux is preferred to UFH in most patients because of lower risk of hemorrhage and mortality. Reduce dosage when CrCl <30 mL/min/1.73 m^2.

- Length of long-term tx is based on cause:
  - Provoked VTE from transient cause (eg, surgery, trauma, prolonged immobility that has resolved): anticoagulate for 3 mo.
  - Unprovoked VTE: anticoagulate for at least 3 mo. Consider treating longer for patients at low bleeding risk.
  - Second unprovoked VTE: anticoagulate indefinitely.
- If warfarin is part of a long-term anticoagulation plan, it may be started the same day as acute anticoagulant. Specific conditions may require a period of overlap when both agents should be used (eg, for DVT or PE, heparin or similar products should be used a minimum of 5 d, including 1–3 d of overlap with therapeutic INR).
- Consider low-dose ASA (100 mg/d) after completion of long-term VTE tx (at least 3 mo of warfarin or other anticoagulant).
- Consider placement of inferior vena cava filter in patients with PE who have an absolute contraindication to anticoagulation.
- Don't reimage DVT in the absence of a clinical change during DVT tx.[CW]
- Acute massive PE (filling defects in ≥2 lobar arteries or the equivalent by angiogram; about 5% of PE cases) associated with hypotension, severe hypoxia, or high pulmonary pressures on echocardiogram should usually be treated with thrombolytic tx within 48 h of onset.
- Submassive PE (about 20–25% of PE cases) is defined as PE with normotension and right ventricular failure; if present, thrombolytic tx should be considered. Submassive PE can be diagnosed by detection of right ventricular failure through:
  - Physical exam (eg, increased jugular venous pressure)
  - ECG (eg, right bundle branch block [RBBB] or t-wave inversions in leads V_1–V_4)
  - Elevated cardiac troponins
  - Echocardiography (eg, right ventricular hypokinesis and dilatation)
  - Chest CT showing right ventricular enlargement
- Don't perform workup for clotting disorder (order hypercoagulable testing) for patients who develop a 1st episode of DVT in the setting of a known cause.[CW]

ANTITHROMBOTIC MEDICATIONS
Antiplatelet Agents

Table 17. Antiplatelet Agents

Agent	Dosage	Formulations	Comments
Aspirin (ASA)[▲]	AF, KR, HR, HFS, SP: 75–325 mg/d Valvular disease: 50–100 mg/d ACS: 162–325 mg initially, followed by 75–160 mg/d CVDP, PAD: 75–100 mg/d	T: 81, 162, 325, 500, 650, 975	Risk of GI bleeding is dose-dependent. Use with caution in adults aged ≥80 for primary prevention of CVD.[BC] (L, K)
Dipyridamole/ ASA *(Aggrenox)*	SP: 1 tablet q12h	T: 200/25	Headache a common side effect. May decrease effectiveness of cholinesterase inhibitors. (L)

(cont.)

Table 17. Antiplatelet Agents (cont.)

Agent	Dosage	Formulations	Comments
Thienopyridines			*Class effect:* increased bleeding risk when given with ASA
Clopidogrel▲	ACS: 300–600 mg initially, followed by 75 mg/d SP, PAD: 75 mg/d	T: 75, 300	Some patients may be poor metabolizers due to low activity of the CYP2C19 liver enzyme; unclear if testing for this enzyme activity is effective for guiding dosage; unclear if PPIs inhibit activity (L, K)
Prasugrel *(Effient)*	ACS: 60 mg initially, followed by 10 mg/d	T: 5, 10	Use with caution in adults aged ≥75.[BC] Consider maintenance dose of 5 mg/d in patients <60 kg (L, K)
Ticagrelor *(Brilinta)*	ACS: 180 mg initially, followed by 90 mg 2x/d	T: 90	Should be used with ASA dosage of 75–100 mg/d (K)

ACS = acute coronary syndrome; CVDP = cardiovascular disease prevention; HFS = hip fracture surgery; HR = hip replacement; KR = knee replacement; SP = secondary stroke prevention after TIA/stroke.

Anticoagulant Agents

Table 18. Anticoagulant Agents

Class, Agent	Dose	Oral Formulation	Comments
Heparin			
Unfractionated heparin *(Hep-Lock)*	VTE prophylaxis: 5000 U SC 2h preop and q12h postop; Acute VTE tx: 5000 U/kg IV bolus followed by 15 mg/kg/h IV; ACS: 60–70 U/kg (max 5000 U) IV bolus, followed by 12–15 U/kg/h IV	NA	Bleeding, anemia, thrombocytopenia, hypertransaminasemia, urticaria (L, K)
LMWH			
Enoxaparin *(Lovenox)*	KR, NOS: 30 mg SC q12h; HR, HFS: 30 mg SC q12h or 40 mg SC 1x/d; AS, MP: 40 mg SC 1x/d; Inpatient VTE tx: 1 mg/kg SC q12h or 1.5 mg/kg SC 1×/d; Outpatient DVT tx: 1 mg/kg SC q12h; Unstable angina, NSTEMI: 1 mg/kg SC q12h; STEMI: 30 mg IV bolus, followed by 1 mg/kg SC q12h; STEMI in patients aged ≥75: 0.75 mg/kg SC q12h (no bolus)	NA	Bleeding, anemia, hyperkalemia, hypertransaminasemia, thrombocytopenia, thrombocytosis, urticaria, angioedema[BC]; lower dose if CrCl <30 (K)

(cont.)

Table 18. Anticoagulant Agents (cont.)

Class, Agent	Dose	Oral Formulation	Comments
Dalteparin *(Fragmin)*	HR: 2500–5000 U SC preop, 5000 U SC 1×/d postop; MP, NOS: 2500–5000 U SC preop and postop; LT VTE tx in cancer patients: 200 U/kg SC q24h × 30 d, followed by 150 U/kg SC q24g for the next 5 mo; ACS: 120 IU/kg SC q12h	NA	Same as above (K)
Tinzaparin *(Innohep)*	Acute VTE tx: 175 anti-Xa IU/ kg SC 1×/d	NA	Same as above; contraindicated in older patients with CrCl <30 (K)
Direct Factor Xa Inhibitors			*Class effect:* monitor patient at least q3mo for bleeding and side effects; follow renal function q6mo in patients aged ≥75.
Apixaban *(Eliquis)*	AF: 5 mg po q12h HR, KR: 2.5 mg po q12h Acute VTE tx: 10 mg po q12h for 7 d, followed by 5 mg po q12h Secondary prevention of VTE recurrence: 2.5 mg po q12h	T: 2.5, 5	Lower dose to 2.5 mg po q12h if patient has 2 of the following: age ≥80, weight ≤60 kg, Cr ≥1.5 mg/dL; not recommended in patients with mechanical heart valves[BC] (L, K)
Betrixaban *(Bevyxxa)*	MP: Initial single dose of 160 mg po, followed by 80 mg po daily for 35–42 d	T: 40, 80	Reduce dose by half if CrCl 15–29 (K)
Edoxaban *(Savaysa)*	AF: 60 mg po 1×/d VTE after patient has been treated for 5–10 d with a parenteral anticoagulant: weight ≤60 kg: 30 mg po 1×/d weight >60 kg: 60 mg po 1×/d	T: 15, 30, 60	Reduce dose to 30 mg/d if CrCl 15–50; do not use if CrCl >95[BC] (K)
Indirect Factor Xa Inhibitors			*Class effect:* monitor patient at least q3mo for bleeding and side effects; follow renal function q6mo in patients aged ≥75.
Fondaparinux *(Arixtra)*	ACS: 2.5 mg SC 1×/d MP, KR, HR, NOS: 2.5 mg SC 1×/d beginning 6–8 h postop; Acute VTE tx: weight <50 kg: 5 mg SC 1×/d weight 50–100 kg: 7.5 mg SC 1×/d, weight >100 kg: 10 mg SC 1×/d	NA	Lower dosage in renal impairment; contraindicated if CrCl <30[BC] (K)

(cont.)

Class, Agent	Dose	Oral Formulation	Comments
Table 18. Anticoagulant Agents (cont.)			
Rivaroxaban *(Xarelto)*	KR, HR, NOS: 10 mg/d po, begin 6–10 h after surgery; AF: 20 mg/d po with evening meal VTE: 15 mg po q12h for 1st 21 d, followed by 20 mg/d po	T: 10, 15, 20	Lower dosage to 15 mg/d in AF patients with CrCl 15–50: contraindicated if CrCl <15; not recommended in patients with mechanical heart valves [BC] (L, K)
Direct Thrombin Inhibitors			
Argatroban	HIT + VTE prophylaxis or tx: 2 mcg/kg/min IV infusion	NA	Lower dosage if hepatic impairment (L)
Bivalirudin *(Angiomax)*	ACS: 0.75 mg/kg bolus, followed by 1.75 mg/kg/h IV	NA	(L, K)
Dabigatran *(Pradaxa)*	AF, HR[OL], KR[OL], VTE after patient has been treated for 5–10 d with a parenteral anticoagulant, secondary prevention of VTE recurrence: 150 mg po q12h	T: 75, 150	Monitor patient at least q3mo for bleeding and side effects; follow renal function q6mo in patients aged ≥75. Reduce dosage to 75 mg po q12h if CrCl = 15–30; contraindicated in patients with mechanical heart valves; use with caution in adults aged >75 or if CrCl <30[BC] (K)
Desirudin *(Iprivask)*	HR: 15 mg SC q12h starting 5–15 min before surgery	NA	If CrCl = 31–60, starting dose is 5 mg; if CrCl <31, starting dose is 1.7 mg (K)
Glycoprotein IIb/IIIa Inhibitors			
Abciximab *(ReoPro)*	ACS: 0.25 mg/kg IV bolus, followed by 0.125 mcg/kg/min (max 10 mcg/min)	NA	
Eptifibatide *(Integrilin)*	ACS: 180 mcg/kg IV bolus, followed by 2 mcg/kg/min IV	NA	
Tirofiban *(Aggrastat)*	ACS: 0.4 mcg/kg/min IV over 30 min, followed by 0.1 mcg/kg/min	NA	

ACS = acute coronary syndrome; AS = Abdominal surgery; HFS = hip fracture surgery; HIT = heparin-induced thrombocytopenia; HR = hip replacement; KR = knee replacement; LT = long-term; MP = medical inpatients at moderate/high risk for VTE; NA = not available; NOS = nonorthopedic surgery at moderate/high risk of VTE; [OL] = off-label use; VTE = venous thromboembolism (DVT/PE). CrCl unit = mL/min/1.73 m².

MANAGEMENT OF BLEEDING WHILE ON ANTICOAGULANTS

- Major bleeding defined as bleeding at a critical site (intracranial or other CNS hemorrhage, pericardial tamponade, airway bleeding, hemothorax, abdominal bleeding, intramuscular or intra-articular bleeding), hemodynamic instability, or Hgb decrease of at least 2 g/dL.
- D/C anticoagulant, employ local bleeding control measures (pressure, packing), give volume resuscitation with IV 0.9% NaCl or Ringer's lactate.
- Use reversal agents in life-threatening bleeding (**Table 19**).

Table 19. Selecting Oral Anticoagulant Reversal Agents

Oral Anticoagulant	Preferred Reversal Agent	Alternate Reversal Agent	Tests to Assess Anticoagulant Drug Level
Apixaban, rivaroxaban	Andexanet alfa *(Andexxa)*: for apixaban dose ≤5 mg or rivaroxaban dose ≤10 mg: 400 mg IV bolus followed by 4 mg/min infusion; for apixaban dose >5 mg or rivaroxaban dose >10 mg: 800 mg IV followed by 8 mg/min infusion [sol: 100-mg single-use vials]	4F-PCC	Anti-Xa assay, PT
Betrixaban, edoxaban	4F-PCC	aPCC	Anti-Xa assay, PT
Dabigatran	Idarucizumab *(Praxbind)*: 5 g IV [sol: 2.5 g/50 mL]	4F-PCC, aPCC	TT, ECT, ECA
Warfarin	INR 3.6–10 without bleeding: omit next 1–2 doses and recheck INR INR >10 without bleeding: omit next 1–2 doses and give Vitamin K 2.5 mg po, recheck INR Any INR with major bleeding: VK 5–10 mg IV + 4F-PCC	Plasma (fresh frozen, frozen, thawed)	INR

4F-PCC = 4-factor prothrombin complex concentrate; aPCC = activated prothrombin complex concentrate; ECA = ecarin chromogenic assay; ECT = ecarin clotting time; PT = prothrombin time; TT = thrombin time; VK = vitamin K.

WARFARIN THERAPY

- For anticoagulation in nonacute conditions, initiate tx by giving warfarin▲ 2–10 mg/d as fixed dose [T: 1, 2, 2.5, 3, 4, 5, 6, 7.5, 10]. The usual starting dose for patients aged >70 is 5 mg/d, adjusted up or down depending on body size, comorbidities, and age.
- INR should be checked every 2–3 d until INR is stable. Reduce dose if INR >2.5 on day 3.
- Half-life is 31–51 h; steady state is achieved on day 5–7 of fixed dose. Genetic tests for VKORC1 (modulates sensitivity to warfarin) and CYP2C9 (modulates metabolism of warfarin) are available to help guide dosing for initiation of warfarin tx; it is unknown if their routine use significantly improves outcomes. Medicare does not cover genetic testing.
- For stable outpatients with INRs in the therapeutic range, routine INR monitoring every 12 wk is reasonable.
- Home INR testing results in similar outcomes (rates of stroke, death, or severe bleeding episodes) compared with monthly testing in an anticoagulation clinic.
- Tx of warfarin overdose, see **Table 19**:
- Warfarin tx is implicated in **many** adverse drug-drug interactions.

- Some drugs that **increase** INR in conjunction with warfarin (type in *italics* = major interaction):
  - alcohol (with concurrent liver disease)
  - amiodarone
  - many antibiotics*
  - APAP (>1.3 g/d for >1 wk)
  - celecoxib
  - *cilostazol*
  - *clofibrate*
  - *duloxetine*
  - flu vaccine
  - INH
  - *ketoprofen*
  - *naproxen*
  - sulindac
  - *tamoxifen*

  * especially fluconazole, itraconazole, ketoconazole, miconazole, ciprofloxacin, erythromycin, *moxifloxacin*, metronidazole, *sulfamethoxazole, trimethoprim*

- Some drugs that **decrease** INR in conjunction with warfarin:
  - carbamazepine
  - cholestyramine
  - dicloxacillin
  - nafcillin
  - rifampin
  - vitamin K

Table 20. Indications for Warfarin Anticoagulation in the Absence of Active Bleeding or Severe Bleeding Risk

Condition	Target INR	Duration of Therapy
Hip fracture or replacement surgery, major knee surgery	2–3	10–35 d
VTE secondary to reversible risk factor	2–3	3 mo
Idiopathic VTE	2–3	At least 3 mo
Recurrent VTE	2–3	Indefinitely
AF with CHADS$_2$ or CHA$_2$DS$_2$–VASc score ≥2[1]	2–3	Indefinitely
Rheumatic mitral valvular disease with hx of systemic embolization, left atrial thrombus, or left atrial diameter >5.5 cm	2–3	Indefinitely
Mitral valve prolapse with documented systemic embolism or recurrent TIAs despite ASA tx	2–3	Indefinitely
Mechanical aortic valve[2]	2–3	Indefinitely
Mechanical mitral valve[2]	2.5–3.5	Indefinitely
Mechanical heart valve with AF, anterior-apical STEMI, left atrial enlargement, hypercoagulable state, or low EF	2.5–3.5	Indefinitely
Bioprosthetic mitral valve	2–3	3 mo
Peripheral arterial embolectomy	2–3	Indefinitely
Cerebral venous sinus thrombosis	2–3	12 mo
MI with large anterior involvement, significant HF, intracardiac thrombosis, or hx of thromboembolic event	2–3	At least 3 mo

[1] See the Atrial Fibrillation section (**Table 31**, p 64) in the chapter on Cardiovascular Diseases for CHA$_2$DS$_2$–VASc scoring. Apixaban, dabigatran, edoxaban, and rivaroxaban are alternate options to warfarin. Patients with CHA$_2$DS$_2$–VASc score = 1 or in whom anticoagulation is contraindicated or not tolerated can be treated with ASA 75–325 mg/d; patients with CHA$_2$DS$_2$–VASc score = 0 should be treated with ASA 75–325 mg/d or receive no tx.

[2] Aspirin 75–100 mg po 1×/d should be added in addition to anticoagulant.

SWITCHING ANTICOAGULANTS

- ***Warfarin to Direct Oral Anticoagulants (DOACs):*** stop warfarin and check INR daily; when INR is ≤2.5 and trending downward, start DOAC.
- ***DOAC to Warfarin:*** D/C DOAC and begin warfarin at what would be the next scheduled DOAC dose. Continue warfarin and bridge with parenteral anticoagulant as indicated (**Table 102**) until INR ≥2.

DIAGNOSIS

Anxiety disorders as a whole are the most common mental disorders in older adults. Some anxiety disorders (panic disorder, social phobia) appear to be less prevalent in older than in younger adults. Generalized anxiety disorder (GAD) and new-onset anxiety in older adults are often secondary to physical illness, poorer health-related quality of life, depression, or AEs of or withdrawal from medications.

DSM-5 Criteria for GAD

- Excessive anxiety and worry on more days than not for ≥6 mo, about a number of events or activities
- Difficulty controlling the worry
- The anxiety and worry are associated with 3 or more of the following symptoms:
  - restlessness or feeling keyed up or on the edge
  - muscle tension
  - being easily fatigued
  - difficulty concentrating
  - irritability
  - sleep disturbance
- Focus of anxiety and worry not confined to features of another primary psychiatric disorder; often, about routine life circumstances; may shift from one concern to another
- Anxiety, worry, or physical symptoms cause clinically significant distress or impairment in social, occupational, or other important areas of functioning
- Disturbance not due to the direct physiologic effects of a drug of abuse or a medication or to a medical condition; does not occur exclusively during a mood disorder, psychotic disorder, or a pervasive development disorder
- Generalized Anxiety Disorder 7-item scale (GAD-7) is a self-reported questionnaire for screening and measuring the severity of GAD. Research suggests that the cutoff score for the GAD-7 for detecting GAD in older adults should be lowered from 10 to 5.

GAD-7 Scale

Over the last 2 weeks, how often have you been bothered by the following problems?	Not at all	Several days	Over half the days	Nearly every day
1. Feeling nervous, anxious, or on edge	0	1	2	3
2. Not being able to stop or control worrying	0	1	2	3
3. Worrying too much about different things	0	1	2	3
4. Trouble relaxing	0	1	2	3
5. Being so restless that it's hard to sit still	0	1	2	3
6. Becoming easily annoyed or irritable	0	1	2	3
7. Feeling afraid as if something awful might happen	0	1	2	3
Add the score for each column		+	+	+
Total Score *(add your column scores)* =				

If you checked off any problems, how difficult have these made it for you to do your work, take care of things at home, or get along with other people?

☐ Not difficult at all ☐ Somewhat difficult ☐ Very difficult ☐ Extremely difficult

Source: Spitzer RL et al. *Arch Intern Med* 2006;116:1092–1097.

DSM-5 recognizes several other anxiety disorders or trauma- and stressor-related disorders:
(Italicized type indicates the most common anxiety disorder in older adults.)

- Agoraphobia
- *Anxiety disorder due to a general medical condition*
- Obsessive-compulsive disorder (OCD)
- Panic attack
- Panic disorder
- Social anxiety disorder (social phobia)
- Substance-induced anxiety disorder
- Acute stress disorder
- Posttraumatic stress disorder (PTSD)

DSM-5 Criteria for Panic Attack

An abrupt surge of intense fear or discomfort with ≥4 of the following (also, must peak within minutes):

- Palpitations, pounding heart, or accelerated HR
- Sweating
- Trembling or shaking
- Sensations of shortness of breath or smothering
- Feelings of choking
- Chest pain or discomfort
- Nausea or abdominal distress
- Feeling dizzy, unsteady, lightheaded, or faint
- Chills or heat sensations
- Paresthesias (numbness or tingling sensations)
- Derealization (feelings of unreality) or depersonalization (being detached from oneself)
- Fear of losing your mind or going crazy
- Fear of dying

DSM-5 Criteria for PTSD

- Exposure to actual or threatened death, serious injury, or sexual violence
- Presence of intrusion symptoms, ie, distressing memories of the event, recurrent distressing dreams related to the event, dissociative reactions (flashbacks), psychological distress or marked physiological reactions to internal or external cues that resemble an aspect of the traumatic event(s)
- Persistent avoidance of stimuli associated with the traumatic event(s)
- Negative altercations in cognitions and mood associated with the traumatic event(s) (eg, dissociative amnesia)
- Marked alterations in arousal and reactivity, ie, irritable behavior and angry outbursts, reckless or self-destructive behavior, hypervigilance, exaggerated startle response, problems with concentration, sleep disturbance
- Duration of disturbance >1 mo (if duration is 3 d to 1 mo after traumatic event, then acute stress disorder)
- Clinically significant impairment in functioning
- Not attributable to the physiological effects of substance abuse or medical condition

Differential Diagnosis

- Physical conditions producing anxiety
  - Cardiovascular: arrhythmias, angina, MI, HF
  - Endocrine: hyperthyroidism, hypoglycemia, pheochromocytoma
  - Neurologic: movement disorders, temporal lobe epilepsy, mild cognitive impairment (MCI), AD, stroke
  - Respiratory: COPD, asthma, PE

- Medications producing anxiety
  - Caffeine
  - Corticosteroids
  - Nicotine
  - Psychotropics: antidepressants, antipsychotics, stimulants
  - Sympathomimetics: pseudoephedrine, β-agonists
  - Thyroid hormones: overreplacement
- Withdrawal states: alcohol, sedatives, hypnotics, benzodiazepines, SSRIs, SNRIs
- Depression

EVALUATION

- Psychiatric hx
- Drug review: prescribed, OTC, alcohol, caffeine
- MSE
- Physical examination: Focus on signs and symptoms of anxiety (eg, tachycardia, tachypnea, sweating, tremor).
- Laboratory tests: Consider CBC, blood glucose, TSH, B_{12}, ECG, oxygen saturation, drug and alcohol screening.

MANAGEMENT

Nonpharmacologic

- CBT may be useful for GAD, panic disorder, and posttramatic stress disorder (PTSD); efficacy in both individual and group formats.
- In view of potential limitations (eg, availability, cost), free online CBT may be considered. See https://ecouch.anu.edu.au.
- Graded desensitization used in panic and phobia relies on gradual exposure with learning to manage resultant anxiety.
- May be effective alone but mostly used in conjunction with pharmacotherapy.
- Requires a cognitively intact, motivated patient.

Pharmacologic (Table 42 for dosing of antidepressants and indication of generic status)

- Panic: sertraline; venlafaxine HCl XR; secondary choices include β-blockers and 2nd-generation antipsychotics
- Social phobia: sertraline, venlafaxine XR
- Generalized anxiety:
  - Suggested order: SNRIs (duloxetine or venlafaxine XR), SSRIs (escitalopram or sertraline), buspirone, pregabalin, benzodiazepines
- PTSD: sertraline
  - Avoid benzodiazepines.[CW]
  - For nightmares, prazosin may be helpful (initiate at 1 mg qhs and titrate slowly to avoid orthostatic syncope).

Buspirone[▲]:

- Serotonin 1A partial agonist effective in GAD and anxiety symptoms accompanying general medical illness (although geriatric evidence is limited)
- Not effective for acute anxiety or panic disorder
- May take 2–4 wk for tx response
- Recommended starting dosage: 7.5–10 mg q12h [T: 5, 10, 15, 30], up to max 60 mg/d
- No dependence, tolerance, withdrawal, or CNS depression

- Risk of serotonin syndrome with SSRIs, MAOIs, TCAs, 5-hydroxytryptamine 1 receptor agonists, ergot alkaloids, lithium, St. John's wort, opioids, dextromethorphan

Pregabalin:
- Although pregabalin is not FDA approved for the tx of GAD, there is limited evidence to support its use as both single and adjunctive tx, including in older adults (Avoid concurrent use with opioids except when transitioning from opioid tx[BC]; reduce dose if CrCl <60 mL/min/1.73 m² because of CNS AEs[BC])
- Onset of tx response may be longer than that observed in younger adults
- Adverse effects are predominantly somnolence and dizziness
- Risk of dependence or withdrawal appears minimal but is Schedule V medication in the US
- Current evidence does not support the use of gabapentin as an alternative to pregabalin to treat anxiety disorders

Benzodiazepines: (Avoid if hx of falls or fractures, or if concurrent use with an opioid.[BC])
- Restrict use to severe GAD unresponsive to other tx[CW] (**Table 21**)
- Preferred: intermediate–half-life drugs inactivated by direct conjugation in liver and therefore less affected by aging (**Table 21**)
- Avoid long-acting benzodiazepines (eg, flurazepam, diazepam, chlordiazepoxide)
- Linked to cognitive impairment, falls, sedation, psychomotor impairment, delirium
- Problems: dependence, misuse (p 349), tolerance, withdrawal, more so with short-acting benzodiazepines; seizure risk with alprazolam withdrawal
- Potentially fatal if combined with alcohol or other CNS depressants
- Only short-term (60–90 d) use recommended
- Refer to deprescribing.org for suggested algorithm for mitigating benzodiazepine use

Table 21. Benzodiazepines for Anxiety for Older Adults		
Drug	**Dosage**	**Formulations**
Lorazepam▲	0.5–2 mg in 2–3 divided doses	T: 0.5, 1, 2; S: 2 mg/mL; inj: 2 mg/mL
Oxazepam▲	10–15 mg q8–12h	T: 10, 15, 30

Nonbenzodiazepine hypnotics should not be used for tx of anxiety disorders (Sleep Disorders, **Table 130**).

CORONARY ARTERY DISEASE

Screening/Calculating Risk in Persons Without History of CVD (2013 ACC/AHA Guidelines)

- Quantify CVD risk: every 4–6 y in persons up to age 79 without hx of CVD by assessing traditional risk factors
  - Traditional risk factors for quantifying risk are: increasing age, male sex, African American race, total cholesterol >170, HDL cholesterol <50, SBP >120, tx for high blood pressure, DM, and current smoking
  - 10-y risk of CVD can be calculated using a downloadable spreadsheet available at https://tools.acc.org/ascvd-risk-estimator-plus/#!/calculate/estimate/
  - If 10-y risk of CVD is elevated (≥7.5%), patient should be considered for intensive lipid management (p 53), lifestyle alteration, and assessment and tx for obesity
- If tx decision based on 10-y CVD risk is uncertain, the presence of one or more of the following other risk factors would suggest further increased risk: 1st-degree relative with hx of premature CVD (male <55, female <65), high-sensitivity CRP >2 mg/L, coronary artery calcium >30 Agatston units or >75th percentile, ABI <0.9.
- Don't order coronary artery calcium scoring for screening purposes on low-risk asymptomatic individuals except those with a family hx of premature CAD.[CW]
- Don't routinely order coronary CT angiography for screening asymptomatic individuals.[CW]

Diagnostic Cardiac Tests

- Cardiac catheterization is the gold standard; cardiac CT angiography is a less invasive, but less accurate, alternative.
- Stress testing: The heart is stressed either through exercise (treadmill, stationary bicycle) or, if the patient cannot exercise or the ECG is markedly abnormal, with pharmacologic agents (dipyridamole, adenosine, dobutamine). Exercise stress tests can be performed with or without cardiac imaging, while pharmacologic stress tests always include imaging. Imaging can be accomplished by echocardiography or single-photon-emission computed tomography (SPECT).
- Don't perform stress cardiac imaging or advanced noninvasive imaging in the initial evaluation of patients without cardiac symptoms unless high-risk markers are present.[CW]
- Don't use coronary artery calcium scoring for patients with known CAD (including stents and bypass grafts).[CW]
- Don't obtain screening exercise ECG testing in individuals who are asymptomatic and at low risk for coronary heart disease.[CW]

Acute Coronary Syndrome (ACS)

- ACS encompasses diagnoses of ST segment MI (STEMI), non-ST segment MI (NSTEMI), and unstable angina.
- Suspect ACS with anginal chest pain or anginal equivalent: arm, jaw, or abdominal pain (with or without nausea); acute functional decline.
- Diagnosis is based on symptoms along with cardiac serum markers and ECG findings:
  - STEMI: elevated serum markers, elevated ST segments
  - NSTEMI: elevated serum markers, depressed ST segments or inverted T-waves
  - Unstable angina: nonelevated serum markers, normal or depressed ST segments, normal or inverted T-waves

- Measuring cardiac serum markers:
  - Most protocols call for checking troponins T or I at presentation and 2 h later.
  - A single negative enzyme measurement, particularly within 6 h of symptom onset, does not exclude MI; 2 negative measurements exclude MI.
  - Sensitivity of troponins is improved with the use of sensitive or ultrasensitive assays.
  - Troponins are not useful for detecting reinfarction within 1st wk of an MI. CK-MB is the preferred marker for early reinfarction.
  - Both CK-MB and cardiac troponins can have false-positive results due to subclinical ischemic myocardial injury or nonischemic myocardial injury.
- Troponin levels can be transiently or persistently minimally elevated by many non-ACS causes, including severe HTN, tachyarrhythmias, coronary spasm, HF, viral myocarditis, endocarditis, myocarditis, pericarditis, malignancy, cancer chemotherapy, trauma, PE, sepsis, renal failure, and stroke. Evaluation (hx, physical exam, assessment of renal function, ECG, echocardiography) should focus on finding and treating the underlying cause. Elevated troponin in the face of normal CK-MB can indicate increased risk of MI in the ensuing 5 y.

Initial Management of ACS (at presentation)

- ASA 162–325 mg initially (have patient chew it if possible), followed by 81–325 mg/d; D/C NSAIDs
- Chair/bed rest with continuous ECG monitoring
- Oxygen to maintain saturation >90%
- If ischemia is ongoing (based on symptoms or ECG changes), give nitroglycerin[A] 0.4 mg sl q5min for a total of 3 doses.
- Nitroglycerin IV is indicated for persistent ischemia, HTN, large anterior infarction, or HF. Begin at 5–10 mcg/min IV and titrate to pain relief while maintaining SBP >90 mmHg, or resolution of ECG abnormalities.
- If chest pain persists on nitroglycerin tx, give morphine sulfate 2–4 mg IV with increments of 2–8 mg IV repeated q5–15 min prn.
- Administer antiplatelet agents, anticoagulants, and glycoprotein IIb/IIIa inhibitors according to reperfusion strategy (**Tables 12, 17**, and **18**):
  - Thrombolytic tx: ASA, clopidogrel or ticagrelor, and an anticoagulant
  - Early invasive tx with planned percutaneous cardiac intervention: ASA, clopidogrel or prasugrel or ticagrelor, an anticoagulant, and a glycoprotein IIb/IIIa inhibitor
  - Medical management: ASA, clopidogrel or ticagrelor, and an anticoagulant; consider adding a glycoprotein IIb/IIIa inhibitor
  - CABG: ASA and UFH

Ongoing Hospital Management of ACS (1st 24–48 h)

- An oral β-blocker should be started within 24 h of symptom onset and continued long-term unless there is acute HF, evidence of a low-output state, pronounced bradycardia, or cardiogenic shock.
- An oral ACEI should be started within 24 h of symptom onset for STEMI patients, for NSTEMI patients with clinical HF or EF <40%, and for NSTEMI patients with HTN, DM, or stable chronic kidney disease (**Table 24**). If patient cannot tolerate ACEIs for reasons other than hypotension, give oral ARB.
- An aldosterone antagonist (spironolactone[BC] or eplerenone, p 59) should be added to the above medications in post-MI patients without significant renal disease (Cr ≤2.5 mg/dL in men and ≤2.0 mg/dL in women), without hyperkalemia (serum potassium ≤5.0 mEq/L), and who have LVEF <40%, DM, or HF.

- A high-intensity statin should be started if there are no contraindications. (Dyslipidemia Management, p 53).
- Anticoagulation with warfarin▲ (p 38), apixaban (**Table 18**), edoxaban (**Table 18**), rivaroxaban (**Table 18**), or dabigatran (**Table 18**) is indicated in post-MI patients with AF (2014 ACC/AHA AF Guidelines, p 64–66). Warfarin is indicated in post-MI patients with left ventricular thrombosis or large anterior infarction (**Table 19**).
- At time of discharge, prescribe rapid-acting nitrates prn: sl nitroglycerin▲ or nitroglycerin spr q5min for max of 3 doses in 15 min (**Table 22**).
- Longer-acting nitrates should be prescribed if symptomatic angina and tx will be medical rather than surgical or angioplasty. May be combined with β-blockers or CCBs, or both (**Table 22**).
- CCBs should be used cautiously for management of angina only in non-Q-wave infarctions without systolic dysfunction and a contraindication to β-blockers.

Table 22. Nitrate Dosages and Formulations		
Medication	**Dosage**	**Formulations**
Oral		
Isosorbide dinitrate▲	10–40 mg 3 ×/d (6 h apart)	T: 5, 10, 20, 30, 40; ChT: 5, 10
Isosorbide dinitrate SR *(Dilatrate SR)*	40–80 mg q8–12h	T: 40
Isosorbide mononitrate▲	20 mg q12h (8 am and 3 pm)	T: 10, 20
Isosorbide mononitrate SR▲	start 30–60 mg/d; max 240 mg/d	T: 30, 60, 120
Nitroglycerin▲	2.5–9 mg q8–12h	T: 2.5, 6.5, 9
Sublingual		
Isosorbide dinitrate▲	1 tab prn	T: 2.5, 5, 10
Nitroglycerin *(Nitrostat)*	0.4 mg prn	T: 0.15, 0.3, 0.4, 0.6
Oral spray		
Nitroglycerin *(Nitrolingual, NitroMist)*	1–2 spr prn; max 3/15 min	0.4 mg/spr
Ointment		
Nitroglycerin 2%▲	start 0.5–4 inches q4–8h	2%
Transdermal		
Nitroglycerin▲	1 pch 12–14 h/d	0.1, 0.2, 0.3, 0.4, 0.6, 0.8

POST-MI AND CHRONIC STABLE ANGINA CARE

- Unless contraindicated, all post-MI patients should be on ASA, a β-blocker, an ACEI, and a statin (high-intensity dose for patients aged <75, medium-intensity dose for patients aged ≥75; see p 53 Dyslipidemia Management).
- Consider tapering and then stopping β-blocker tx after 1–3 y in patients with normal LVEF and without angina or signs of ischemia.
- Dual antiplatelet therapy (DAPT): in addition to ASA, give clopidogrel or ticagrelor (**Table 17**) for at least 12 mo in patients receiving stents, on medical tx, or undergoing CABG. Consider continuing DAPT beyond 12 mo if bleeding risk is low and there have been no significant bleeding events. Prasugrel (**Table 17**) can be given as an alternative to clopidogrel. Prasugrel should be considered only in patients aged <75 without hx of TIA or stroke.[BC] ASA dosage in DAPT should be 75–100 mg/d.

- Angina management:
  - If β-blockers are contraindicated, use long-acting nitrates or long-acting CCBs for chronic angina.
  - For refractory chronic angina despite tx with β-blocker, CCB, or nitrates, consider the addition of ranolazine *(Ranexa)* 500–1000 mg po q12h [T: 500]; contraindicated in patients with QT prolongation or on QT-prolonging drugs, with hepatic impairment, or on CYP3A inhibitors, including diltiazem (p 61).
  - Use sl or spr nitroglycerin for acute angina.
- Treat HTN (p 56).
- Treat DM; see p 106 for target goals. Consider adding empagliflozin (**Table 48**) in patients with DM.
- Weight reduction in obese individuals; initial tx goal is 5–10% reduction with ultimate goal of BMI <25 kg/m^2.
- Aerobic exercise 30–60 min/d, at least intermediate intensity (eg, brisk walking).
- Smoking cessation.
- Encourage adoption of DASH (Dietary Approaches to Stop Hypertension) or Mediterranean diet.
- Consider supplementation with omega-3 polyunsaturated fatty acid (inconsistent data supporting effectiveness for reducing outcomes).
- Consider placement of ICD (p 71) in patients with LVEF ≤30% at least 40 d after MI or 3 mo after CABG.
- Don't perform routine annual stress testing after coronary artery revascularization.[CW]
- Avoid NSAIDs other than ASA.

HEART FAILURE (HF; 2017 ACC/AHA GUIDELINES)

Evaluation and Assessment

- All patients initially presenting with overt HF should have an echocardiogram to evaluate left ventricular function. An EF of ≤40% indicates systolic dysfunction and a diagnosis of HF with reduced EF (HFrEF). An EF ≥50% indicates diastolic dysfunction and a diagnosis of HF with preserved EF (HFpEF). An EF of 41–49% is a midrange classification (sometimes indicated as HFmEF) but patients usually resemble those with HFpEF.
  - Echocardiography can also evaluate cardiac dyssynchrony (**Table 23**) in patients with a wide QRS complex on ECG.
  - Echocardiography with tissue doppler imaging may be helpful in diagnosing diastolic dysfunction.

Table 23. Heart Failure Staging and Management

Clinical Profile	ACC/AHA Staging	NYHA Staging	Management
Asymptomatic but at high risk of developing HF (eg, HTN, DM, CAD present)	Stage A	—	RFR, E
Asymptomatic with structural disease: LVH, low EF, prior MI, or valvular disease	Stage B	Class I	RFR, E, ACEI (or ARB if unable to tolerate ACEI), BB
Normal EF; current or prior symptoms (HFpEF)	Stage C	Class I-IV	RFR, drug tx for symptomatic HF, control of ventricular rate
Low EF[1]; currently asymptomatic but with hx of symptoms	Stage C	Class I	RFR, E, DW, SR, ACEI (or ARB if unable to tolerate ACEI), BB

(cont.)

Table 23. Heart Failure Staging and Management (cont.)

Clinical Profile	ACC/AHA Staging	NYHA Staging	Management
Low EF[1]; patient comfortable at rest but symptomatic on normal physical activity	Stage C	Class II	Class II–IV: RFR, E, DW, SR, drug tx for symptomatic HF (below), consider biventricular pacing if cardiac dyssynchrony is present, consider placement of ICD if LVEF ≤35% (see p 71)
Low EF[1]; patient comfortable at rest but symptomatic on slight physical activity	Stage C	Class III	
Low EF[1]; patient symptomatic at rest	Stage C	Class IV	
Refractory symptoms at rest in hospitalized patient requiring specialized interventions (eg, transplant) or hospice care	Stage D	Class IV	Decide on care preference; above measures or hospice as appropriate

RFR = cardiac risk factor reduction; E = exercise (regular walking or cycling); BB = β-blocker, DW = measurement of daily weight; SR = salt restriction (≤3 g/d if severe HF).

[1] Low EF = EF ≤40%

- Other routine initial assessment: orthostatic BPs, height, weight, BMI calculation, ECG, CXR, CBC, UA, electrolytes, calcium, magnesium, Cr, BUN, lipid profile, fasting glucose, LFTs, TSH, functional status.
- Measurement of plasma brain natriuretic peptide (BNP) or N-terminal prohormone brain natriuretic peptide (NT-proBNP) can aid in diagnosis of HF in patients presenting with acute dyspnea.
  - BNP and NT-proBNP levels increase with age.
  - In dyspneic patients aged >70:
    - HF very unlikely (likelihood ratio negative = 0.1) if BNP <125 pg/mL or if NT-proBNP < 35 pg/mL)
    - HF very likely (likelihood ratio positive = 6) if BNP >500 pg/mL (110 mmol/L) or if NT-proBNP >1200 pg/mL (140 mmol/L)
  - Other conditions causing increased BNP or NT-proBNP levels include ACS, heart muscle disease, valvular disease, pericardial disease, AF, anemia, impaired renal function, pulmonary disease, pulmonary HTN, OSA, critical illness, severe burns, and sepsis.
- Optional: Radionuclide ventriculography, which measures EF more precisely, provides a better evaluation of right ventricular function, and is more expensive than echocardiography.
- If HF is accompanied by angina or signs of ischemia, coronary angiography should be strongly considered.
- Consider coronary angiography if HF presents with atypical chest pain or in patients who have known or suspected CAD.
- Consider stress testing if HF presents in patients at high risk (ie, numerous risk factors) for CAD.
- Drugs to be avoided in patients with HF:
  - Thiazolidinediones[BC] **(Table 48)**, NSAIDs, and COX-2 inhibitors[BC]
  - Dronedarone and most antiarrhythmic agents (amiodarone preferred if necessary)
  - Nondihydropyridine CCBs in patients with HFrEF[BC]
- Use metformin with caution.
- Cilostazol is contraindicated in decompensated HF.[BC]

Drug Therapy for Symptomatic HFrEF (AHA Stage C and D, NYHA Class II–IV)

For information on drug dosages and AEs not listed below, see **Table 28**. Efficacy of different medications may vary significantly across racial and ethnic groups; eg, blacks may require higher doses of ACEIs and β-blockers and may benefit from isosorbide dinitrate combined with hydralazine tx.

- Diuretics if volume overload. In patients with normal renal function, the IV dose of furosemide is about twice as potent as the oral dose. The IV and oral potencies of bumetanide and torsemide are about equal, and these 2 agents have a shorter half-life than furosemide. In refractory acute decompensated HF, consider continuous infusion of loop diuretics, supplemented by metolazone.
- ARB, ACEI, or combination ARB-neprilysin inhibitor (ARNI: sacubitril/valsartan [*Entresto*; T: 24/26, 49/51, 97/103]) to target doses (**Table 24**). ARNI is contraindicated in patients with a hx of angioedema. ARBs have been shown to improve HFrEF outcomes in older adults, while ACEIs have been found to improve outcomes in subjects aged <75 but not in those older than 75.
- In NYHA Class II and III patients on ACEI or ARB who are chronically symptomatic, replacing ACEI or ARB with ARNI can be beneficial.
- β-blocker to target dose (**Table 24**) after volume status is stabilized

Table 24. Target Dosages of ACEIs, Angiotensin II Receptor Blockers, and β-Blockers in Patients with HFrEF

Agent	Starting Dosage	Target Dosage
ACEIs[1,BC]		
Benazepril▲	2.5 mg/d	40 mg/d
Captopril▲	6.25 mg q8h	50 mg q8h
Enalapril▲	2.5 mg q12h	10–20 mg q12h
Fosinopril▲	5 mg/d	40 mg/d
Lisinopril▲	2.5 mg/d	20–40 mg/d
Perindopril	2 mg/d	8–16 mg/d
Quinapril▲	5 mg q12h	20 mg q12h
Ramipril▲	1.25 mg/d	10 mg/d
Trandolapril▲	1 mg/d	4 mg/d
Angiotensin II Receptor Blockers (ARBs)[1,BC]		
Candesartan	4 mg/d	32 mg/d
Losartan▲	12.5 mg/d	100 mg/d
Valsartan	20 mg q12h	160 mg q12h
Angiotensin Receptor-Neprilysin Inhibitor (ARNI)[BC]		
Sacubitril/Valsartan	49/51 mg q12h	97/103 mg q12h
β-Blockers		
Bisoprolol▲	1.25 mg/d	10 mg/d
Carvedilol▲	3.125 mg q12h	25 mg q12h
Carvedilol ER	10 mg/d	80 mg/d
Metoprolol XR▲	12.5–25 mg/d	200 mg/d
Nebivolol	1.25 mg/d	10 mg/d

[1] Check Cr and electrolytes 1–2 wk after initiating tx. Titrate to target dosage by gradually increasing or doubling the dose every 2 wk as tolerated.

- Adding an aldosterone antagonist can reduce mortality in patients with NYHA Class II–IV failure. Use either spironolactone▲ BC 25 mg/d po [T: 25] (Avoid if CrCl <30 mL/min/1.73 m².BC) or eplerenone *(Inspra)* 25–50 mg/d po [T: 25, 50, 100]. Monitor serum potassium carefully and avoid these medications if Cr >2.5 mg/dL in men or >2 mg/dL in women, or serum K+≥5.0 mEq/L.
- Adding a combination of isosorbide dinitrate and hydralazine (**Table 22** and **Table 28**; also available as a single preparation: *BiDil* 1–2 tabs po q8h [T: 20/37.5]) can be helpful for patients, particularly African Americans, with persistent symptoms. Use vasodilators with caution in patients with hx of syncope.
- For patients with EF ≤35%, with stable symptoms, and in sinus rhythm with HR ≥70 who are taking maximally tolerated doses of β-blockers or intolerant to β-blockers, consider adding ivabradine *(Corlanor)* [T: 5, 7.5] to reduce risk of hospitalization for HF.
- Consider low-dose digoxin▲ [T: 0.125, 0.25; S: 0.05 mg/mL]; 0.0625–0.125 mg/d (target serum levels 0.5–0.8 mg/dL) if HF is not controlled on diuretics and ACEIs, with or without an aldosterone antagonist. Avoid doses >0.125 mg/d.BC Digoxin may be less effective and even harmful in women and has been associated with increased mortality in patients with AF.
  - Digoxin concentration must be monitored with concomitant administration of many other medications.
    - The following **increase** digoxin concentration or effect, or both:

amiodarone	esmolol	tetracycline
diltiazem	ibuprofen	verapamil
erythromycin	spironolactone	

    - The following **decrease** digoxin concentration or effect, or both:

aminosalicylic acid	colestipol	sulfasalazine
antacids	kaolin pectin	St. John's wort
antineoplastics	metoclopramide	
cholestyramine	psyllium	

- Consider adding omega-3 polyunsaturated fatty acid supplements as adjunctive tx for symptomatic patients.
- Correct iron deficiency using IV iron (**Table 67**) with or without anemia.
- Concomitant HTN should be treated with goal SBP <130 mmHg.
- Class I antiarrhythmics are not indicated.

Drug Therapy for Symptomatic HFpEF

- For acute HFpEF with volume overload, loop diuretics and vasodilation with nitroglycerin are indicated. Parenteral nitroglycerin can cause hypotension in HFpEF patients without elevated BP, so use it cautiously if BP is normal or low.
- For HFpEF without volume overload, pharmacologic management focuses on control of HTN (goal SBP <130 mmHg); rate control, especially in patients with AF; and avoidance of digoxin.

LEG EDEMA

Differential

- Acute (<72 h) unilateral: DVT (by far most common and must be ruled out), ruptured Baker's cyst, ruptured medial head of the gastrocnemius
- Acute bilateral: acute worsening of HF, renal disease
- Chronic unilateral: venous insufficiency, secondary lymphedema (from tumor, radiation tx, surgery), cellulitis (warmth, erythema that does not resolve on raising leg), reflex sympathetic dystrophy
- Chronic bilateral: venous insufficiency (most common of all causes), HF, pulmonary HTN, drugs (see below), idiopathic edema, obesity, renal disease, liver disease, primary lymphedema, secondary lymphedema (from tumor, radiation tx, surgery)
- Drugs commonly causing edema include:
  - Antihypertensives: CCBs, β-blockers, clonidine, hydralazine
  - Hormones: corticosteroids, sex hormones
  - NSAIDs

Evaluation

- History: duration and location of edema; overnight improvement (less likely in lymphedema), presence of pain (more likely in DVT, reflex sympathetic dystrophy); medication review; hx of heart, kidney, or liver disease; hx of cancer and/or radiation tx; sleep apnea (increases likelihood of pulmonary HTN)
- Physical exam: BMI; location of edema; tenderness (more likely in DVT); skin changes; signs of heart, kidney, or liver disease; pelvic exam if suspect pelvic tumor
- Diagnostic studies: CBC, UA, electrolytes, Cr, BUN, glucose, TSH, albumin. See p 31 for workup of possible DVT. Other tests obtained according to hx and physical exam findings.

Treatment

- Venous insufficiency: leg elevation, skin care (daily mild soap and moisturizers), and compression stockings worn during the day (**Table 25**).
  - Below-the-knee stockings are usually sufficient. Above-the-knee stockings are appropriate for more extensive edema and for patients with orthostatic hypotension.
  - ABI measurement should precede use of compression stockings.
  - Compression stockings are not covered under traditional Medicare Part B unless an ulcer is present. Other insurance plans may cover them and require a doctor's prescription for coverage (although a prescription is not required to obtain them).
  - Antiembolism stockings (eg, T.E.D.™) are not designed for managing venous insufficiency.
  - Intermittent pneumatic compression pumps can be tried for recalcitrant edema.
  - Compression wraps can be used in patients who have difficulty donning compression stockings.
  - Diuretics should be used only for short-term tx of severe cases; chronic use can lead to intravascular dehydration and electrolyte imbalances.

Table 25. Prescribing Compression Stockings			
Stocking Class (Compression Grade)	**Pressure Delivered (mmHg)**	**Indications**	**Appropriate ABI Range**
1 (mild)	10–20	Mild edema Varicose veins	>0.5[1]
2 (moderate-firm)	20–30	Moderate edema Pigmentation	>0.8
3 (firm-extra firm)	30–50	Severe edema Lymphedema	>0.8

[1] Use with great caution in patients with ABI of 0.5–0.8.

- Complex decompression physiotherapy is an intensive multiweek intervention that is covered by Medicare for lymphedema.
- See **Table 16** and p 30 for DVT tx.
- Other tx should be directed at the underlying cause.

DYSLIPIDEMIA MANAGEMENT
Nonpharmacologic

A cholesterol-lowering diet should be considered initial tx for dyslipidemia and should be used as follows:

- The patient should be at low risk of malnutrition.
- The diet should be nutritionally adequate, with sufficient total calories, protein, calcium, iron, and vitamins, and low in saturated fats (<7% of total calories), trans-fatty acids, and cholesterol.
- The diet should be easily understood and affordable (a dietitian can be very helpful).
- Plant stanol/sterols (2 g/d), found in many fruits, vegetables, vegetable oils, nuts, seeds, cereals, and legumes, can lower LDL.
- Cholesterol-lowering margarines can lower LDL cholesterol by 10% to 15% (*Take Control* 1–2 tbsp/d, 45 calories/tbsp; *Benecol* 3 servings of 1.5 tsp each/d, 70 calories/tbsp).

Pharmacologic

- 2013 ACC/AHA indications for evidence-based statin tx to reduce cardiovascular risk:
  - Statins are dosed according to intensity of lipid lowering: high-intensity (usually lowers LDL ≥50%), moderate-intensity (usually lowers LDL 30–49%), and low-intensity (usually lowers LDL <30%). See **Table 27** for dosages. The LDL-lowering target should be the percentage of lowering rather than an absolute LDL target value.
  - Patients over age 75:
    - For those with CVD (prior MI, angina, ACS, coronary revascularization, stroke, TIA, or PAD), a moderate-intensity statin is recommended.
    - For those without CVD, one study (secondary analysis of the ALLHAT-LLT trial) showed a nonsignificant trend toward increased mortality with rosuvastatin tx compared to placebo in participants aged ≥75.
  - Patients aged 40–75:
    - For those with CVD or LDL ≥190, a high-intensity statin is recommended.
    - For those with DM, a moderate-intensity statin is recommended unless they also have a 10-y CVD risk of ≥7.5% (risk calculator at my.americanheart.org/cvriskcalculator), in which case a high-intensity statin is recommended.

- For those without CVD and a 10-y CVD risk of ≥7.5%, clinicians should have a discussion with patient about statin tx, assessing CVD risk factors, adverse effects of tx, and patient preferences. If statin tx is elected, a moderate- or high-intensity statin is recommended. The USPSTF recommends tx with a moderate-intensity statin for those without CVD and a 10-y CVD risk of ≥10%, and recommends selective use of low- or moderate-intensity statins in those without CVD and a 10-y CVD risk of 7.5%–10%.
  - Some experts are concerned that the risk calculator designates many more older adults as being eligible for primary prevention with statin tx than previous guidelines. For example, the calculator assesses a 10-y CVD risk of ≥7.5% in all men aged 63–75 and all women aged 71–75 with optimal values for other risk factors.
- Prescribing statins:
  - Tx is focused more on choice of statin intensity and percentage of LDL lowering rather than targeting a specific LDL level.
  - Check fasting lipids, measure ALT, and screen for DM before initiating tx. If ALT is normal, there is no need to recheck LFTs unless hyperbilirubinemia, jaundice, or clinically apparent hepatic disease occurs.
  - Statins should be taken in the evening.
  - Check fasting lipid profile 4–12 wk after statin initiation to assess adherence and response (see above for expected percentage of LDL lowering by intensity).
  - About 10% of patients on statins will report myalgias. Severe myopathy with CK levels >10× normal are very rare (about 1 in 10,000 cases).
  - If severe muscle pain develops after initiation, D/C statin immediately and check creatine kinase, Cr, and a UA for myoglobinuria. Most benign myalgias will resolve within weeks of statin cessation.
  - Statin tx has been uncommonly associated with increases in A1c and fasting glucose.
- A PCSK9 inhibitor (**Table 27**) can be added to statin tx to further lower LDL and cardiovascular risk.
- There are no updated guidelines regarding management of hypertriglyceridemia or mixed dyslipidemia. **Table 26** lists suggested tx choices for these conditions.

Table 26. Treatment Choices for Dyslipidemia			
	Type of Dyslipidemia		
Agent	↑**LDL**	↑**TG**	↑ **LDL** + ↑**TG** + ↓**HDL**
Statin	1	3	1
Fibrate		1	2
Ezetimibe	3		2, C
Niacin	2	2, C	
Bile Acid Sequestrant	2		2, C
Omega-3 Fatty Acid		2, 3, C	
PCSK9 Inhibitor	C		C

1 = 1st-line tx; 2 = 2nd-line tx; 3 = 3rd-line tx; C = appropriate for combined tx with another agent.

Table 27. Medications for Dyslipidemia

Class	Medication	Dosage[1]	Formulations
Statin (HMG-CoA reductase inhibitor)[2]	Atorvastatin▲	H: 40–80 mg/d; M: 10–20 mg/d	T: 10, 20, 40, 80
	Fluvastatin▲	M: 40 mg q12h or 80 mg XL/d; L: 20–40 mg/d	C: 20, 40; T: ER 80
	Lovastatin▲[3]	M: 40 mg/d; L: 10–20 mg/d	T: 10, 20, 40; T: ER 10, 20, 40, 60
	Pitavastatin *(Livalo)*	M: 2–4 mg/d; L: 1 mg/d	T: 1, 2, 4
	Pravastatin▲	M: 40–80 mg/d; L: 10–20 mg/d	T: 10, 20, 40, 80
	ASA/pravastatin *(Pravigard PAC)*	1 tab/d	T: 81/20, 81/40, 81/80, 325/20, 325/40, 325/80
	Rosuvastatin▲[4]	H: 20–40 mg/d; M: 5–10 mg/d	T: 5, 10, 20, 40
	Simvastatin▲	M: 20–40 mg/d; L: 10 mg/d	T: 5, 10, 20, 40, 80
Fibrate (fibric acid derivative)	Fenofibrate▲[5]	48–200 mg/d	T: 48, 54, 145, 160 C: 43, 67, 130, 134, 200
	Fenofibrate delayed release *(Trilipix)*	45–135 mg/d	C: 45, 135
	Gemfibrozil▲[6]	300–600 mg po q12h	T: 600
Cholesterol absorption inhibitor	Ezetimibe *(Zetia)* [7]	10 mg/d	T: 10
Nicotinic acid	Niacin▲[8]	100 mg q8h to start; increase to 500–1000 mg q8h; ER 150 mg qhs to start, increase to 2000 mg qhs prn	T: 25, 50, 100, 250, 500; ER: 150, 250, 500, 750, 1000 C: TR 125, 250, 400, 500
	Niacin ER▲[8]	500–2000 mg/d	T: 500, 750, 1000
Bile acid sequestrant[9]	Colesevelam *(Welchol)*	Monotx: 1850 mg po q12h; combination tx: 2500–3750 mg/d in single or divided doses	T: 625
	Colestipol▲	5–30 g mixed with liquid in 1 or more divided doses	Pks or scoops: 5 g, 7.5 g T: 1 g

(cont.)

Table 27. Medications for Dyslipidemia (cont.)

Class	Medication	Dosage[1]	Formulations
Fatty acid	Omega-3-acid ethyl esters (Omacor, Lovaza)	4 g/d in single or divided doses	C: 1 g
Combination preparations	Ezetimibe/simvastatin combination[2] (Vytorin)[2,7] Lovastatin/niacin combination[2,3,8] (Advicor)	10 mg/10 mg to 10 mg/40 mg qhs 20 mg/500 mg qhs to start; max dose 40 mg/2000 mg	T: 10/10, 10/20, 10/40, 10/80 T: 20/500, 20/750, 20/1000, 40/1000
	Simvastatin/niacin combination[2,8] (Simcor)	20 mg/500 mg qhs to start; max dose 40 mg/2000 mg	T: 20/500, 20/750, 20/1000
PCSK9 (Proprotein convertase subtilisin kexin type 9) inhibitor[10]	Alirocumab (Praluent)	75–150 mg SC q2wk	Inj: 75 mg/mL, 150 mg/mL
	Evolocumab (Repatha)	140 mg SC q2wk or 420 mg SC q1mo	Inj: 140 mg/mL

H = high-intensity statin dose, M = moderate-intensity statin dose, L = low-intensity statin dose

[1] Dosage ranges for statins are listed as high-intensity (usually lowers LDL ≥50%), moderate-intensity (usually lowers LDL 30–49%), and low-intensity (usually lowers LDL <30%)

[2] See p 53 for prescribing information.

[3] Numerous drug interactions warranting contraindication or dose adjustment of lovastatin; see package insert for details.

[4] Maximum dose is 10 mg/d if CrCl <30 mL/min/1.73 m^2.

[5] Measure Cr level at baseline, within 3 mo of initiating tx, and q6mo thereafter. Reduce dose if CrCl <60 mL/min/1.73 m^2; do not use if CrCl <30 mL/min/1.73 m^2.

[6] Contraindicated with concomitant statin tx.

[7] Use as monotx only in patients unable to tolerate statins, niacin, or a bile acid sequestrant (colesevelam, colestipol) and who have not reached LDL-lowering goal.

[8] Obtain baseline and q6mo LFTs, fasting blood glucose, or A1c, and uric acid. Monitor for flushing, pruritus, nausea, gastritis, ulcer. Dosage increases should be spaced 1 mo apart. ASA 325 mg po 30 min before 1st niacin dose of the day is effective in preventing AEs.

[9] Do not use if fasting TG >300 mg/dL. Use with caution if fasting TG is 250–299 mg/dL.

[10] Adjunctive tx for LDL lowering in patients with homozygous familial hypercholesterolemia and in patients with atherosclerotic vascular disease on maximally tolerated doses of a statin. Very expensive.

HYPERTENSION

Goal BP

• For older adults with HTN and multiple comorbidities, limited life expectancy, or both, goal BP should be individualized to consider benefits and side effects of tx and to reflect patient goals.

• The 2017 ACC/AHA guidelines recommend a tx goal BP of <130/80 mmHg for most older adults, including those with CVD, DM, or CKD.

Definition

- Elevated BP: SBP 120–129 mmHg and DBP <80 mmHg
- HTN Stage 1: SBP 130–139 mmHg or DBP 80–89 mmHg
- HTN Stage 2: SBP ≥140 or DBP ≥90

The above definitions classify about 80% of person aged 65+ as having HTN.

Evaluation and Assessment

- Measure both standing and sitting BP after 5 min of rest.
- Base diagnosis on 2 or more readings at each of 2 or more visits. After diagnosis is made, evaluation includes:
  - Assessment of cardiac risk factors: smoking, dyslipidemia, obesity, DM are important in older adults
  - Routine laboratory tests: CBC, UA, electrolytes, Cr, A1c, total cholesterol, HDL cholesterol, and ECG
  - Assessment of end-organ damage as guided by clinical judgment: testing for HF/LVH, CAD, cerebrovascular disease, nephropathy, PAD, retinopathy
  - Consider renal artery stenosis (RAS) if new onset of diastolic HTN, sudden rise in BP in previously well controlled HTN, HTN despite tx with maximal dosages of 3 antihypertensive agents, or azotemia induced by ACEI/ARB tx.
    - RAS diagnostic test options include renal artery duplex ultrasonography, CT angiography, or MRA.
    - Don't screen for RAS in patients without resistant HTN and with normal renal function, even if known atherosclerosis present.[CW]
    - Medical tx for RAS includes aggressive management of vascular risk factors and antihypertensive regimens that include an ACEI or ARB (monitor Cr closely).
    - Renal artery angioplasty and/or stenting can be considered in patients for whom medical tx has failed (refractory HTN, worsening renal function, intractable HF) or who have nonatherosclerotic disease such as fibromuscular dysplasia.

Aggravating Factors

- Amphetamines/stimulants
- Atypical antipsychotics (clozapine, olanzapine)
- Decongestants
- Emotional stress
- Excessive alcohol intake
- Excessive salt intake
- Lack of aerobic exercise
- Low potassium intake
- Low calcium intake
- Nicotine
- NSAIDs
- Obesity
- SNRIs
- Systemic corticosteroids

Management

- Initiate pharmacologic tx if goal BP (see above) has not been attained using nonpharmacologic methods.
- Clinic-based BP measurements are usually consistent with home-based readings for BPs <140/90 mmHg. Patients whose clinic-based BP readings are >140/90 mmHg will often have lower home-based readings.
- For patients with suspected "white coat" HTN, 24-h ambulatory blood pressure monitoring (covered by Medicare if office-based BP is >140/90 mmHg) can produce more reliable readings than office-based measurements.

Nonpharmacologic:
- Adequate dietary potassium intake; goal 3500–5000 mg/d.
- Aerobic and resistance exercise: 90–150 min/wk for each.
- Diet rich in fruits, vegetables, whole grains, and low-fat dairy projects; reduced intake of saturated and total fat.
- Moderation of alcohol intake: limit to 1 drink/d for women, 2 drinks/d for men.
- Moderation of dietary sodium: watch for volume depletion with diuretic use. Goal: reduction of 1 g Na+/d, optimal total intake of ≤1.5 g Na+/d.
- Smoking cessation
- Weight reduction if obese: even a 10-lb weight loss can significantly lower BP. Goal: BMI <25 kg/m^2.

Pharmacologic: **Table 28** lists commonly used antihypertensives.
- Use antihypertensives carefully in patients with orthostatic BP drop.
- Base tx decisions on standing BP.
- First-line drugs: a thiazide diuretic, an ACEI, an ARB, or a CCB.
- Follow-up BP measurements monthly until target BP is attained.
  - If BP is not at target, clinician has the option of increasing the dose of the initial drug or adding a 2nd drug from the 1st-line list above.
  - Many patients require 2 or more drugs to achieve goal BP.
- Visits may be q3–6mo if BP is stable at target goal.
- If coexisting conditions, tx can be individualized (**Table 29**).
- Available dose formulations of oral potassium supplements▲: [T (mEq): 6, 7, 8, 10, 20; S (mEq/15 mL): 20, 40; pwd (mEq/pk): 15, 20, 25]

Hypertensive Emergencies and Urgencies:
- Elevated BP alone without symptoms or target end-organ damage does not require emergent BP lowering.
- Emergent BP lowering is indicated with BP >180/120 **_and_** signs of new or worsening end-organ damage.
- Conditions requiring emergent BP lowering with goal of BP ≤160/100–110 mmHg in the 1st hour, hypertensive encephalopathy, intracranial hemorrhage, unstable angina, acute MI, acute left ventricular failure with pulmonary edema, acute renal failure; most common initial tx for emergent BP lowering is IV sodium nitroprusside▲ 0.3–10 mcg/kg/min.
- Aortic dissection warrants emergent BP lowering with goal of SBP ≤120 mmHg in the 1st hour; IV esmolol or labetalol are preferred agents.
- For BP management of acute ischemic stroke or ICH, see Neurologic Disorders, p 234.
- Nonemergent (ie, urgent) BP lowering is indicated only in cases in which BP needs to be lowered for procedures or tx (such as β blockade before surgery, p 283) or in asymptomatic people with SBP >210 mmHg or DBP >120 mmHg.
  - Administer standard dose of a recommended antihypertensive orally (**Table 28**) or an extra dose of patient's usual antihypertensive.
  - If the patient is npo, give **low**-dose antihypertensive IV, titrating upward **slowly**. Options include β-blocker (eg, labetalol 20 mg), ACEI (eg, enalapril at 0.625 mg over 5 min), or diuretic (eg, furosemide 10 mg).

Table 28. Commonly Prescribed Oral Antihypertensive Agents

Class, Medication	Geriatric Dosage Range, Total mg/d (times/d)	Formulations	Comments (Metabolism, Excretion)
Diuretics			↓ potassium, Na, magnesium levels; ↑ uric acid, calcium, cholesterol (mild), and glucose (mild) levels
Thiazides			
✓Chlorothiazide▲	125–500 (1)	T: 250, 500	
✓Chlorthalidone▲	12.5–25 (1)	T: 25, 50	↑ AEs at >25 mg/d (L)
✓HCTZ▲	12.5–25 (1)	T: 25, 50, 100; S: 50 mg/mL; C: 12.5	↑ AEs at >25 mg/d (L)
✓Indapamide▲	0.625–2.5 (1)	T: 1.25, 2.5	Less or no hypercholesterolemia (L)
✓Metolazone *(Mykrox)*	0.25–0.5 (1)	T rapid: 0.5	Monitor electrolytes carefully (L)
✓Metolazone▲	2.5–5 (1)	T: 2.5, 5, 10	Monitor electrolytes carefully (L)
✓Polythiazide *(Renese)*	1–4 (1)	T: 1, 2, 4	
Loop diuretics			
♥Bumetanide▲	0.5–4 (1–3)	T: 0.5, 1, 2	Short duration of action, no hypercalcemia (K)
♥Furosemide▲	20–160 (1–2)	T: 20, 40, 80; S: 10, 40 mg/5 mL	Short duration of action, no hypercalcemia (K)
♥Torsemide▲	2.5–50 (1–2)	T: 5, 10, 20, 100	Short duration of action, no hypercalcemia (K)
Potassium-sparing drugs			
Amiloride▲	2.5–10 (1)	T: 5	Avoid in patients with CrCl <30 (↑ potassium, ↓ sodium)[BC] (L, K)
Triamterene▲	25–100 (1–2)	T: 50, 100	Avoid in patients with CrCl <30 (increased risk of kidney injury; ↑ potassium, ↓ sodium)[BC]; avoid in patients with CKD Stage 4 or 5.[BC] (L, K)
Aldosterone-receptor blockers			
♥Eplerenone *(Inspra)*	25–100 (1)	T: 25, 50, 100	(L, K)
♥Spironolactone▲	12.5–50 (1–2)	T: 25, 50, 100	Gynecomastia; Avoid if CrCl <30.[BC] (L, K)

(cont.)

✓ = preferred for treating older adults; ♥ = useful in treating HFrEF; CrCl unit = mL/min/1.73 m^2.

[1]See **Table 24** for target dosages in treating HF.

Note: Listing of AEs is not exhaustive, and AEs are for the drug class except when noted for individual drugs.

Table 28. Commonly Prescribed Oral Antihypertensive Agents (cont.)

Class, Medication	Geriatric Dosage Range, Total mg/d (times/d)	Formulations	Comments (Metabolism, Excretion)
Adrenergic Inhibitors			
α1-Blockers[BC]			Avoid as antihypertensive unless patient has BPH; avoid in patients with syncope; avoid in patients with HF.
Doxazosin▲	1–16 (1)	T: 1, 2, 4, 8	(L)
Prazosin▲	1–20 (2–3)	T: 1, 2, 5	(L)
Terazosin▲	1–20 (1–2)	T: 1, 2, 5, 10; C: 1, 2, 5, 10	(L, K)
Central α2-agonist			
Clonidine▲	0.1–1.2 (2–3) *or* 1 pch/wk	T: 0.1, 0.2, 0.3▲; pch: 0.1, 0.2, 0.3 mg/d	Sedation, dry mouth, bradycardia, withdrawal HTN. Avoid as 1st-line antihypertensive.[BC] Continue oral for 1–2 d when converting to patch (L, K)
β-Blockers[1]			Bronchospasm, bradycardia, acute HF, may mask insulin-induced hypoglycemia; less effective for reducing HTN-related endpoints in older vs younger patients; lipid solubility is a risk factor for delirium
✓Acebutolol▲	200–800 (1)	C: 200, 400	β1, low lipid solubility, intrinsic sympathomimetic activity (L, K)
✓Atenolol▲	12.5–100 (1)	T: 25, 50, 100	β1, low lipid solubility (K)
✓Betaxolol▲	5–20 (1)	T: 10, 20	β1, low lipid solubility (L, K)
✓♥Bisoprolol▲	2.5–10 (1)	T: 5, 10	β1, low lipid solubility (L, K)
✓Metoprolol tartrate (immediate-release)▲	25–400 (2)	T: 25, 50, 100	β1, moderate lipid solubility (L)
✓♥Metoprolol succinate (sustained-release)▲	50–400 (1)	T: 25, 50, 100, 200	β1, moderate lipid solubility (L)
Nadolol▲	20–160 (1)	T: 20, 40, 80, 120, 160	β1, β2, low lipid solubility (K)
✓♥Nebivolol *(Bystolic)*	2.5–40 (1)	T: 2.5, 5, 10	β1, low lipid solubility (L, K)
Penbutolol *(Levatol)*	10–40 (1)	T: 20	β1, β2, high lipid solubility, intrinsic sympathomimetic activity (L, K)
Pindolol▲	5–40 (2)	T: 5, 10	β1, β2, moderate lipid solubility, intrinsic sympathomimetic activity (K)

(cont.)

✓ = preferred for treating older adults; ♥ = useful in treating HFrEF; CrCl unit = mL/min/1.73 m^2.

[1]See **Table 24** for target dosages in treating HF.

Note: Listing of AEs is not exhaustive, and AEs are for the drug class except when noted for individual drugs.

Table 28. Commonly Prescribed Oral Antihypertensive Agents (cont.)

Class, Medication	Geriatric Dosage Range, Total mg/d (times/d)	Formulations	Comments (Metabolism, Excretion)
Propranolol▲	20–160 (2)	T: 10, 20, 40, 60, 80, 90; S: 4, 8, 80 mg/mL	β1, β2, high lipid solubility (L)
Long-acting▲	60–180 (1)	C: 60, 80, 120, 160	β1, β2, high lipid solubility (L)
Timolol▲	10–40 (2)	T: 5, 10, 20	β1, β2, low to moderate lipid solubility (L, K)
Combined α- and β-blockers[1]			Postural hypotension, bronchospasm
✓♥Carvedilol▲	3.125–25 (2)	T: 3.125, 6.25, 12.5, 25	β1, β2, high lipid solubility (L)
✓♥Extended-release (Coreg CR)	10–80 (1)	C: 10, 20, 40, 80	Multiply regular daily dose of carvedilol by 1.6 to convert to CR dose; do not take within 2 h of alcohol ingestion
✓Labetalol▲	100–600 (2)	T: 100, 200, 300	β1, β2, moderate lipid solubility (L, K)
Direct Vasodilators			Headaches, fluid retention, tachycardia
♥Hydralazine▲	25–100 (2–4)	T: 10, 25, 50, 100	Lupus syndrome; used in combination with isosorbide dinitrate for HF in blacks (L, K)
Minoxidil▲	2.5–50 (1)	T: 2.5, 10	Hirsutism (K)
Calcium Antagonists			
Nondihydropyridines			Conduction defects, worsening of systolic dysfunction,[BC] gingival hyperplasia
✓Diltiazem SR▲	120–360, max 480	C: 120, 180, 240, 300, 360, 420; T: 120, 180, 240, 300, 360	Nausea, headache (L)
✓Verapamil SR▲	120–360 (1–2)	T: 120, 180, 240; C: 100, 120, 180, 200, 240, 300, 360	Constipation, bradycardia (L)
Dihydropyridines			Ankle edema, flushing, headache, gingival hypertrophy
✓Amlodipine▲	2.5–10 (1)	T: 2.5, 5, 10	(L)
✓Felodipine▲	2.5–20 (1)	T: 2.5, 5, 10	(L)
✓Isradipine SR (DynaCirc CR)	2.5–10 (1)	T: 5, 10	(L)

(cont.)

✓ = preferred for treating older adults; ♥ = useful in treating HFrEF; CrCl unit = mL/min/1.73 m².
[1]See **Table 24** for target dosages in treating HF.
Note: Listing of AEs is not exhaustive, and AEs are for the drug class except when noted for individual drugs.

Table 28. Commonly Prescribed Oral Antihypertensive Agents (cont.)

Class, Medication	Geriatric Dosage Range, Total mg/d (times/d)	Formulations	Comments (Metabolism, Excretion)
✓ Nicardipine SR▲	30–120	T: 30, 45	(L)
✓ Nifedipine SR▲	30–60 (1)	T: 30, 60, 90	(L)
✓ Nisoldipine▲	10–40 (1)	T: ER 10, 20, 30, 40	(L)
ACEIs[BC, 1]			Cough (common), angioedema (rare), hyperkalemia, rash, loss of taste, leukopenia
✓ ♥Benazepril▲	2.5–40 (1–2)	T: 5, 10, 20, 40	(L, K)
✓ ♥Captopril▲	12.5–150 (2–3)	T: 12.5, 25, 50, 100	(L, K)
✓ ♥Enalapril▲	2.5–40 (1–2)	T: 2.5, 5, 10, 20	(L, K)
✓ ♥Fosinopril▲	5–40 (1–2)	T: 10, 20, 40	(L, K)
✓ ♥Lisinopril▲	2.5–40 (1)	T: 2.5, 5, 10, 20, 30, 40	(K)
✓ Moexipril▲	3.75–30 (1)	T: 7.5, 15	(L, K)
✓ ♥Perindopril▲	4–8 (1–2)	T: 2, 4, 8	(L, K)
✓ ♥Quinapril▲	5–40 (1)	T: 5, 10, 20, 40	(L, K)
✓ ♥Ramipril▲	1.25–20 (1)	T: 1.25, 2.5, 5, 10	(L, K)
✓ ♥Trandolapril▲	1–4 (1)	T: 1, 2, 4	(L, K)
Angiotensin II Receptor Blockers (ARBs)[BC, 1]			Angioedema (very rare), hyperkalemia
✓ Azilsartan *(Edarbi)*	20–80 (1)	T: 40, 80	(L, K)
✓ ♥Candesartan *(Atacand)*	4–32 (1)	T: 4, 8, 16, 32	(K)
✓ Eprosartan *(Teveten)*	400–800 (1–2)	T: 400, 600	(biliary, K)
✓ Irbesartan *(Avapro)*	75–300 (1)	T: 75, 150, 300	(L)
✓ ♥Losartan▲	12.5–100 (1–2)	T: 25, 50, 100	(L, K)
✓ Olmesartan *(Benicar)*	20–40 (1)	T: 5, 20, 40	Severe GI symptoms (rare) (L, K)
✓ Telmisartan *(Micardis)*	20–80 (1)	T: 20, 40, 80	(L)
✓ ♥Valsartan *(Diovan)*	40–320 (1)	T: 40, 80, 160, 320; C: 80, 160	(L, K)
Renin Inhibitor[BC]			
Aliskiren *(Tekturna)*	150–300 (1)	T: 150, 300	Monitor electrolytes in patients with renal disease; contraindicated in patients with DM who are also taking an ACEI or ARB

✓ = preferred for treating older adults; ♥ = useful in treating HFrEF

[1]See **Table 24** for target dosages in treating HF.

Note: Listing of AEs is not exhaustive, and AEs are for the drug class except when noted for individual drugs.

Table 29. Choosing Antihypertensive Therapy on the Basis of Coexisting Conditions		
Condition	**Appropriate for Use**	**Avoid or Contraindicated**
Angina	β, CA	
Atrial tachycardia and fibrillation	β, NDCA	
Bronchospasm		β, αβ
CKD	AA, ACEI[1], ARB[1]	
DM	ACEI, ARB, β, T[2]	T[1]
Dyslipidemia		β, T[3]
Essential tremor	β	
Gout		L, T
HFrEF	AA, ACEI, ARB, β, αβ, L	NDCA
Hyperthyroidism	β	
MI	β, AA, ACEI, ARB	CA
Osteoporosis	T	
Prostatism (BPH)	α	
Urge UI	CA	L, T

AA = aldosterone antagonist; α = α-blocker; β = β-blocker; αβ = combined α- and β-blocker; CA = calcium antagonist; NDCA = nondihydropyridine calcium antagonist; L = loop diuretic; T = thiazide diuretic.

[1] Use with great caution in renovascular disease.

[2] Low-dose diuretics probably beneficial in type 2 DM; high-dose diuretics relatively contraindicated in types 1 and 2.

[3] Low-dose diuretics have a minimal effect on lipids.

PULMONARY ARTERIAL HYPERTENSION (PAH)

Evaluation and Assessment

- PAH can be primary (unexplained) or secondary to underlying conditions.
- Almost all cases in older adults are secondary, most commonly associated with chronic pulmonary and/or cardiac disease, including COPD, interstitial lung disease, obstructive sleep apnea, pulmonary emboli, HF, and mitral valvular disease.
- Early symptoms are often nonspecific and include dyspnea on exertion, fatigue, and vague chest discomfort.
- Late symptoms include severe dyspnea on exertion, cyanosis, syncope, chest pain, HF, arrhythmias.
- Physical examination findings relate to manifestations of the associated conditions mentioned above.
- Diagnostic tests:
  - ECG may show right-axis deviation, right atrial and ventricular hypertrophy, T-wave changes
  - CXR may show large right ventricle, dilated pulmonary arteries
  - Echocardiography estimates pulmonary arterial pressure and evaluates possible valvular disease
  - Right heart catheterization is gold standard, with PAH defined as mean pulmonary arterial pressure >25 mmHg at rest or >30 mmHg during exercise.
- Additional tests (eg, pulmonary function tests, sleep study) may clarify severity of coexisting conditions.

Management

- Correct/optimize underlying conditions.
- Supplemental oxygen for chronic hypoxemia
- Diuretics for volume overload from HF
- Avoid CCBs unless they have been shown to be of benefit from a right heart catheterization vasodilator challenge study.
- Other agents have been studied mainly in primary PAH and are of uncertain effectiveness and safety in secondary PAH:
  - Warfarin (p 38)
  - Prostacyclins: epoprostenol *(Flolan)* by continuous IV infusion, treprostinil *(Remodulin)* by continuous SC infusion, treprostinil or iloprost *(Ventavis)* by inhalation, or selexipag *(Uptravi)* 200–1600 mcg q12h
  - Endothelial receptor antagonists: ambrisentan *(Letairis)* 5–10 mg/d; bosentan *(Tracleer)* 62.5 mg q12h × 4 wk, then 125 mg q12h; macitentan *(Opsumit)* 10 mg/d
  - Guanylate cyclase stimulator: riociguat *(Adempas)*, 0.5 mg q8h, increase dose gradually to maximum of 2.5 mg q8h
  - Sildenafil *(Revatio, Viagra)* po 20–25 mg q8h, tadalafil *(Cialis)* po 40 mg/d

ATRIAL FIBRILLATION (AF)

Evaluation and Assessment

Causes:

- Cardiac disease: cardiac surgery, cardiomyopathy, HF, hypertensive heart disease, ischemic disease, pericarditis, valvular disease
- Noncardiac disease: alcoholism, chronic pulmonary disease, infections, pulmonary emboli, thyrotoxicosis

Standard testing: ECG, CBC, electrolytes, Cr, BUN, TSH, echocardiogram

Management (2014 ACC/AHA Guidelines)

- Correct precipitating cause.
- Patients presenting with AF and hypotension, severe angina, or advanced HF should be strongly considered for acute direct-current cardioversion.
- For acute management of AF with rapid ventricular response in patients who do not receive or respond to cardioversion, ventricular rate should be acutely lowered with one or more of the following medications:
  - β-Blockers, eg, metoprolol[▲] 2.5–5 mg IV bolus over 2 min; may repeat twice
  - Diltiazem[▲] 0.25 mg/kg IV over 2 min
  - Verapamil[▲] 0.075–0.15 mg/kg IV over 2 min
- For patients with minimal symptoms or in whom sinus rhythm cannot be easily achieved, rate control (target <110 bpm in asymptomatic patients with normal EF, <80 bpm for symptomatic patients or reduced EF) plus antithrombotic tx is the preferred tx strategy.
  - In patients without left ventricular dysfunction or without HFrEF, rate control can be achieved with oral metoprolol or other β-blocker, diltiazem, or verapamil.
  - In patients with left ventricular dysfunction or with HFrEF, 1st-line tx for rate control is a β-blocker after fluid status is stabilized; digoxin[▲BC] in combination with a β-blocker or amiodarone[BC] (**Table 30**) can be used as alternatives for rate control. Digoxin has been associated with increased mortality in observational studies of patients with AF. Avoid dronedarone.[BC]

- In patients with preexcitation and AF, digoxin, nondihydropyridine calcium antagonists, and amiodarone are contraindicated.
- For symptomatic patients in whom ventricular rate does not respond to pharmacologic tx, AV node ablation with pacemaker placement can effectively control rate. Anticoagulation should continue for at least 2 mo postablation; long-term postablation anticoagulation decisions should be based on stroke risk, bleeding risk, and patient preference (see below).
- Antithrombotic tx should be individualized to balance reduced stroke risk vs increased bleeding risk. Except in patients with advanced frailty or with severe bleeding risks, the benefits of anticoagulation outweigh the risks.
  - Two risk scoring instruments are commonly used for assessing stroke risk while bleeding risk can be assessed using the HAS-BLED score (**Table 31**). The CHA_2DS_2–VASc is generally preferred over the $CHADS_2$ by cardiologists. The CHA_2DS_2–VASc classifies many more older adults (including everyone aged 75 and older) as warranting anticoagulant tx than the $CHADS_2$.
  - Direct-acting oral anticoagulants (DOACs; apixaban, dabigatran, edoxaban, rivaroxaban) and warfarin can be used in AF. Compared to warfarin, DOAC use lowers rates of all-cause mortality, hemorrhagic stroke, ischemic stroke, and major bleeding. Dabigatran and rivaroxaban have been associated with higher rates of nonmajor GI bleeding compared to warfarin.
  - If anticoagulation is contraindicated or not tolerated in patients with $CHADS_2$ or CHA_2DS_2–VASc scores ≥1, use ASA 81–325 mg/d. Addition of clopidogrel 75 mg/d to ASA lowers stroke risk but also increases risk of major hemorrhage. Both ASA and clopidogrel are less effective for stroke prevention in patients aged ≥75. An additional option is percutaneous left atrial appendage occlusion, which has been shown to reduce the risk of hemorrhagic stroke when compared to warfarin tx.

Table 30. Selected Medications for Rhythm Control in AF

Medication	Maintenance Dosage	Formulations	Comments (Metabolism)
Amiodarone▲BC	100–200 mg/d	T: 200, 400	Most effective antifibrillatory agent; avoid as 1st-line tx for AF unless patient has HF or LVH; numerous AEs, including pulmonary and hepatic toxic effects, neurologic and dermatologic AEs, hypothyroidism, hyperthyroidism, corneal deposits, warfarin▲ interaction (L)
Propafenone▲ Immediate-release	150–300 mg q8h	T: 150, 225, 300	Contraindicated in patients with ischemic and structural heart disease; AEs include VT and HF (L)
Sustained-release (*Rythmol SR*)	225–425 q12h	C: 225, 325, 425	
Sotalol▲	40–160 mg q12h	T: 80, 120, 160, 240	Prolongs QT interval; AEs include torsades de pointes, HF, exacerbation of COPD/ bronchospasm (K)

Note: pretx (30 min before antiarrhythmic administration) with β-blocker, diltiazem, or verapamil is recommended.

Table 31. Risk Instruments to Guide Antithrombotic Treatment in AF

Instrument	What is Assessed	Score Calculation	Antithrombotic Tx by Score		
			0	1	≥2
CHA$_2$DS$_2$–VASc	Stroke risk	1 point each for HF, HTN, DM, vascular disease, age ≥65 y, female sex; 2 points each for age ≥75 y, hx of stroke	ASA or no tx	ASA or Anticoagulant[1] or no tx	Anticoagulant[1]
HAS-BLED	Bleeding risk of anticoagulant tx	1 point each for HTN, abnormal renal function, abnormal liver function, prior stroke, prior major bleeding, labile INRs, age ≥65, alcohol use, drug use	If CHADS$_2$ or CHA$_2$DS$_2$–VASc score is 1, the risk of bleeding with anticoagulant tx may outweigh the risk of stroke if the HAS-BLED score is >2. If CHADS$_2$ or CHA$_2$DS$_2$–VASc score is ≥2, the risk of bleeding from anticoagulant tx may outweigh the risk of stroke if the HAS-BLED score exceeds the CHADS$_2$ or CHA$_2$DS$_2$–VASc score.		

[1] Apixaban, dabigatran, edoxaban, rivaroxaban, or warfarin; see **Tables 18** and **19** for dosing, p 30 for selection of anticoagulant.

- For patients with unpleasant symptoms or decreased exercise tolerance on rate control tx, rhythm control via direct-current or pharmacologic cardioversion is the preferred tx strategy.
  - For direct-current cardioversion, 3 methods may be used:
    - Early cardioversion (<48 h from onset): proceed with cardioversion; use adjunctive anticoagulation based on risk of thromboembolism (eg, CHA$_2$DS$_2$–VASc score).
    - Delayed cardioversion (≥48 h from onset or unknown duration) with transesophageal echocardiography (TEE): perform TEE to exclude intracardiac thrombus; if no thrombus, begin anticoagulation and cardiovert.
    - Delayed cardioversion (≥48 h from onset or unknown duration) without TEE: anticoagulate for at least 3 wk with INR ≥2 before cardioversion; continue anticoagulation after cardioversion.
  - For pharmacologic cardioversion and rhythm maintenance (recommended only if AF produces symptoms significantly impairing quality of life), rhythm control drugs may be tried (**Table 30**).
  - Stroke risk should be assessed (**Table 31**), and if indicated, antithrombotic tx should be continued indefinitely after cardioversion due to the high risk for recurrent AF.
  - In selected patients with symptomatic AF refractory to antiarrhythmic drugs, catheter or surgical AF ablation may be considered.

AORTIC STENOSIS (AS)

Evaluation and Assessment

- Presence of symptoms—angina, syncope, HF (frequently HFpEF)—indicates severe disease and a life expectancy without surgery of <2 y.
- Echocardiography is essential to measure mean aortic valve gradient (AVG) and aortic valve area (AVA).
  - Moderate AS is indicated by an AVG of 20–39 mmHg and by an AVA of 1–1.5 cm^2.
  - Severe AS is indicated by an AVG ≥40 mmHg and by an AVA ≤1 cm^2.

- For asymptomatic cases, echocardiography should be repeated annually for moderate AS and q6–12 mo for severe AS.
- Don't perform echocardiography as routine follow-up for mild, asymptomatic native valve disease in adult patients with no change in signs or symptoms.[CW]
- ECG and CXR should be obtained initially to look for conduction defects, LVH, and pulmonary congestion.

Treatment
- Aortic valve replacement (AVR)
  - AVR alleviates symptoms and improves ventricular functioning.
  - In most cases, perform AVR promptly *after* symptoms have appeared.
  - Surgical AVR (SAVR) vs transcatheter AVR (TAVR; a percutaneous procedure in the catheterization lab in which an artificial valve is implanted via a catheter):
    - Both methods result in comparable mortality.
    - Compared to SAVR, TAVR results in fewer major bleeding episodes, less new-onset AF, and a higher stroke rate.
    - Based on limited data, dual platelet tx with ASA 75–100 mg/d and clopidogrel 75 mg/d is recommended for 6 mo after TAVR, followed by ASA 75–100 mg/d for life.
- Avoid vasodilators if possible, unless used with invasive hemodynamic monitoring in patients with acute decompensated severe AS and NYHA class IV HF.

ABDOMINAL AORTIC ANEURYSM (AAA)
- Ultrasound should be performed if aortic diameter is felt to be >3 cm on physical examination.
- Ultrasonographic screening for AAA is recommended once for men between age 65 and 75 if former or current smoker.
- Management is based on diameter of AAA:
  - <4.5 cm: ultrasound q12mo
  - 4.5–5.4 cm: ultrasound q3–6mo
  - >5.4 cm: surgical referral
- Endovascular repair is associated with significantly less perioperative morbidity and mortality up to 3 y.

PERIPHERAL ARTERIAL DISEASE (PAD)

Evaluation
Hx should include inquiry regarding the following:
- Lower extremity exertional fatigue or pain, or pain at rest
- Poorly healing or nonhealing wounds
- Cardiac risk factors

Physical examination should include the following:
- Palpation of pulses (brachial, radial, ulnar, femoral, popliteal, posterior tibial, and dorsalis pedis)
- Auscultation for abdominal, flank, and femoral bruits
- Inspection of feet
- Skin inspection for distal hair loss, trophic skin changes, and/or hypertrophic nails

Diagnosis established by ABI <0.9 or other test (**Table 32**).

Table 32. Management of PAD

Signs and Symptoms	Useful Tests	Treatment (see below)
Asymptomatic; diminished or absent peripheral pulses	ABI[1]	Risk factor reduction[2]
Atypical leg pain	ABI[1], SABI	Risk factor reduction, antiplatelet tx[2]
Claudication: exertional fatigue, discomfort, pain relieved by rest	ABI[1], SABI, Doppler ultrasound, pulse volume recording, segmental pressure measurement	Risk factor reduction, antiplatelet tx, claudication tx; consider endovascular or surgical revascularization if symptoms persist[2]
Rest pain, nonhealing wound (see also p 331), gangrene	ABI[1], Doppler ultrasound, angiography (MRI, CT, or contrast)	Risk factor reduction, antiplatelet tx, claudication tx, endovascular or surgical revascularization[2]

SABI = stress test (exercise treadmill test or reactive hyperemia for those who cannot walk on a treadmill) with ABI measurement.

[1] Abnormal is <0.9; <0.4 is critical. An ABI >1.40 is also considered abnormal, possibly due to calcified arteries, and may require further testing to rule out arterial stenosis.

[2] Refrain from percutaneous or surgical revascularization of peripheral artery stenosis in patients without claudication or critical limb ischemia.[CW]

Treatment

Risk Factor Reduction
- Smoking cessation
- Lipid-lowering tx (Dyslipidemia Management, p 53)
- HTN tx (p 56)
- DM tx (Endocrine chapter, p 101)

Antiplatelet Therapy
- ASA▲ 75–325 mg/d
- Clopidogrel *(Plavix)* 75 mg/d [T: 75] if no response or intolerant of ASA

Claudication Therapy
- Walking program (goal: 50 min of intermittent walking 3–5 ×/wk)
- Cilostazol▲ 100 mg q12h, 1 h before or 2 h pc (contraindicated in patients with Class III or IV HFrEF[BC]); 2nd-line alternative tx is pentoxifylline▲ 400 mg q8h [T: 400]
- If ACEI not contraindicated, routine use is recommended to prevent adverse cardiovascular events in patients with claudication.

SYNCOPE

Table 33. Classification of Syncope

Cause	Frequency (%)	Features	Increased Risk of Death
Vasovagal	21	Preceded by lightheadedness, nausea, diaphoresis; recovery gradual, frequently with fatigue	No
Cardiac	10	Little or no warning before blackout, rapid and complete recovery	Yes
Orthostatic	9	Lightheaded prodrome after standing, recovery gradual	No

(cont.)

Table 33. Classification of Syncope (cont.)

Cause	Frequency (%)	Features	Increased Risk of Death
Medication-induced	7	Lightheaded prodrome, recovery gradual	No
Seizure	5	No warning, may have neurologic deficits, slow recovery	Yes
Stroke, TIA	4	Little or no warning, neurologic deficits	Yes
Other causes	8	Preceded by cough, micturition, or specific situation	No
Unknown	37	Any of the above	Yes

Source: Adapted from Soteriades ES et al. *N Engl J Med* 2002;347:878–885.

Evaluation

- Focus hx on events before, during, and after loss of consciousness; hx of cardiac disease (significantly worsens prognosis of syncope of all causes); careful medication review.
- Focus on cardiovascular and neurologic systems in physical examination.
- ECG and orthostatic BP or pulse check for all patients.
- Characteristics associated with serious outcomes and likely to require urgent/emergent further testing and hospital admission with monitoring include:
  - advanced age, especially >90
  - male sex
  - abnormal ECG
  - exertional syncope
  - hx of palpitations
  - syncope without prodrome
  - hx of HF
  - hx of arrhythmia (VT, symptomatic supraventricular tachycardia, 3rd-degree or Mobitz II AV block, sinus pause >3 sec, symptomatic bradycardia)
  - structural heart disease
  - dyspnea
  - abnormal troponin I
  - persistent abnormal vital signs (eg, SBP <90 mmHg or >160 mmHg)
  - significant comorbidity (eg, electrolyte imbalance, severe anemia)
- Additional testing as suggested by initial evaluation:
  - Ambulatory ECG monitoring for further evaluation of arrhythmia
  - Stress testing to investigate ischemic heart disease
  - Echocardiography to investigate structural heart disease
  - Electrophysiologic studies in patients with prior MI or structural heart disease
  - Tilt-table testing for suspected vasovagal cause
  - Head imaging, EEG for suspected neurologic cause
  - Don't perform imaging of the carotid arteries for simple syncope without other neurologic symptoms.[CW]
  - In the evaluation of simple syncope and a normal neurological examination, don't obtain brain imaging studies (CT or MRI).[CW]
  - If suspected orthostatic cause, evaluation for Parkinson disease, autonomic neuropathy, DM, hypovolemia.

Management

- Patients with cardiac syncope require immediate hospitalization on telemetry; exclude MI and PE.
- Strongly consider hospital admission for patients with syncope due to neurologic or unknown causes, particularly if concurrent heart disease.
- Patients with syncope due to vasovagal, orthostatic, medication-induced, or other causes can usually be managed as outpatients, particularly if there is no hx of heart disease.
- Tx is correction of underlying cause.

ORTHOSTATIC (POSTURAL) HYPOTENSION

See also **Table 56**.

Evaluation and Assessment

- Associated with the following symptoms usually after standing: lightheadedness, dizziness, syncope, blurred vision, diaphoresis, head or neck pain, decreased hearing
- Diagnosis: ≥20 mmHg drop in SBP or ≥10 mmHg in DBP within 3 min of rising from lying to standing
- Causes
  - Medications, including antihypertensives, antipsychotics, TCAs, MAOIs, acetylcholinesterase inhibitors, SGLT2 inhibitors, anti-Parkinsonian drugs, PDE5 inhibitors (for erectile dysfunction)
  - Autonomic dysregulation (suggested by lack of compensatory rise in HR with postural hypotension): age-related decreased baroreceptor sensitivity, Parkinson disease and related disorders, peripheral neuropathy, prolonged bed rest
  - Hypovolemia
  - Anemia

Management

- Correct underlying disorder, particularly by discontinuing medications that could exacerbate hypotension
- Alter movement behavior: educate patients to rise slowly, flex calf and forearm muscles when standing, stand with one foot in front of other, avoid straining, and elevate head of bed
- Dietary changes: avoid alcohol, maintain adequate fluid intake, increase salt and caffeine intake
- Above-the-knee compression stockings (at least medium compression strength, eg, Jobst)
- Pharmacologic interventions:
  - First-line: fludrocortisone▲: 0.1–0.2 mg q8–24h [T: 0.1]; use with caution in patients with HF, cardiac disease, HTN, renal disease, esophagitis, peptic ulcer disease, or ulcerative colitis; watch for fluid overload and hypokalemia.
  - Midodrine▲: 2.5–10 mg q8–24h [T: 2.5, 5]; use with caution in patients with HTN, DM, urinary retention, renal disease, hepatic disease, glaucoma, BPH.
  - Pyridostigmine▲: 60 mg q24h [T: 60]; can be used in combination with midodrine 2.5–5 mg/d.
  - Caffeine: 1 cup of caffeinated coffee q8–12h; alternatively, caffeine tabs 100–200 mg q8–12h; useful for postprandial hypotension when taken with meals. Avoid in patients with insomnia.[BC]
  - Droxidopa *(Northera):* 100–600 mg q8h [T: 100, 200, 300]; use with caution in patients with HTN, cardiac disease, HF, mild cognitive impairment, dementia, Parkinson disease on carbidopa tx.
  - Erythropoietin can be useful for hypotension secondary to anemia if Hb <10 mg/dL.

IMPLANTABLE CARDIAC DEFIBRILLATOR (ICD) PLACEMENT

Indications

- Carefully consider age, life expectancy, and comorbid status for deciding ICD placement. Data are limited in patients aged >65 and suggest no all-cause mortality benefit in patients aged >75.
- Established indications:
  - Cardiac arrest due to VF or VT
  - Spontaneous sustained VT with structural heart disease
  - Spontaneous sustained VT without structural heart disease not alleviated by other tx
  - Unexplained syncope with hemodynamically significant VF or VT inducible by electrophysiologic study when drug tx is ineffective, not tolerated, or not preferred
  - Nonsustained VT, CAD, and inducible VF by electrophysiologic study that is not suppressed by Class I antiarrhythmic
  - LVEF ≤30%, NYHA Class II or III HF, and CAD >40 d after MI
  - ICD + biventricular pacing for advanced HF (NYHA Class III or IV), LVEF ≤35%, and QRS interval ≥120 millisec or mild HF (NYHA Class I or II), LVEF <30%, and QRS interval ≥130 millisec

Contraindications

- Terminal illness with life expectancy <6 mo
- Unexplained syncope without inducible VT or VF and without structural heart disease
- VT or VF due to transient or easily reversible disorder
- End-stage HF (ACC/AHA Stage D) not awaiting cardiac transplant

Complications

- Surgical: infection (1–2%), hematoma, pneumothorax
- Device-related: lead dislodgement or malfunction, connection problems, inadequate defibrillation threshold
- Tx-related: frequent shocks (appropriate or inappropriate), acceleration of VT, anxiety and other psychological stress
- End-of-life planning: discuss and document the circumstances in which the patient would desire the ICD to be turned off. ICDs can be turned off by the cardiologist or the device manufacturer's representative. Don't leave an ICD activated when it is inconsistent with the patient/family goals of care.**CW**

DELIRIUM

DIAGNOSIS

Diagnostic Criteria—Adapted from *DSM-5*

- Core symptom: disturbed consciousness (ie, decreased attention, environmental awareness)
- Cognitive change (eg, memory deficit, disorientation, language disturbance) or perceptual disturbance (eg, visual illusions, hallucinations)
- Three subtypes: hyperactive, hypoactive, and apparently normal alertness but cannot attend
- Rapid onset (hours to days) and fluctuating daily course
- Evidence of a causal physical condition

Predisposing Factors

- Major or Mild Neurocognitive Disorder (Dementia or MCI)
- Advanced age, hearing and visual impairment
- Hospitalization and/or surgery (Postoperative Delirium, p 288)

Prediction of Delirium Risk in Hospitalized Older Patients

- Physical restraints; >3 new medications; Foley catheter; malnutrition; any iatrogenic event
- 1 point each for any, likelihood of delirium based on total: 0 points: 4%; 1–2 points: 20%; ≥3 points: 35%

Evaluation

- Assume reversibility unless proven otherwise.
- Thoroughly review prescription and OTC medications, and alcohol usage.
- Exclude infection and other medical causes.
- 4AT is a screening instrument for rapid initial assessment of delirium and cognitive impairment, but is not diagnostic.
- Confusion Assessment Method (CAM): Both acute onset and fluctuating course and inattention and either disorganized thinking or altered level of consciousness. CAM–S allows for scoring of delirium severity. For nonverbal patients, use CAM-ICU to assess attention and level of consciousness.
- Laboratory studies may include CBC, electrolytes, LFTs, ammonia, thyroid function tests, renal function tests, serum albumin, B_{12}, serum calcium, serum glucose, UA, oxygen saturation, ABG levels, CXR, and ECG.
- Brain imaging and EEG typically not helpful unless there is evidence of cerebral trauma, possible stroke, focal neurologic signs, or seizure activity.

Mnemonic for Delirium Etiology

D Drugs
E Electrolyte disturbances
L Lack of drugs (withdrawal of sedatives, alcohol, opioids)
I Infection
R Reduced sensory input
I Intracranial disorders
U Urinary and fecal disorders
M Myocardial and pulmonary disorders

CAUSES

(Italicized type indicates the most common causes in older adults.)

Medications (Table 34 and Table 35)

- *Anticholinergics* (Avoid[BC])
- Anti-inflammatory agents, including prednisone
- Benzodiazepines[BC] or alcohol: either acute toxicity or withdrawal
- Cardiovascular (eg, digoxin, antihypertensives, diuretics)
- Lithium
- Opioid analgesics, especially meperidine (Avoid[BC])

Table 34. Potentially Differentiating Features of Medication-induced Delirium

Medication type	Early	Late
Anticholinergic	Visual impairment, dry mouth, constipation, urinary retention	↑ HR, mydriasis, ↓ bowel sounds
Serotonin syndrome	Tremor, diarrhea	Hyperreflexia, clonus, myoclonic jerks, ↑ bowel sounds, diaphoresis
Neuroleptic malignant syndrome	↑ EPS	Marked rigidity, bradyreflexia, hyperthermia

Note: The use of urinary catecholamines and/or metabolics as diagnostic aids require further evaluation.

Table 35. Some Drugs with Strong Anticholinergic Properties[BC]

Antidepressants

Amitriptyline	Doxepin (>6 mg)	Protriptyline
Amoxapine	Imipramine	Trimipramine
Clomipramine	Nortriptyline	
Desipramine	Paroxetine	

Antihistamines

Brompheniramine	Dexbrompheniramine	Hydroxyzine
Carbinoxamine	Dexchlorpheniramine	Meclizine
Chlorpheniramine	Dimenhydrinate	Pyrilamine
Clemastine	Diphenhydramine	Triprolidine
Cyproheptadine	Doxylamine	

Antimuscarinics (urinary incontinence)

Darifenacin	Oxybutynin	Trospium
Fesoterodine	Solifenacin	
Flavoxate	Tolterodine	

Antiparkinson agents

Benztropine	Trihexyphenidyl

Antipsychotics

Chlorpromazine	Olanzapine	Thioridazine
Clozapine	Perphenazine	Trifluoperazine
Loxapine	Promethazine	

(cont.)

Table 35. Some Drugs with Strong Anticholinergic Properties[BC] (cont.)

Antispasmodics

Atropine products (excludes ophthalmics)	Dicyclomine	Methscopolamine
Belladonna alkaloids	Homatropine (excludes ophthalmics)	Propantheline
Chlordiazepoxide-clidinium	Hyoscyamine products	Scopolamine (excludes ophthalmics)

Skeletal Muscle Relaxants

Cyclobenzaprine	Orphenadrine

Note: AGS updated Beers Criteria for potentially inappropriate medication use in older adults.[BC] American Geriatrics Society 2015 Beers Criteria Update Expert Panel. *J Am Geriatr Soc* 2015:63(11):2227–2246.

Infections

Respiratory, skin, urinary tract, others

Metabolic Disorders

Acute blood loss, *dehydration, electrolyte imbalance,* end-organ failure (hepatic, renal), hyperglycemia, *hypoglycemia, hypoxia*

Cardiovascular

Arrhythmia, *HF, MI,* shock

Neurologic

CNS infections, head trauma, seizures, stroke, subdural hematoma, TIAs, tumors

Miscellaneous

Fecal impaction, *postoperative state,* sleep deprivation, urinary retention, pain, immobility

PREVENTIVE MEASURES

Delirium can be prevented in 30% of cases. (https://www.nice.org.uk/about/nice-communities/social-care/quick-guides/recognising-and-preventing-delirium#preventing)

Table 36. Preventive Measures for Delirium[1]

Target for Prevention	Intervention
Cognitive impairment	Orientation protocol: board with names, daily schedule, and reorienting communication Therapeutic activities: stimulating activities 3×/d
Sleep deprivation	Nonpharmacologic: warm milk/herbal tea, music, massage Noise reduction: schedule adjustments and unit-wide noise reduction 0.5 mg melatonin or 8 mg ramelteon may prevent delirium in acute care
Immobility	Early mobilization: ambulation or range of motion 3×/d, minimal immobilizing equipment
Visual impairment	Visual aids and adaptive equipment
Hearing impairment	Amplification, cerumen disimpaction, special communication techniques
Dehydration	Early recognition and volume repletion
Infection, HF, hypoxia, pain	Identify and treat medical conditions

[1] May also be valuable for management

MANAGEMENT

Nonpharmacologic

- Identify and correct underlying cause or contributing factors.
- Relieve distress and maintain safety and vital functions.
- Use families or sitters as 1st line.
- Physical restraints can lead to serious injury or death and may worsen agitation and delirium.[CW] Use soft physical restraints or mitts only as last resort to maintain patient safety (eg, to prevent patient from pulling out tubes or catheters).

Pharmacologic

Avoid antipsychotics for behavioral problems unless nonpharmacological options (eg, behavioral interventions) have failed or are not possible, and the older adult is threatening substantial harm to self or others.[BC]

For acute agitation or aggression that impairs care or safety (other than delirium due to alcohol or benzodiazepine withdrawal), choose from one of the following:

Haloperidol[BC]

- The most often recommended and studied agent in intensive care; controls symptoms and may reduce duration and severity of delirium.
- Because of the risk of QTc prolongation, the IV route is not recommended. *Caution:* If the patient is taking other medications that prolong QTc (**Table 11**), D/C all if possible. Obtain an ECG before the 1st dose (if possible) or as soon as the patient is calm enough to tolerate the procedure. If QTc exceeds 500 millisec, *do not* administer any antipsychotic; all may prolong QTc. If QTc >460 millisec, correct any deficiency of Mg^{++} and K^+ and recheck.
- The standard dose is 0.5–1 mg po [T: 0.5, 1, 2, 5, 10, 20; S: 2 mg/mL]; evaluate effect in 1–2 h.
- If patient is not able to take medications po, haloperidol 0.5–1 mg IM [5 mg/mL] (twice as potent as po, peak effect 20–40 min). Reevaluate q30–60min for continued significant agitation. Most older patients respond to 1–2 mg total dose.
- Maintain effective dose for 2–3 d.
- Slowly taper and D/C haloperidol over 3–5 d while monitoring for recurrence of symptoms. If necessary, continue the minimal dose necessary to control symptoms.
- EPS will develop with prolonged use. If use exceeds 1 wk, switch to a 2nd-generation antipsychotic agent.

Quetiapine[BC]

- The drug of choice for patients with LBD, Parkinson disease, AIDS-related dementia, or EPS
- Initial dosage 12.5–25 mg po daily or q12h, increase q2d prn to a max of 100 mg/d (50 mg/d in frail older adults). Once symptoms are controlled, administer half the dose needed to control symptoms for 2–3 d; then taper as described above.

Cholinesterase inhibitors

- Contraindicated for adjunctive tx of delirium in intensive care (may increase mortality).

Alcohol/Benzodiazepine withdrawal

- Benzodiazepine (eg, lorazepam) in dosages of 0.5–2 mg IV q30–60min or po q1–2h titrated to effect
- Validated scales are used to guide dosing of benzodiazepines in alcohol withdrawal (ci2i. research.va.gov/paws/support_site/HOWTO/detoxification.html).
- Because these agents themselves may cause delirium, gradual withdrawal and discontinuation are desirable.
- If delirium is secondary to alcohol, also use thiamine at 100 mg/d (po, IM, or IV).

PROGNOSIS

- Weeks or months to resolve
- Waxing and waning mental status continues as patient improves, but there will be a general trend toward improvement.
- Persistent symptoms at discharge: 44.7%; at 1 mo: 32.8%; at 3 mo: 25.6%; at 6 mo: 21%.
- Accelerated cognitive decline: Patients with AD may experience a faster rate of cognitive decline after an episode of delirium.
- Prolonged delirium is associated with higher risk of death (2.5× more likely within 1 y compared to those whose delirium has resolved).

DEMENTIA SYNDROME (*DSM-5:* MAJOR NEUROCOGNITIVE DISORDER)

Definition

Chronic acquired decline in one or more cognitive domains (learning and memory, complex attention, language, visual-spatial, executive) sufficient to affect daily life.

Estimated Frequencies of Causes of Dementia

- AD: 60–70%
- Other progressive disorders: 15–30% (eg, vascular, Lewy body [LBD], frontotemporal [FTD] including primary progressive aphasia [PPA])
- Completely reversible dementia (eg, drug toxicity, metabolic changes, thyroid disease, subdural hematoma, normal-pressure hydrocephalus): 2–5%

Screening

- Dementia is largely unrecognized and underdiagnosed. Clinicians should have a low threshold for triggering an investigation for possible cognitive impairment.
- The value of dementia screening in older adults is controversial. Some professional organizations strongly endorse screening while others do not recommend it, citing lack of evidence of benefit. USPSTF 2014 concluded that evidence was insufficient to recommend either for or against dementia screening.
- Screening for cognitive impairment is a required element of the initial and subsequent Medicare Annual Wellness Visit.
- Suitable screening tests in primary care include the Mini-Cog (p 5), the Memory Impairment Screen (MIS), General Practitioner Assessment of Cognition (GPCOG), the Informant Questionnaire on Cognitive Decline in the Elderly (IQCODE), the Self Administered Gerocognitive Examination (SAGE), and the AD8 Dementia Screening Interview.

EVALUATION

Although completely reversible dementia (eg, drug toxicity) is rare, identifying and treating secondary physical conditions may improve function.

- Hx: Obtain from family or other caregiver
- Physical and neurologic examination
- Assess functional status: ADLs, IADLs, or using a home-based caregiver scale such as the Dementia Severity Rating Scale (DSRS)
- Assess for depression (PHQ-9, GDS)
- Evaluate mental status for attention, immediate and delayed recall, remote memory, and executive function. Useful assessment instruments include MoCA or MoCA-B (for illiterate patients and those with less than a gradeschool education) and SLUMS (medschool.slu.edu/agingsuccessfully/pdfsurveys/slumsexam_05.pdf) to evaluate attention, immediate and delayed recall, remote memory, and executive function. Use MMSE, CDR, or FAST [p 78] for staging.
- Comprehensive evaluation can be billed using cognition and functional assessment code 99483 (see Appendix)

Clinical Features Distinguishing AD and Other Types of Dementia

- AD: Memory, language, visual-spatial disturbances, indifference, delusions, agitation
- FTD: Personality change, executive dysfunction, hyperorality, relative preservation of visual-spatial skills

- LBD: visual hallucinations, delusions, EPS, fluctuating mental status, increased ADRs to antipsychotic medications
- Vascular dementia: abrupt onset, stepwise deterioration, prominent aphasia, motor signs

Laboratory Testing
- Routine testing: CBC, TSH, homocysteine, MMA, serum calcium, liver and kidney function tests, electrolytes; HIV, and serologic test for syphilis (selectively)
- Used for research but not clinical practice: genetic testing, commercial "Alzheimer blood tests," and CSF levels (tau and beta-amyloid) are not currently recommended for clinical use.

Neuroimaging

The likelihood of detecting structural lesions is increased with:
- Onset age <60
- Focal (unexplained) neurologic signs or symptoms
- Abrupt onset or rapid decline (weeks to months)
- Predisposing conditions (eg, metastatic cancer or anticoagulants)

Neuroimaging may detect the 5% of cases with clinically significant structural lesions that would otherwise be missed.

American Academy of Neurology (AAN) recommends at least one structural scan (CT or MRI) in the routine evaluation of dementia.

FDG-PET scans approved by Medicare for atypical presentation or course of AD in which FTD is suspected. See cms.gov/medicare-coverage-database/details/nca-decision-memo.aspx?NCAId=104.

Florbetapir F18 *(Amyvid)* has been approved by the FDA for the detection of amyloid plaques. A positive scan does not establish diagnosis. Medicare will not cover.

REISBERG FUNCTIONAL ASSESSMENT STAGING (FAST) SCALE

This 16-item scale is designed to parallel the progressive activity limitations associated with AD. Stage 7 identifies the threshold of activity limitation that would support a prognosis of ≤6 mo remaining life expectancy.

FAST Scale Item	Activity Limitation Associated with AD
Stage 1	No difficulty, either subjectively or objectively
Stage 2	Complains of forgetting location of objects; subjective work difficulties
Stage 3	Decreased job functioning evident to coworkers; difficulty in traveling to new locations
Stage 4	Decreased ability to perform complex tasks (eg, planning dinner for guests, handling finances)
Stage 5	Requires assistance in choosing proper clothing
Stage 6	Decreased ability to dress, bathe, and toilet independently
Substage 6a	Difficulty putting clothing on properly
Substage 6b	Unable to bathe properly, may develop fear of bathing
Substage 6c	Inability to handle mechanics of toileting (ie, forgets to flush, does not wipe properly)
Substage 6d	Urinary incontinence
Substage 6e	Fecal incontinence

(cont.)

FAST Scale Item	Activity Limitation Associated with AD
Stage 7	Loss of speech, locomotion, and consciousness
Substage 7a	Ability to speak limited (1–5 words a day)
Substage 7b	All intelligible vocabulary lost
Substage 7c	Nonambulatory
Substage 7d	Unable to sit up
Substage 7e	Unable to smile
Substage 7f	Unable to hold head up

Source: Sclan S et al. Int *Psychogeriatr* 1992;4(Suppl 1):55–69.

DSM-5 CRITERIA FOR MILD NEUROCOGNITIVE DISORDER (aka Mild Cognitive Impairment [MCI])

- Evidence of modest cognitive decline from a previous level of performance in one or more cognitive domains (**Tables 37 and 38**)
  - concern of the individual, a knowledgeable informant, or the clinician that there has been a mild decline in cognitive function, and
  - a modest impairment in cognitive performance, preferably documented by standardized neuropsychological testing or, in its absence, another quantified clinical assessment

Table 37. Cognitive Domains

Domain	Example of associated skill
Complex attention	Selective and sustained attention
Executive function	Decision making; flexibility; planning; working memory
Language	Object naming; word retrieval; use of speech
Learning and memory	Episodic and semantic memory; short-term and long-term recall
Perceptual/motor	Visual discrimination; spatial ability; hand-eye and body-eye coordination
Social cognition	Nonverbal communication; emotional recognition and regulation

Table 38. Major and Mild Neurocognitive Disorder

	Normal	Mild	Major
Memory complaints	+	+	+
Decline in objective cognition	-	+	+
Functional impairment	-	-	+

- The cognitive deficits do not interfere with one's capacity for independence in everyday activities (ie, complex IADLs such as paying bills or managing medications are preserved), but greater effort, compensatory strategies, or accommodation may be required.
- The cognitive deficits do not occur exclusively in the context of a delirium.
- The cognitive deficits are not better explained by another mental disorder (eg, major depressive disorder, schizophrenia).
- In addition to the above, NIA-AA criteria for diagnosis of Mild Neurocognitive Disorder (aka MCI) requires at least 2 abnormal neuropsychological test scores (–1.0 to –2.0 SD) based on published norms, corrected for age, education, and premorbid IQ.

- MCI diagnoses may be further classified as amnestic MCI if at least one episodic memory test score is abnormal. If no memory test scores are abnormal, the MCI diagnosis is classified as nonamnestic MCI.
- Demarcations between normal cognition and MCI can be difficult, requiring clinical judgment.
- 12–15% annual conversion of MCI to dementia syndrome; some cases may not progress.
- Depression frequently coexists with MCI, remains underdiagnosed and undertreated, and may contribute to dementia progression.

Table 39. Progression of Alzheimer Disease

Functional Impairment	Cognitive Changes	Behavioral Issues	Complications	Score			
				MMSE	CDR	DSRS	FAST
Mild Cognitive Impairment (preclinical)				26–30	0.5	5–10	3
None	Report by patient or caregiver of memory loss Objective signs of memory impairment Mild construction, language, or executive dysfunction	—	—				
Early, Mild Impairment (y 1–3 from onset of symptoms)				21–25	1	11–24	4
Managing finances Driving Managing medications	Decreased insight Short-term memory deficits Poor judgment	Social withdrawal Mood changes: apathy, depression	Poor financial decisions AEs due to medication errors				
Middle, Moderate Impairment (y 2–8)				11–20	2	25–35	5–6
IADL Difficulty with some ADLs Gait and balance	Disoriented to date and place Worse memory Getting lost in familiar areas Repeating questions	Delusions, agitation, aggression Apathy, depression Restlessness, anxiety, wandering	Inability to remain at home, ALF Falls				
Late, Severe Impairment (y 6–12)				0–10	3	36–54	7
ADLs including continence Mobility Swallowing	Little or unintelligible verbal output Loss of remote memory Inability to recognize family/friends	Motor or verbal agitation, aggression Apathy, depression Sundowning	Pressure sores Contractures Aspiration, pneumonia				

CDR = Clinical Dementia Rating Scale; DSRS = Dementia Severity Rating Scale; FAST = Reisberg Functional Assessment Staging Scale (p 78); MMSE = Mini-Mental State Examination.

Prognosis

- Among nursing-home residents with advanced dementia, 71% die within 6 mo of admission.
- Distressing conditions common in advanced dementia include pressure ulcers, constipation, pain, and shortness of breath.

NONCOGNITIVE SYMPTOMS

Psychotic Symptoms (eg, delusions, hallucinations)
- Seen in about 20% of AD patients
- Delusions may be paranoid (eg, people stealing things, spouse unfaithful)
- Hallucinations (~11% of patients) are more commonly visual

Depressive Symptoms
- Seen in up to 40% of AD patients; may precede onset of AD
- May cause acceleration of decline if untreated
- Suspect if patient stops eating or withdraws

Apathy
- High prevalence and persistence throughout course of AD
- Causes more impairment in ADL than expected for cognitive status
- High overlap with depressive symptoms but lacks depressive mood, guilt, and hopelessness

Agitation or Aggression
- Seen in up to 80% of patients with AD
- A leading cause of nursing-home admission
- Consider superimposed delirium
- Consider pain as a cause in moderate or severe dementia and possible trial of analgesics (Pain chapter, p 252)

RISK AND PROTECTIVE FACTORS FOR DEMENTIA

Definite Risks	Possible Risks	Possible Protections
Age	DM	Mediterranean diet, DASH diet
APOE-E4 (whites)	Delirium	Physical activity
Atrial fibrillation	Head trauma	
Depression	Heavy smoking	
Down syndrome	Hypercholesterolemia	
Family hx	HTN	
	Lower educational level	
	Other genes	
	Postmenopausal HT	
	Sleep apnea	

TREATMENT

Primary goals of tx are to improve quality of life and maximize functional performance by enhancing cognition, mood, and behavior.

General Treatment Principles
- Identify and treat comorbid physical illnesses (eg, HTN, DM).
- Promote brain health by exercise, balanced diet, stress reduction.
- Supervised exercise, whether individual or group, slows disability and prevent falls.

- A large 2-y RCT (FINGER)—a multidomain intervention of diet, exercise, cognitive training, vascular risk monitoring—suggests that cognitive functioning in at-risk older people may be improved or maintained.
- Vitamin E at 1000 IU 2×/d found to delay functional decline in mild to moderate AD. *Note:* The USPSTF recommends against the use of vitamin E for the prevention of CVD or cancer.
- Avoid anticholinergic medications (**Table 35**).
- Set realistic goals.
- Limit prn psychotropic medication use.
- Maximize and maintain functioning.
- Identify, quantify, and examine the context of any problematic behaviors (is it harmful to patient or others) and environmental triggers (eg, overstimulation, unfamiliar surroundings, frustrating interactions); exclude underlying physical discomfort (eg, illnesses or medication); consider nonpharmacologic strategies.
- Consider referral to hospice (FAST=7; diminished speech, movement, and consciousness; see Palliative Care and Hospice chapter).
- The Dementia Management Quality Measurement Set developed by the AAN and the American Psychiatric Association serves as a useful guideline (www.psychiatry.org/psychiatrists/practice/quality-improvement/quality-measures-for-mips-quality-category/dementia-updates).

Caregiver Issues
- Establish and maintain alliance with patient.
- Discuss with patient and family concerns (eg, driving).
- Intervene to decrease hazards of wandering.
- Advise family about sources of care and support, financial and legal issues.
- Over 50% develop depression.
- Physical illness, isolation, anxiety, and burnout are common.
- Intensive education and support of caregivers may delay institutionalization.
- Adult day care for patients and respite services may help.
- Alzheimer's Association offers support, education services (eg, Safe Return).
- Family Caregiver Alliance offers support, education, information for caregivers.
- Information about clinical studies can be found at alz.org/research.

Nonpharmacologic Approaches for Problem Behaviors
To improve function:
- Behavior modification, scheduled toileting, and prompted toileting (p 168) for UI
- Graded assistance (as little help as possible to perform ADLs), practice, and positive reinforcement to increase independence

For problem behaviors:
- Music during meals, bathing
- Walking or light exercise
- Simulate family presence with video or audio tapes
- Pet tx
- Speak at patient's comprehension level
- Bright light, "white" noise (ie, low-level, background noise)

Approaches for assessment and management of behavioral symptoms of dementia can be found on the UCLA Alzheimer's and Dementia Care Program website (uclahealth.org/dementia).

The evidence base for specific nonpharmacological approaches using a person-centered approach to care is growing. A nonpharmacological toolkit for reducing antipsychotic use in nursing homes can be found at: nursinghometoolkit.com.

Pharmacologic Treatment of Cognitive Dysfunction

- Patients with a diagnosis of mild or moderate AD should receive a trial of a cholinesterase inhibitor; donepezil also approved for severe AD (**Table 40**).
  - Cholinesterase inhibitors should be prescribed with periodic assessment for cognitive benefits and adverse gastrointestinal effects.[CW] Patients should be monitored for weight loss.
  - Only 10–25% of patients taking cholinesterase inhibitors show modest global improvement, but many more have less rapid cognitive decline.
  - Initial studies show benefits of cholinesterase inhibitors for patients with dementia associated with LBD, Parkinson disease, and mixed dementia (AD and vascular). May worsen behavioral variant FTD.
  - Cholinesterase inhibitors may attenuate noncognitive symptoms and delay nursing-home placement.
  - AEs increase with higher dosing. Possible AEs include nausea, vomiting, diarrhea, dyspepsia, anorexia, weight loss, leg cramps, bradycardia, syncope, insomnia, and agitation.
- Patients with moderate to severe AD may benefit from a trial of memantine *(Namenda)*.
  - Side effects minimal (confusion, dizziness, constipation, headache)
  - A controlled trial did not demonstrate significant advantage to the combination of memantine and donepezil compared with donepezil alone in patients with severe dementia.
  - To evaluate response:
    - Elicit caregiver observations of patient's behavior (alertness, initiative) and follow functional status (ADLs and IADLs).
    - Follow cognitive status (eg, improved or stabilized) by caregiver's report or serial ratings of cognition (eg, Mini-Cog [p 5]; MMSE).
- D/C cognitive enhancers when FAST = 7 (p 78).

Table 40. Cognitive Enhancers		
Medication	**Formulations**	**Dosing (Metabolism)**
Cholinesterase Inhibitors		*Class effects:* Avoid if hx of syncope.[BC]
Donepezil[▲ 1,2]	T: 5[▲], 10[▲], 23 ODT: 5, 10 S: 5 mg/mL	Start at 5 mg/d, increase to 10 mg/d after 1 mo (CYP2D6, -3A4); must be on 10 mg/d ≥3 mo to consider increasing to 23 mg/d in moderate to severe AD (L)
Galantamine[▲ 1,3]	T: 4, 8, 12 S: 4 mg/mL	Start at 4 mg q12h, increase to 8 mg q12h after 4 wk; recommended dosage 8 or 12 mg q12h (CYP2D6, -3A4) (L)
(Razadyne ER)	C: 8, 16, 24	Start at 1 capsule daily, preferably with food; titrate as above. Rare complication: Stevens-Johnson syndrome
Rivastigmine[▲] *(Exelon)* [1]	C[▲]: 1.5, 3, 4.5, 6 S[▲]: 2 mg/mL pch: 4.6, 9.5, 13.3	Start at 1.5 mg q12h and gradually titrate up to minimally effective dosage of 3 mg q12h; continue up to 6 mg q12h as tolerated; for pch, start at 4.6 mg/d, may be increased after ≥4 wk to 9.5 mg/d (recommended effective dosage; value of increase to 13.3 mg/d is not established): retitrate if drug is stopped (K)

(cont.)

Table 40. Cognitive Enhancers (cont.)		
Medication	**Formulations**	**Dosing (Metabolism)**
NMDA antagonist[2]		
Memantine▲ [4]	T: 5, 10 S: 2 mg/mL	Start at 5 mg/d, increase by 5 mg at weekly intervals to max of 10 mg q12h; if CrCl <30 mL/min/1.73 m^2, max of 5 mg q12h (K)
(Namenda XR)	C: 7, 14, 21, 28	Start at 7 mg/d, increase by 7 mg at weekly intervals to max of 28 mg; if severe renal impairment, max of 14 mg daily (L)
(Namzaric)	C: 28/10, 14/10	Fixed-dose combination of donepezil and memantine for patients previously stabilized on combination tx of both individual drugs

[1] Cholinesterase inhibitors. Continue if improvement or stabilization occurs; stopping medications can lead to rapid decline.

[2] Approved by FDA for moderate to severe AD.

[3] Increased mortality found in controlled studies of mild cognitive impairment.

[4] Patients can switch directly from *Namenda* IR 20 mg (10 mg tabs 2×/d) to *Namenda* XR capsules 28 mg 1×/d on the day after the last dose of a 10-mg IR tab. Patients with severe renal impairment on *Namenda* IR 5 mg 2×/d tabs can be switched to *Namenda* XR 14 mg 1×/d capsule.

- Ginkgo biloba is not generally recommended (p 27).
- *Axona* (medium-chain TG) has insufficient evidence to support its value in preventing or treating AD, and long-term effects are uncertain.

Treatment of Agitation

- Consider nonpharmacologic approaches first before pharmacologic tx (**Table 41**).
- Steps to reduce nonverbalized pain (p 252).
- Cognitive enhancers may slow deterioration, and agitation may worsen if discontinued.
- Low doses of antipsychotic medications have limited role but may be necessary.[BC,CW] Note that this use is off-label and increases risk of death compared with placebo in patients with AD. CATIE-AD trial showed modest tx benefit compared with placebo for olanzapine and risperidone that was mitigated by greater EPS, sedation, and confusion. In this trial, quetiapine did not appear to be efficacious compared with placebo but caused greater sedation (**Table 107** and **Table 108**).
- CATIE-AD reported 2nd-generation antipsychotics cause weight gain, particularly in women treated with olanzapine or quetiapine; olanzapine tx was also associated with decreased HDL cholesterol.
- In a placebo-controlled randomized trial, citalopram was found to significantly reduce agitation and caregiver distress. Cognitive and cardiac (QT interval prolongation) AEs at the study dose of 30 mg/d limits practical application. Appropriate trials for escitalopram have not yet been conducted.
- Limited evidence supports use of dextromethorphan-quinidine *(Nuedexta)*[BC] 20 mg/10 mg 1×/d.
- Behavioral variant FTD: consider memantine or SSRI.

Treatment of Apathy

- Assess and treat underlying depression.
- Cholinesterase inhibitors help.
- Methylphenidate (5–20 mg/d), very limited data, may cause agitation and psychosis.

Table 41. Pharmacologic Treatment of Agitation

Symptom	Medication	Dosage	Formulations
Agitation in context of psychosis	Aripiprazole[1,2,BC] *(Abilify)*	2.5–12.5 mg/d	T: 5, 10, 15, 20, 30
	Olanzapine[1,2,BC] *(Zyprexa) (Zydis)*	2.5–10 mg/d	T: 2.5, 5, 7.5, 10, 15, 20 ODT: 5, 10, 15, 20
	Quetiapine[1,2,BC] *(Seroquel)*	12.5–100 mg/d	T: 25, 100, 200, 300
	Risperidone[▲1,2,BC]	0.25–3 mg/d	T: 0.25, 0.5, 1, 2, 3, 4 S: 1 mg/mL
Agitation in context of depression	SSRI[BC], eg, citalopram[▲], escitalopram[▲], sertraline[▲]	10–20 mg/d (citalopram) 5–10 mg/d (escitalopram) 25–100 mg/d (sertraline)	T: 20, 40 S: 2 mg/mL
Anxiety, mild to moderate irritability	Buspirone[▲], Trazodone[▲]	15–60 mg/d[3] 50–100 mg/d[4]	T: 5, 7.5, 10, 15, 30 T: 50, 100, 150, 300
Refractory agitation or aggression	Carbamazepine[▲BC]	300–600 mg/d[5]	T: 200; ChT: 100 S: sus 100/5 mL
	Divalproex sodium[▲BC]	500–1500 mg/d[6]	T: 125, 250, 500 S: syr 250 mg/mL sprinkle capsule: 125
	Olanzapine[2,7,BC] *(Zyprexa Intramuscular)*	2.5–5 mg IM	Inj
Sexual aggression, impulse-control symptoms in men	SSRIs[BC], 2nd-generation antipsychotic[BC] or divalproex[▲BC]	See dosages above	
	If no response, estrogen[▲]	0.625–1.25 mg/d	T: 0.3, 0.625, 0.9, 1.25, 2.5
	medroxyprogesterone[▲]	100 mg IM/wk	Inj
	or		
	Leuprolide acetate *(Lupron Depot)*	**Table 106**	

[1] Avoid.[BC]

[2] Increased risk of mortality and cerebrovascular events compared with placebo; use with particular caution in patients with cerebrovascular disease or hypovolemia.

[3] Can be given q12h; allow 2–4 wk for adequate trial.

[4] Small divided daytime dosage and larger bedtime dosage; watch for sedation and orthostasis.

[5] Monitor serum levels; periodic CBCs, platelet counts secondary to agranulocytosis risk. Beware of drug-drug interactions.

[6] Can monitor serum levels; usually well tolerated; check CBC, platelets for agranulocytosis, thrombocytopenia risk in older adults.

[7] For acute use only; initial dose 2.5–5 mg, 2nd dose (2.5–5 mg) can be given after 2 h, max of 3 injections in 24 h (max daily dose 20 mg); should not be administered for >3 consecutive d.

EVALUATION AND ASSESSMENT

Major depression occurs in approximately 2% of people aged ≥55 and increases with age; 15% may have clinically significant depressive symptoms without major depression.

Recognizing and diagnosing late-life depression can be difficult. Older adults may complain of lack of energy or other somatic symptoms, attribute symptoms to old age or other physical conditions, or neglect to mention them to a healthcare professional.

Consider screening with Patient Health Questionnaire 2 (PHQ-2):

• Over the past 2 wk, have you often had little interest or pleasure in doing things?

• Over the past 2 wk, have you often been bothered by feeling down, depressed, or hopeless?

Score each item: 0 = not at all, 1 = several days, 2 = more than half the days, 3 = nearly every day; a score ≥3 indicates high probability of depressive disorder.

Follow-up and/or assess tx with structured self-assessment scale such as the GDS or the PHQ-9.

Medical Evaluation

TSH, B$_{12}$, calcium, liver and kidney function tests, electrolytes, UA, CBC

DSM-5 Criteria for Major Depressive Disorder (Abbreviated)

Five or more of the following criteria have been present during the same 2-wk period and represent a change from previous functioning; at least one of the symptoms is either depressed mood *or* loss of interest or pleasure. Do not include symptoms that are clearly due to a medical condition.

• Depressed mood

• Loss of interest or pleasure in activities

• Significant weight loss or gain (not intentional), or decrease or increase in appetite

• Insomnia or hypersomnia

• Psychomotor agitation or slowing

• Fatigue or loss of energy

• Feelings of worthlessness or excessive or inappropriate guilt

• Diminished ability to think or concentrate, or indecisiveness

• Recurrent thoughts of death; suicidal ideation, attempt, or plan

The *DSM-5* criteria are not specific for older adults; cognitive symptoms may be more prominent, and concurrent medical disorders are common.

Subsyndromal Depression

Subsyndromal depression does not meet full criteria for major depressive disorder and may include adjustment disorders and milder depression with anxiety symptoms but can be serious and associated with functional impairment. In older adults, subsyndromal depression may actually reflect major depression not diagnosed by current diagnostic criteria and may require pharmacologic and nonpharmacologic intervention.

MANAGEMENT

Tx should be individualized on the basis of hx, past response, and severity of illness as well as concurrent illnesses.

Nonpharmacologic

For mild to moderate depression (PHQ-9 scores 4–9) or in combination with pharmacotherapy: CBT, mindfulness-based CBT, interpersonal tx, problem-solving tx, or repetitive transcranial magnetic stimulation (rTMS) (p 90), bright light tx in morning for seasonal depression.

Recently, mindfulness-based CBT performed via Internet or by phone has been found to reduce the risk of relapse in patients with MDD.

For patients with major depression with mild to moderate dementia, problem adaptive therapy (PATH) may be helpful. PATH is a home-based tx that integrates problem-solving approaches with alternate strategies, environmental adaptations, and caregiver participation to improve the regulation of emotion. Supportive tx for cognitively impaired patients focuses on expression of affect, understanding, and empathy.

For severe pharmacological-resistant or psychotic depression, consider electroconvulsive tx (ECT) (p 89).

Pharmacologic

For mild, moderate, or severe depression: the duration of tx should be at least 6–12 mo after remission for patients experiencing their 1st depressive episode. Most older adults with major depression require maintenance antidepressant tx. Ensure an adequate initial trial of 4–6 wk after titrating up to therapeutic dosage; if inadequate response, consider switching to a different 1st-line agent of a different class or 2nd-line tx or psychiatric referral/consult. Combining antidepressants can lead to significant adverse effects. SSRIs may increase hemorrhagic stroke risk; low initial dosages and monitoring are recommended, especially in patients at risk of stroke. Check serum sodium before starting SSRI and after a few weeks of tx; high index of suspicion for hyponatremia. SSRIs are also associated with increased risk of GI and postsurgical bleeding.

Choosing an Antidepressant (Table 42 and list on p 89)

First-line Therapy: SSRI[BC] (consider sertraline), bupropion[▲], or SNRI[BC] (desvenlafaxine, duloxetine, venlafaxine[▲])

Second-line Therapy: Consider mirtazapine[▲] or vilazodone.

Third-line Therapy: Consider augmentation of 1st- or 2nd-line antidepressants with 2nd-generation atypical antipsychotics[BC] (aripiprazole, quetiapine), buspirone[▲], bupropion[▲], or lithium[BC] (Table 43).

Maintenance Treatment

After symptoms have remitted, pharmacotherapy should be maintained for 1 y after a single episode of depression, 2 y after 2 episodes, and at least 3 y for 3 or more episodes or consider indefinite maintenance.

- When stopping antidepressants, a gradual reduction in dose over at least 1 mo is recommended.
- Patients should be monitored carefully for discontinuation symptoms (flu-like syndrome, hyperarousal) or depression relapse.
- Discontinuation symptoms may be severe if medication is stopped abruptly or has a short half-life.

Table 42. Antidepressants Used for Older Adults

Class, Medication	Initial Dosage	Usual Dosage	Formulations	Comments (Metabolism, Excretion)
SSRIs	*Class AEs*: EPS, hyponatremia, increased risk of upper GI bleeding, suicide (early in tx), lower BMD and fragility fractures, risk of toxicity if methylene blue or linezolid co-administered. Avoid if hx of falls or fracture; caution if hx of SIADH.[BC] (L, K [10%])			
Citalopram▲	10–20 mg qam	20 mg/d	T: 20, 40, 60 S: 5 mg/10 mL	20 mg/d is max dosage in adults aged >60; risk of QTc prolongation
Escitalopram▲	10 mg/d	10 mg/d	T: 10, 20	10 mg/d is max dosage in adults aged >60; risk of QTc prolongation
Fluoxetine▲	5 mg qam	5–60 mg/d	T: 10 C: 10, 20, 40 S: 20 mg/5 mL C: SR 90 (weekly dose)	Long half-lives of parent and active metabolite may allow for less frequent dosing; may cause more insomnia than other SSRIs; CYP2D6, -2C9, -3A4 inhibitor (L)
Fluvoxamine▲	25 mg qhs	100–300 mg/d	T: 25, 50, 100	Not approved as an antidepressant in US; greater likelihood of GI AEs; CYP1A2, -3A4 inhibitor (L)
Paroxetine▲	5 mg	10–40 mg/d	T: 10, 20, 30, 40	Increased risk of withdrawal symptoms (dizziness); anticholinergic AEs; CYP2D6 inhibitor (L)
Paroxetine hydrochloride▲	12.5 mg/d	12.5–37.5 mg/d	T: ER 12.5, 25, 37.5 S: 10 mg/5 mL	Increase by 12.5 mg/d no faster than 1×/wk (L)
Sertraline▲	25 mg qam	50–200 mg/d	T: 25, 50, 100 S: 20 mg/mL	Greater likelihood of GI AEs (L)
SNRIs				Avoid if hx of falls or fracture; caution if hx of SIADH.[BC]
◆Duloxetine *(Cymbalta)*	20 mg/d, then 20 mg q12h	40–60 mg q24h or 30 mg q12h	C: 20, 30, 60	Most common AEs: nausea, dry mouth, constipation, diarrhea, urinary hesitancy; contraindicated if CrCl <30
Venlafaxine▲	25–50 mg q12h	75–225 mg/d in divided doses	T: 25, 37.5, 50, 75, 100	Low anticholinergic activity; minimal sedation and hypotension; may increase BP and QTc; may be useful when somatic pain present; EPS, withdrawal symptoms, hyponatremia (L)
(Effexor XR▲)	75 mg qam	75–225 mg/d	C: 37.5, 75, 150	Same as above
Desvenlafaxine *(Pristiq)*	50 mg/d	50 mg; max 400 mg	SR tab: 50, 100	Active metabolite of venlafaxine; adjust dosage when CrCl <30 (L, K 45%)

(cont.)

Table 42. Antidepressants Used for Older Adults (cont.)

Class, Medication	Initial Dosage	Usual Dosage	Formulations	Comments (Metabolism, Excretion)
Additional Medications				
Bupropion▲	37.5–50 mg q12h	75–150 mg q12h	T: 75, 100	Consider for SSRI, TCA nonresponders; safe in HF; may be stimulating; can lower seizure threshold. Avoid.[BC] (L)
Bupropion hydrochloride SR▲	100 mg q12h or q24h	100–150 mg q12h	T:100, 150, 200	
Bupropion hydrochloride *ER*▲	150 mg/d	300 mg/d	T: 150, 300	
Levomilnacipran *(Fetzima)*	20 mg q24h × 2 d	40 mg q24h max; 120 mg/d	C: ER 20, 40, 80	SNRI (L, K 58%)
Lithium▲	150 mg/d	300–900 mg/d Levels 0.4–0.8 mEq/L	T: 300 T: ER 300 T: CR 450 C: 150, 300, 600 syr 300 mg/mL	Risk of CNS toxicity; cognitive impairment; hypothyroidism; interactions with diuretics, ACEIs, CCBs, NSAIDs[BC]
Methylphenidate▲[BC]	2.5–5 mg at 7 AM and noon	5–10 mg at 7 AM and noon	T: 5, 10, 20	Short-term tx of depression or apathy in physically ill older adults; used as an adjunct. Avoid if insomnia (L)
Mirtazapine▲	7.5 mg qhs	15–45 mg/d	T: 15, 30, 45	May be quite sedating but this may diminish as dosage is increased; increased appetite; ODT (SolTab) available (L)
Vilazodone *(Viibryd)*	10 mg/d for 7 d, then 20 mg/d	40 mg/d	T: 10, 20, 40	Metabolized by CYP3A4; limited geriatric data; AEs: diarrhea and nausea
Vortioxetine *(Trintellix)*		5–10 mg q24h max; 20 mg/d	T: 5, 10, 20	SSRI with 5-HT1A agonist and 5-HT3 antagonist activity (L)
TCAs				Avoid.[BC]
◆Desipramine▲	10–25 mg qhs	50–150 mg/d	T: 10, 25, 50, 75, 100, 150	Therapeutic serum level >115 ng/mL (L)
◆Nortriptyline▲	10–25 mg qhs	75–150 mg/d	C: 10, 25, 50, 75 S: 10 mg/5 mL	Therapeutic window (50–150 ng/mL) (L)

◆ = Also has primary indication for neuropathic pain. CrCl unit = mL/min/1.73 m^2

Antidepressants to Avoid in Older Adults to Avoid Excessive AEs or Drug Interactions[BC]

- Amitriptyline▲
- Amoxapine▲
- Doxepin▲
- Imipramine▲
- Ketamine
- Maprotiline▲
- Protriptyline▲
- St. John's wort
- Trimipramine

Electroconvulsive Therapy (ECT)

Generally safe and very effective. Potential complications include temporary confusion, anterograde and retrograde amnesia, arrhythmias, aspiration, falls.

Indications: Severe depression when a rapid onset of response is necessary; when depression is resistant to drug tx; for patients who are unable to tolerate antidepressants, have previous response to ECT, have psychotic depression, severe catatonia, or depression with Parkinson disease.

Evaluation: Before ECT, perform CXR, ECG, serum electrolytes, and cardiac examination. Additional tests (eg, stress test, neuroimaging, EEG) are used selectively.

Contraindications:

- Increased intracranial pressure
- Intracranial tumor
- MI within 3 mo (relative)
- Stroke within 1 mo (relative)

Consider Maintenance ECT:

- Hx of ECT-responsive illness
- Resistance or intolerance to medications alone
- Serious medical comorbidity
- More effective than pharmacotherapy after successful ECT

Repetitive Transcranial Magnetic Stimulation (rTMS)

- Series of magnetic pulses directed to brain at frequency of 1–20 stimulations per sec. Each tx session lasts ~30 min, and a full course of tx may be as long as 30 sessions.
- Placebo-controlled studies have demonstrated moderate effect sizes for tx-resistant depression in younger adults and appears safe with minimal adverse effects.
- Limited experience with rTMS in tx-resistant late-life depression; rTMS tx parameters may need to be optimized to address age-related changes such as prefrontal cortical atrophy.

Depression and Parkinson Disease

Patients with Parkinson disease and depression may benefit more from nortriptyline than SSRIs. Pramipexole may also reduce depressive symptoms independent of effect on motor symptoms (also p 238).

Psychotic Depression

- Psychosis accompanying major depression; increased disability and mortality
- ECT is the tx of choice
- Olanzapine 15–20 mg/d added to sertraline 150–200 mg/d significantly improves remission rate vs placebo.

BIPOLAR DISORDER

See **Table 43**.

- 5–19% of mood disorders in older adults.
- Usually begins in early adulthood, family hx.
- 10% may develop after age 50.
- Distinct period of abnormally and persistently elevated, expansive, or irritable mood for longer than 1 wk.
- Symptoms may include racing thoughts, pressured speech, decreased need for sleep, distractibility, grandiose delusions.
- A single manic episode is sufficient for a diagnosis if secondary causes are excluded.
- Late-onset mania may be secondary to head trauma, stroke, delirium, other neurologic disorders, alcohol abuse, or medications (eg, corticosteroids, L-dopa, thyroxine).
- Use aripiprazole, lurasidone, olanzapine, quetiapine, risperidone▲, or ziprasidone for acute mania (**Table 107**) and D/C antidepressants if taking.

- If depression emerges in bipolar disorder, lamotrigine▲ may be helpful.
- Initiate long-term tx (**Table 43**) as soon as patient is able to comply with oral tx.

Table 43. Medications for Management of Bipolar Disorders

Medication	Mania		Depression	
	Acute	*Maintenance*	*Acute*	*Maintenance*
Atypical antipsychotics	All +	Aripiprazole + Olanzapine +/–	Quetiapine + Olanzapine +/– Lurisadone+	Olanzapine +/–
Mood stabilizers				
Lithium▲	+	+	+	+
Valproate▲	+	+/–	–	+/–
Lamotrigine▲	–	+/–	+	+
Carbamazepine▲	+	+/–	?	+/–
Antidepressants				
SSRIs	Avoid	Avoid	+	+
TCAs	Avoid	Avoid	–	–

+ = evidence to support use; +/– = some evidence to support use; – = evidence does not support use; ? = has not been studied.

Table 44. Long-term Treatment of Bipolar Disorders[1]

Medication	Initial Dosage	Usual Dosage	Formulation	Comments
Lithium▲	150 mg/d	300–900 mg/d Levels 0.4–0.8 mEq/L	T: 300 T: ER 300 T: CR 450 C: 150, 300, 600 syr 300 mg/mL	Risk of CNS toxicity; cognitive impairment; hypothyroidism; interactions with diuretics, ACEIs, CCBs, NSAIDs[BC]
Carbamazepine▲	100 mg q12h	800–1200 mg/d Levels 4–12 mcg/L	T: 100, 200, 400	Many drug interactions; may cause SIADH[BC]; risk of leukopenia, neutropenia, agranulocytosis, thrombocytopenia; monitor CBC; drowsiness, dizziness
Valproic acid▲	125 mg q12h	750 mg/d in divided doses Levels 50–125 mcg/L	T: 125, 250, 500	Can cause weight gain, tremor, several drug interactions; risk of hepatotoxicity, pancreatitis, neutropenia, thrombocytopenia; monitor LFTs and platelets. Avoid concurrent use of ≥1 CNS agents.[BC]
Lamotrigine▲	25 mg/d	100–200 mg/d	T: 25, 100, 150, 200	D/C if rash; interaction with valproate (when used together, begin at 25 mg q48h, titrate to 25–100 mg q12h); prolongs PR interval; somnolence, headache common

[1] Limited evidence base in older adults. See healthquality.va.gov (also **Table 92**).

DERMATOLOGIC CONDITIONS COMMON IN OLDER ADULTS

For numerous dermatologic images, see https://medicine.uiowa.edu/dermatology/education/clinical-skin-disease-images.

Skin Cancers and Precancerous Conditions

Actinic Keratosis

Erythematous, flat, rough, scaly papules 2–6 mm; may be easier felt than seen; precancerous (can develop into squamous or basal cell carcinoma); cutaneous horn may develop; affects sun-exposed areas, including lips (actinic cheilitis)

Risk Factors: UV light exposure (amount and intensity), increased age, fair coloring, immunosuppression

Prevention: Limit UV light exposure, use sunscreen with UVA and UVB coverage, wear protective clothing

Treatment

- Topical 5-fluorouracil *(Carac* crm 0.5% or *Tolak* crm 4% daily × 4 wk, *Efudex* crm 5% q12h × 2–4 wk, *Fluoroplex* crm 1% to face, 5% elsewhere, q12h × 2–6 wk) to entire area affected
- Imiquimod 2.5% and 3.75% pk *(Zyclara).* Apply 1 or 2 pk to face or scalp (not both) qhs × 14 d, wash off with soap and water after 8 h. Rest 14 d, then repeat another 14 d. Max 56 pk/2 cycles
- Imiquimod 5% pk *(Aldara).* Apply 1 or 2 pk to face or scalp (not both) qhs × 16 d, wash off with soap and water after 8 h. Rest 14 d, then repeat another 14 d. Max 56 pk/2 cycles
- Diclofenac 3% gel *(Solaraze)* applied q12h × 60–90 d
- Ingenol mebutate 0.015% gel *(Picato).* Face and scalp: apply q24h × 3 d; trunk and extremities: apply q24h × 2 d. Allow gel to dry × 15 min, do not wash or touch for 6 h
- Cryosurgery
- Aminolevulinic acid *(Levulan Kerastick* 20%) applied to lesions with red light or blue light illumination after 14–18 h, repeat in 8 wk. Curettage with or without electrosurgery
- Chemical peels (trichloroacetic acid), dermabrasion, laser tx

Basal Cell Carcinoma

Can affect any body surface exposed to the sun, most often head and neck

Types

- Nodular: pearly papule or nodule over telangiectases with a rolled border; may contain melanin; most common type
- Superficial: scaly erythematous patch or plaque, may contain melanin
- Morpheaform: indurated, whitish, scar-like plaque with indistinct margins

Risk Factors

- Exposure to UV radiation (sun or tanning beds), especially intense intermittent exposure during childhood or adolescence
- Physical factors: fair skin, light eye color, red or blonde hair
- Exposure to ionizing radiation, arsenic, psoralen, UVA radiation, smoking
- Immunosuppression (eg, after solid-organ transplant)

Prevention: Avoid sun exposure, use sunscreen with UVA and UVB coverage, wear protective clothing

Treatment: (localized control)
- As with any cancer, the course of tx should be balanced with the patient's wishes, current quality of life, and life expectancy (eg, Mohs surgery in the last year of life)
- Surgical: Mohs micrographic surgery (1st-line for facial lesions), cryosurgery, excision, curettage and electrodessication
- Nonsurgical: radiotherapy, imiquimod 5% crm *(Aldara)* applied 5 d/wk × 6 wk (not for use on face, hands, or feet); photodynamic tx; 5-fluorouracil 5% crm or sol q12h × 3–6 wk or longer; vismodegib *(Erivedge)* 150 mg q24h until disease progresses or unacceptable toxicity (L, F 92% [C: 150])

Melanoma

Less common than nonmelanoma lesions; usually asymptomatic

Clinical Features

Asymmetry: a line down the center of the lesions does not create a mirror image

Border: irregular, ragged, fuzzy, or scalloped

Color: nonuniform throughout the lesion; red, blue, black, gray, or white

Diameter: >6 mm (considered relatively insensitive as an independent factor)

Types: ulcer biopsy can be performed by PCP
- Lentigo maligna: most often located on atrophic, sun-damaged skin; irregular-shaped tan or brown macule; slow growing
- Superficial spreading: occur anywhere; irregular-shaped macule, papule, or plaque; coloration varies
- Nodular: a rapidly growing, often black or gray papule or nodule
- Acral lentiginous: located on the palms, soles, or nail beds; dark brown or black patch; more common in Hispanic, black, and Asian individuals

Risk Factors
- Very fair skin type
- Family hx
- Dysplastic or numerous nevi
- Sun exposure; blistering sunburns as a child

Prevention: Avoid sun exposure, use sunscreen with UVA and UVB coverage, wear protective clothing

Treatment: Surgical excision; advanced: ipilimumab, vemurafenib, dabrafenib plus trametinib, pembrolizumab, nivolumab

Squamous Cell Carcinoma (SCC)
- Erythematous papule, plaque, or nodule with keratotic scale; maybe tender
  - Scaling or crusting may be present.
  - May develop in nonhealing wounds or scars (Marjolin ulcers)

Risk Factors: cumulative sun exposure, age, immunosuppression, exposure to ionizing radiation or arsenic

Treatment
  - Surgical excision, cryotherapy, electrosurgery

- Ionizing radiation is an alternative.
- 5-fluorouracil 5% crm or sol q12h × 4–8 wk or longer (off-label) tx for SCC in situ (Bowen disease); not for invasive cutaneous SCC.
- Imiquimod 5% for Bowen disease: apply q24h × 5 d/wk, before normal sleeping hours × 6 wk; leave on skin for ~8 h, then remove with mild soap and water. Maximum to be prescribed: 36 packets during the 6-wk tx period.
- As with any cancer, the course of tx should be balanced with the patient's wishes, current quality of life, and life expectancy (eg, Mohs surgery in the last year of life)

Infectious Conditions

Cellulitis

Ill-defined erythema, pain, blisters, and exudates; most often affects lower dermis and subcutaneous tissue, commonly the legs; group A streptococci and *Staphylococcus aureus* most frequent pathogens

Treatment

- Antistaphylococcal penicillin, amoxicillin-clavulanate[▲] × 10 d
- Macrolide (eg, erythromycin[▲BC]), 1st-generation cephalosporin (eg, cephalexin[▲]), or tetracycline[▲] if penicillin allergy
- MRSA suspected or known
  - Oral empiric options: amoxicillin plus doxycycline or minocycline; clindamycin, TMP/SMX, or linezolid
  - Tailor tx to culture and sensitivity results when available
- Drain abscess

Folliculitis

Multiple small, erythematous papules and pustules surrounding a hair; most often affects areas with coarse, short hair (ie, neck, beard, buttocks, thighs)

Treatment

- Mild localized cases—topical antibiotic: mupirocin 2%[▲], erythromycin, or clindamycin
- Extensive or severe cases—oral antistaphylococcal penicillin, amoxicillin-clavulanate, or erythromycin

Impetigo

Very contagious; nonbullous and bullous variants; honey-colored crusts on face around nose and mouth

Treatment

- Small, localized lesions: topical mupirocin 2%[▲] q8h × 7–10 d, topical retapamulin 1% oint *(Altabax)* q12h × 5 d
- Widespread: oral antistaphylococcal penicillin, erythromycin, or a cephalosporin × 10 d

Rosacea

Vascular and follicular dilatation; mild to moderate; can accompany seborrhea; can affect face (nose, chin, cheeks, forehead) or eyes (dryness, blepharitis, conjunctivitis)

Prevention: Avoid triggers (stress, prolonged sun exposure and exercise, hot and humid environment, alcohol, hot drinks, spicy foods); may be worsened by vasodilators, niacin, or topical corticosteroids. Wear sunscreen with UVA and UVB coverage (SPF ≥15) or sunblock with titanium and zinc oxide. See rosacea.org.

Treatment

- Topical (for mild cases and maintenance)
  - Azelaic acid 15% gel *(Finacea)* q12–24 h or 20% crm *(Azelex, Finevin)* q12h
  - Brimonidine 0.5% gel *(Mirvaso)* q24h
  - Benzoyl peroxide 2.5, 5, 10% crm, gel, wash, soap q12–24h
  - Ivermectin 1% crm *(Soolantra)* q24h
  - Metronidazole 0.75% crm▲ q12h or 1% crm or gel *(Noritate, MetroGel)* q24h
  - Sodium sulfacetamide 10% + sulfa 5% (*Rosula* aqueous gel, *Clenia* crm, foaming wash) q12–24h, avoid if sulfa allergy or kidney disease (K)
  - Erythromycin 2% sol▲ q12h
  - Tretinoin▲ 0.025% crm or liq, 0.01% gel qhs
  - Oxymetazoline 1% crm *(Rhofade)* q24h for persistent facial erythema
- Oral (for moderate to severe papulo-pustular rosacea)
  - Tetracycline▲ 250–500 mg q8–12h × 6–12 wk
  - Doxycycline▲ 50–100 mg q12–24h × 6–12 wk
  - Minocycline▲ 50–100 mg q12h × 6–12 wk
  - Clarithromycin▲ᴮᶜ 250–500 mg q12h × 6–12 wk
  - Metronidazole▲ 200 mg q12–24h × 4–6 wk
  - Erythromycin▲ᴮᶜ 250–500 mg q12–24h × 6–12 wk
  - Azithromycin▲ 250–500 mg q24h × 6–12 wk

Scabies

Burrows, erythematous papules or rash, dry or scaly skin, pruritus (worse at night); spread by close, skin-to-skin or sexual contact; can affect interdigital webs, flexor aspects of wrists, axillae, umbilicus, nipples, genitalia. Diagnostic confirmation by microscopic exam of skin scrapings in mineral oil.

Treatment

- Infestation can result in epidemics; treat all contacts including family members and treat environment
- Oatmeal baths, topical corticosteroids, or emollient creams for symptom relief
- Apply topical products from head to toe:
  Preferred tx
  - Permethrin 5% crm▲, wash off after 8–1 h, repeat in 7–10 d if symptomatic or if live mites were found
  - Ivermectin *(Stromectol)* 200 mcg/kg po, may repeat 1× in 1 or 2 wk [T: 3, 6]
  Alternative tx
  - Crotamiton 10% crm, lot *(Eurax)*, less effective, leave on 48 h, repeat in 7–10 d if necessary

Inflammatory Conditions

Atopic dermatitis (Eczema)

Chronic and pruritic with dry skin, erythema, oozing, crusting, and lichenification.

Treatment

- Avoid environmental triggers (eg, heat and low humidity), harsh soaps, detergents, and contact allergens.
- Maintain skin hydration with barrier creams or ointments (eg, petrolatum based) that have little or no water content.

- Topical corticosteroids applied 1 or 2×/d
  - Mild eczema: lowest to low potency corticosteroid cream or ointment (**Table 46**)
  - Reserve moderate and high potency corticosteroids for moderate disease and flare-ups.
  - Avoid applying moderate- and higher-potency corticosteroids to the face and skin folds; if needed, no more than 5–7 d. Skin atrophy can result.
- Topical tacrolimus▲ 0.1% or 0.03% ointment 2×/d or pimecrolimus 1% *(Elidel)* crm 2×/d for patients who do not respond or cannot tolerate topical corticosteroids
- Treat skin infections (eg, Staph aureus and herpes simplex)
- Treat pruritus with oral antihistamines.
- Phototherapy (eg, UV light), oral cyclosporine, dupilumab are reserved for severe cases.

Neurodermatitis

Generalized or localized itching, redness, scaling; can affect any skin surface

Treatment: Mid- to higher-potency topical corticosteroids (**Table 46**); exclude other causes, (eg, allergies, irritants, xerosis)

Psoriasis

Well-defined, erythematous plaques covered with silver scales; severity varies; can affect all skin areas, nails (pitting)

Treatment

- Topical corticosteroids, UV light, PUVA, methotrexate, cyclosporine, etretinate, sulfasalazine, tacrolimus, pimecrolimus *(Elidel)*, tazarotene gel 0.05%, 0.1%, anthralin preparations, and tar + 1–4% salicylic acid
- Calcipotriene for nonfacial areas
- Cyclosporine, methotrexate, and biological agents for extensive and recalcitrant disease

Seborrheic Dermatitis

Greasy, yellow scales with or without erythematous base; common in Parkinson disease and in debilitated patients; can affect nasal labial folds, eyebrows, hairline, sideburns, posterior auriculare, and midchest

Treatment

- Hydrocortisone 1% or 2% crm▲ q12h or triamcinolone 0.1% oint q12h × 2 wk
- Scalp: shampoo containing selenium sulfide, zinc, or tar
- Ketoconazole 2% crm▲ for severe conditions if *Pityrosporum orbiculare* infection suspected

Urticaria

Hives

- Uniform, red edematous plaques surrounded by white halos, can affect any skin surface
- Treatment
  - Identify cause
  - Oral H$_1$ antihistamines (**Table 114**) or oral H$_2$ antihistamines (**Table 58**)
  - Oral glucocorticoids[BC] (eg, prednisone 40 mg q24h)
  - Doxepin▲[BC] (po or topical 5%) for refractory cases

Angioedema

- Larger, deeper than hives; can affect lips, eyelids, tongue, larynx, GI tract
- Treatment
  - Oral H₁ antihistamines (**Table 114**)
  - Oral glucocorticoids[BC]
  - For severe reactions, epinephrine 0.3 mL of a 1:1000 dilution *(EpiPen)* SC

Cholinergic

- Round, red papular wheals; can affect any skin surface
- Treatment
  - Hot shower may relieve itching
  - Oral H₁ antihistamines (**Table 114**) 1 h before exercise

Fungal Conditions

Candidiasis

Erythema, pustules, or cheesy, whitish matter in body folds; satellite lesions

Treatment: See intertrigo; topical antifungals (**Table 45**)

Intertrigo

Moist, erythematous lesions with local superficial skin loss; satellite lesions caused by *candida*; can affect any place 2 skin surfaces rest against one another (eg, under breasts, between toes)

Treatment

- Keep area dry.
- Topical antifungals (**Table 45**), absorbent pwd, 1–2% hydrocortisone[▲] or 0.1% triamcinolone[▲] crm q12h × 1–2 d if inflamed

Onychomycosis

Thickening and discoloration; affects nails *(Tinea unguium); Tinea rubrum* most common in people with DM; candida, mold, and bacteria are other causes

Treatment: Obtain nail specimens for laboratory culture to confirm diagnosis before prescribing itraconazole or terbinafine. Treat affected family members to decrease risk of reinfection.

- Itraconazole[▲] (C: 100; S: 100 mg/mL), contraindicated in HF (L), mycologic cure rate on pulse tx 63%
  - Toenails: 200 mg po q24h × 3 mo—23% complete cure rate (negative mycologic analysis and normal nail) reported with this regimen, or 200 mg po q12h × 1 wk/mo × 3 mo
  - Fingernails: 200 mg po q12h × 1 wk/mo × 2 mo ("Pulse Therapy") or 200 mg q24h × 12 wk
- Fluconazole[▲] (T: 50, 100, 150, 200; S: 10, 40 mg/mL) (L), mycologic cure rate 48%
  - Toenails: 150 or 300 mg po/wk × 6–12 mo
  - Fingernails: 150 or 300 mg po/wk × 3–6 mo
- Efinaconazole (*Jublia* [Sol: 10%])
  - Toenails: apply q24h × 48 wk
- Terbinafine[▲] (T: 250), avoid if CrCl <50 mL/min/1.73 m², active or chronic liver disease; mycologic cure rate 76%; choice for diabetics
  - Toenails: 250 mg po q24h × 12–16 wk—48% complete cure rate reported with this regimen
  - Fingernails: 250 mg po q24h × 6 wk

- Ciclopirox▲: Toenails and fingernails—apply lacquer q12h to nails and adjacent skin; remove with alcohol q7d—8% complete cure rate reported with this regimen; Duration: fingernails 24 wk, toenails 48 wk
- Tavaborole 5% sol *(Kerydin):* Toenails—apply daily × 48 wk; affective against *T. rubrum* and *mentagrophytes sp.*
- OTC lacquers (eg, *Fungi-Nail*) treat the fungus around the nail but do not penetrate the nail
- Laser tx: improves appearance; not covered by insurance

Other Conditions

Skin Maceration

Erythema; abraded, excoriated skin; blisters; white and silver patches; can affect any area constantly in contact with moisture, covered by occlusive dressing or bandage; skin folds, groin, buttocks

Prevention and Treatment
- Eliminate cause of moisture.
  - Toileting program for incontinence (p 164)
  - Condom catheter
  - Indwelling catheter (reserve for most intractable conditions)
  - FI collector
- Protect skin from moisture.
  - Clean gently with mild soap after each incontinent episode.
  - Apply moisture barrier (eg, *Vaseline, Proshield, Smooth and Cool, Calmoseptine*).
  - Use disposable briefs that wick moisture from the skin; use linen incontinence pads when disposable briefs worsen perineal dermatitis.

Xerosis

Dull, rough, flaky, cracked; nummular; can affect all skin surfaces

Treatment
- Increase humidity
- Avoid excess bathing, sponges, brushes, and use of bath oils, which can lead to falls from slippery feet
- Tepid water in baths or showers
- Oatmeal baths
- Apply emollient oint (eg, *Aquaphor*) or crm (eg, *Eucerin*) immediately after bathing
- Hydrocortisone 1% oint

DERMATOLOGIC MEDICATIONS

Table 45. Topical Antifungal Medications

Medication	Formulation	Dermatologic Indications	Dosing Frequency
Butenafine▲OTC	1% crm	*Tinea pedis, T cruris, T corpis, T versicolor*	q24h × 2–4 wk
Ciclopirox▲	0.77% crm, gel, lot, sus; 1% shp; 8% lacquer	*Tinea pedis, T cruris, T corpis, T versicolor;* candidiasis; scalp seborrhea; onychomycosis	q12–24h × 4 wk; shp /× 3 wk; lacquer qhs
Clotrimazole▲OTC	1% crm, oint, sol	Candidiasis, dermatophytoses; superficial mycoses	q12h
Econazole nitrate	1% crm▲ 1% foam	Candidiasis; *Tinea cruris, T corpis, T versicolor*	q12–24h × 2–4 wk
Ketoconazole▲	2% crm, foam, gel, shpOTC	Candidiasis; seborrhea; *Tinea cruris, T corpis, T versicolor*	q12–24h × 2–4 wk; shp 2×/wk
Luliconazole▲	1% crm	*Tinea pedis, T crusis*	q24h × 1–2 wk
Miconazole▲OTC	2% crm, lot, pwd, spr, tinc	*Tinea cruris, T corpis, T pedis*	q12h × 2–4 wk
Naftifine	1%▲ and 2% crm▲; 1% and 2% gel	*Tinea cruris, T corpis, T pedis*	1% crm and gel q24h up to 4 wk 2% crm and gel q24h up to 4 wk
Nystatin▲	100,000 U/g crm, oint, pwd	Mucocutaneous candidiasis	q8–12h up to 4 wk
Oxiconazole *(Oxistat)*	1% crm▲, lot	*Tinea corpis, T cruris, T pedis, T versicolor*	q12–24h × 2–4 wk
Sertaconazole *(Ertaczo)*	2% crm	*Tinea pedis*	q12h × 4 wk
Sulconazole *(Exelderm)*	1% crm, sol	*Tinea corpis, T cruris, T versicolor*	q12–24h × 3–4 wk
Terbinafine▲OTC	1% crm▲, gel, spr	*Tinea cruris, T corpis, T pedis, T versicolor*	crm q12h; gel, spr q124h × 1–4 wk
Tolnaftate▲OTC	1% crm▲, gel, S▲, pwd▲, spr	*Tinea cruris, T corpis, T pedis*	q12h × 2–4 wk
Undecylenic acid *(Fungi-Nail*OTC*, MycoNail)*	25% sol, oint	*Tinea pedis,* ringworm (except nails and scalp)	q12h × 2–4 wk
Topical Antifungal Medication plus Corticosteroid			
Clotrimazole 1% Betamethasone 0.05%▲	crm, lot	*Tinea corporis, T pedis, T cruris*	q12h × 1 wk
Iodoquinol 1%, 2% plus Hydrocortisone 1%▲	crm, 1% and 2% gel		q6–8h
Nystatin 100,000 U▲ Triamcinolone 0.1%	crm, oint	*Cutaneous candida*	q12h, max 25 d

[1] Dosing frequency and tx duration can vary by indication and formulation. Consult prescribing information.

Table 46. Topical Corticosteroids

Medication	Strength and Formulations	Frequency of Applications
Lowest Potency		
Hydrocortisone▲	0.5%[OTC], 1%, 2.5% crm, oint, lot, sol	q6–8h
Low Potency		
Alclometasone dipropionate▲¹	0.05% crm, oint	q8–12h
Desonide▲	0.05% crm, oint	q6–12h
Fluocinolone acetonide▲	0.01% crm, sol	q6–12h
Midpotency		
Betamethasone dipropionate▲	0.05% lot	q6–12h
Betamethasone valerate▲	0.1% crm	q6–12h
Clocortolone butyrate	0.05% crm	q8h
Clocortolone pivalate▲	0.1% crm	q8h
Desoximetasone▲	0.05% crm	q12h
Fluocinolone acetonide▲	0.025%[OTC] crm, oint	q6–12h
Flurandrenolide (Cordran)	0.05%[OTC] crm▲, oint▲, lot▲, tape	q12–24h
Fluticasone propionate▲	0.05% crm, lot, 0.005% oint	q12h
Hydrocortisone butyrate▲	0.1% oint	q12–24h
Hydrocortisone valerate▲	0.2% crm, oint	q6–8h
Mometasone furoate▲¹	0.1% crm, lot, oint	q24h
Prednicarbate▲	0.1% crm, oint	q12h
Triamcinolone acetonide▲	0.025%, 0.1% crm, oint, lot	q8–12h
Higher Potency		
Amcinonide▲	0.1%, crm, oint, lot	q8–12h
Betamethasone dipropionate▲	0.05% augmented crm	q6–12h
Betamethasone dipropionate▲	0.05%, crm, oint	q6–12h
Betamethasone valerate▲	0.1% oint	q6–12h
Desoximetasone▲	0.25% crm, oint, spr; 0.05% gel	q12h
Diflorasone diacetate▲	0.05%, crm, oint	q6–12h
Fluocinonide▲	0.05% crm, oint, gel	q6–12h
Halcinonide▲	0.1% crm, oint	q8–24h
Triamcinolone acetate▲	0.5% crm, spr	q8–12h
Super Potency		
Betamethasone dipropionate▲	0.05% oint, lot, gel (augmented)	q6–12h
Clobetasol propionate▲	0.05% crm▲, oint▲, lot, gel▲, shp, spr	q12h
Diflorasone diacetate▲	0.05% optimized oint	q8–24h
Halobetasol propionate▲	0.05% crm, oint	q12h

¹ Hydrocortisone (all forms), alclometasone, and mometasone are nonfluorinated.

HYPOTHYROIDISM

Common Causes

- Autoimmune (primary thyroid failure)
- After tx for hyperthyroidism
- Pituitary or hypothalamic disorders (secondary thyroid failure)
- Medications, especially amiodarone (rare after 1st 18 mo of tx) and lithium

Screening for hypothyroidism in asymptomatic older persons is controversial

Evaluation

TSH (up to 7.5 mU/L is normal in adults aged 80 and older), and if high, repeat TSH and free T_4

Pharmacotherapy

- Tx of subclinical hypothyroidism (TSH 5–10 mIU/L, normal free T_4 concentration, and no overt symptoms) does not improve hypothyroid symptoms, tiredness, cognitive function, depression, or quality of life. Most experts recommend treating if TSH ≥10 mIU/L.
- Levothyroxine▲ (T_4 [T: 25, 50, 75, 88, 100, 112, 125, 137, 150, 175, 200, 300 mcg]) given on empty stomach and waiting for 1 h before eating or hs (4 h after last meal), which is more potent. Start at 25–50 mcg and increase by 12- to 25-mcg intervals q6wk with repeat TSH testing until TSH is in normal range. Prescribe product from same manufacturer for individual patients for consistent bioavailability. Recheck TSH in 6 wk if there is a change in formulation. If adherence is a problem, can be given weekly or twice-weekly.
- Combinations of levothyroxine and L-triiodothyronine (T_3) are not recommended.
- For myxedema coma: Load T_4 400 mcg IV or 100 mcg q6–8h for 1 d, then 100 mcg/d IV (until patient can take orally) and give stress doses of corticosteroids (p 113); then start usual replacement regimen.
- Thyroid USP is not recommended. (Avoid.[BC]) To convert thyroid USP to thyroxine: 60 mg USP = 100 mcg thyroxine.
- If patients are npo and must receive IV thyroxine, dose should be half usual po dose.
- If tx has been interrupted for <6 wk and without an intercurrent cardiac event or marked weight loss, previous full replacement dose can be resumed.
- Monitor TSH level at least q12mo (ASCE/ATA) in patients on chronic thyroid replacement tx. Don't measure total or free T_3.[CW]
- Normal TSH ranges are higher in older persons and higher target (eg, 4–7.5 mIU/L) may be appropriate.

HYPERTHYROIDISM

Common Causes

- Graves disease
- Toxic nodule
- Toxic multinodular goiter
- Medications, especially amiodarone (can occur any time during tx)

Evaluation

Older persons are less likely to have heat intolerance, tremor, nervousness, or goiter but more likely to have weight loss, dyspnea, constipation, AF, and moderate to severe ophthalmopathy.

TSH (biotin supplements can interfere with assay, suggesting hyperthyroidism), free T_4

- If TSH is low and free T_4 is normal, recheck TSH in 4–6 wk; if TSH is still low, check free T_3.
- If TSH is low and free T_4 or free T_3 is high, check radioactive iodine uptake and, if thyroid nodularity, thyroid scan.
- If TSH is low, high T_4, and normal free T_3 suggests concurrent nonthyroidal illness, amiodarone tx, or exogenous T_4 administration.
- If cause is not obvious, check thyrotropin receptor antibodies (TRAb), radioactive iodine uptake, or thyroidal blood flow on ultrasonography.

Pharmacotherapy

- β-blockers (p 60) if symptomatic hyperthyroidism; may add methimazole if severe symptoms or risk of hyperthyroid complications.
- Radioactive iodine ablation is usual tx of choice for older persons, but surgery (works faster but more likely to become hypothyroid) or medical tx are options. Pretreat with methimazole and β-blockers before iodine ablation if symptomatic or if free T_4> 2–3× normal. Monitor free T_4 and total T_3 within 1–2 mo after tx. Pretreat with methimazole and β-blockers before surgery. Give potassium iodide in immediate preoperative period. After surgery, measure calcium or intact PTH, stop antithyroid drugs, and taper β-blockers.
- Methimazole▲ [T: 5, 10]: 1st-line drug tx; start 5–20 mg po q8h, then adjust. If used as primary tx, continue for 12–18 mo then DC or taper if TSH is normal. Check CBC, LFTs before starting.
- Propylthiouracil (PTU [T: 50]): Use only if allergic to or intolerant of methimazole; can cause serious liver injury; start 100 mg po q8h, then adjust up to 200 mg po q8h prn. Check CBC, LFTs before starting.
- When dose has stabilized, follow TSH per hypothyroid monitoring.
- In older adults, treat both symptomatic hyperthyroidism and subclinical hyperthyroidism (low TSH and normal serum-free T_4 and T_3 concentrations confirmed by repeat testing in 3–6 mo) if TSH <0.1 mIU/L or if TSH 0.1–0.5 mIU/L and underlying CVD or low BMD.

EUTHYROID SICK SYNDROME
Definition
Abnormal thyroid function tests in nonthyroidal illness

Evaluation
- Do not assess thyroid function in acutely ill patients unless thyroid dysfunction is strongly suspected.
- Low T_3, high reverse T_3, low T_4, low or high TSH may be seen.
- If TSH is very low (<0.1 mIU/L in high-sensitivity assays), then hyperthyroidism is likely.
- If TSH is very high (>20 mIU/L), then hypothyroidism is likely.
- Do not treat low T_3 or T_4 in absence of clinical symptoms.
- If thyroid disease is not strongly suspected, recheck in 3–6 wk.

SOLITARY THYROID NODULE (ATA)
Evaluation
- Ultrasound of thyroid
- TSH
  - If TSH is normal or high, perform fine-needle aspirate biopsy if nodule ≥1 cm if high- or intermediate-suspicion pattern, ≥1.5 cm if low-suspicion pattern, and ≥2 cm if very low-suspicion pattern on ultrasound. Simple cysts do not require biopsy. Do not perform radionuclide scan.[CW]

○ If TSH is low, perform radionuclide scan; if "hot," then rarely cancer and manage as described below; if "cold" (ie, nonfunctioning), perform fine-needle aspirate.

Management is based on cytology, except for "hot" nodules.

- "Hot" nodules: radioactive iodine or surgery
- Benign nodules (2.5% cancer risk): follow clinically and with ultrasound q12–24mo initially
- Malignant nodules (99% cancer risk), suspicious for malignancy (70% cancer risk): surgery
- Follicular neoplasm or suspicious for follicular neoplasm (25% cancer risk); surgery (preferred) or molecular testing
- Atypical cells of undetermined significance (ACUS) or follicular lesions of undetermined significance (14% cancer risk). If low suspicion, gene expression classifier. If suspicion is high, check for molecular abnormalities.
- Nondiagnostic (20% cancer risk): repeat fine-needle aspirate with ultrasound guidance

HYPERCALCEMIA

Common Causes

- Primary hyperparathyroidism
- Malignancy
- Thyrotoxicosis
- Increased calcium intake (rare unless also CKD or milk-alkali syndrome)
- Hypervitaminosis D
- Lithium
- Thiazide diuretics
- Granulomatous diseases

Evaluation

- Ionized calcium or calcium corrected for albumin
- Intact PTH
  ○ If high, measure urinary calcium excretion. If high, then primary hyperparathyroidism. If low, then familial hypocalciuric hypercalcemia.
  ○ If low, measure PTHrP, 1,25(OH)2D, and 25(OH)D. If PTHrP is high, workup for malignancy. If normal and 1,25(OH)2D is high, get CXR to look for granulomatous diseases. If normal and 25(OH)D is high, probably due to medications, vitamins, supplements. If all are normal, consider other causes (eg, myeloma, vitamin A toxicity).

Management

Treat underlying cause, if possible.

Nonpharmacologic

Asymptomatic: surgery if any of the following: serum calcium >1.0 mg/dL above upper limits of normal, eGFR <60 mL/min/1.73 m^2, BMD T score <-2.5 or prior vertebral fracture, 24h Ca excretion >400 mg/d, nephrolithiasis. If no surgery, avoid thiazide diuretics, dehydration, bedrest, or physical inactivity.

Pharmacologic

If symptomatic or Ca >14 mg/dL:
- Isotonic saline 200–300 mL/h and then adjusted to maintain 100–150 mL/h urine output
- Calcitonin 4 (IU/kg), short term
- Zoledronic acid (4 mg over 15 min) or pamidronate (50–90 mg over 2 h)

- Saline and calcitonin will lower calcium within 12–48 h. Zoledronic acid/pamidronate will be effective by 48–96 h.
- Other tx are reserved for refractory hypercalcemia (eg, denosumab, cinacalcet) or specific causes (glucocorticoids for some lymphomas and granulomatous disease). Denosumab may be valuable but if CrCl <30 mL/min/1.73 m^2 may precipitate hypocalcemia.

DIABETES MELLITUS
Definition and Classification (ADA)
DM is a group of metabolic diseases characterized by hyperglycemia resulting from defects in insulin secretion, insulin action, or both.

Type 1: Caused by an absolute deficiency of insulin secretion.

Type 2: Caused by a combination of resistance to insulin action and an inadequate compensatory insulin secretory response. Type 2 DM is a progressive disorder requiring higher dosages or additional medications over time.

Screening—Screen asymptomatic adults aged ≥45; repeat at 3-y intervals (only if overweight or obese [USPSTF]).

Criteria for Diagnosis—One or more of the following:
- Symptoms of DM (eg, polyuria, polydipsia, unexplained weight loss) plus casual plasma glucose concentration ≥200 mg/dL
- Fasting (no caloric intake for ≥8 h) plasma glucose ≥126 mg/dL
- 2-h plasma glucose ≥200 mg/dL during an OGTT
- Unless hyperglycemia is unequivocal, diagnosis should be confirmed by repeat testing.
- A1c >6.5. *Note:* A1c can be falsely lowered by any condition that shortens erythrocyte survival or decreases mean erythrocyte age (eg, hemolysis, tx for iron, B$_{12}$, folate deficiency, or erythropoietin tx) and falsely increased when RBC turnover is low (eg, iron, B$_{12}$, or folate deficiency, anemia), asplenia; CKD can increase or decrease A1c.

Prediabetes—Any of the following:
- Impaired fasting glucose: defined as fasting plasma glucose ≥100 and <126 mg/dL
- Impaired glucose tolerance: 2-h plasma glucose 140–199 mg/dL
- A1c 5.7–6.4%

Prevention/Delay of Type 2 DM in Patients with Prediabetes
- Lifestyle modification (most effective)
  ○ Weight loss (target 7% loss) if overweight
  ○ Reduction in total and saturated dietary fat
  ○ High dietary fiber (14 g fiber/1000 kcal) and whole grains
  ○ Mediterranean diet and extra-virgin olive oil
  ○ Exercise (at least 150 min/wk of moderate activity, such as walking)
  ○ Medicare Diabetes Prevention Program for persons without DM or ESRD who have BMI ≥25 (≥23 if Asian) and have A1c 5.7%–6.4%, fasting glucose 100–125 mg/dL, or 2-h plasma glucose of 140–199 mg/dL. Program includes a minimum of 10 intensive core sessions of a CDC-approved curriculum over 6 mo in a group-based, classroom-style setting followed by less intensive follow-up meetings monthly for 1–2 y to help ensure that the participants maintain healthy behaviors. Monitor A1c at least yearly.
- Pharmacologic (typically combined with lifestyle modifications). Drugs may be helpful in preventing type 2 DM, but the impact on future CVD events is unclear; it is unknown whether early tx confers benefit versus withholding tx until DM develops.

- Metformin (850 mg q12h) (best long-term evidence but less effective than lifestyle modification)
- Valsartan[BC] (beginning 80 mg/d and increased to 160 mg/d after 2 wk as tolerated) slightly reduces risk of developing DM but does not reduce rate of cardiovascular events.
- Acarbose (100 mg q8h) (less effective than lifestyle modification)
- Liraglutide SC 3.0 mg/d
- Orlistat 120 mg q8h
- Phentermine-topiramate ER 7.5 mg/46 mg/d or 15 mg/92 mg/d

Management of Diabetes

Hospital

- Target glycemic control:
  - If critically ill, 140–180 mg/dL, which usually requires IV insulin infusion.
  - If noncritically ill, there are no clear evidence-based guidelines, but fasting <140 mg/dL and random <180 mg/dL are suggested (might be relaxed if severe comorbidities [ADA]).
  - If good nutritional intake, scheduled basal and prandial insulin doses with correction doses with rapid-acting analog (aspart, glulisine, or lispro).[BC]
    - If npo or poor oral intake, basal plus correction dose only.
  - If insulin-naive, patient can initiate insulin at total daily dose of 0.3 U/kg, half as long-acting (basal) and half as rapid-acting before each meal.
- Correction dose for older persons is 1 unit for every 40–50 mg/dL in excess of 140 mg/dL.
- Point-of-care blood glucose monitoring is used to guide insulin dosing.

Nursing home: Do not use sliding-scale insulin in chronic glycemic management.[BC, CW]

Outpatient Settings

Evaluate and Treat Comorbid Conditions and Provide Preventive Care (AGS, ADA):
Depression (p 86), polypharmacy (p 19), cognitive impairment (p 77), UI (p 161), falls (p 123), pain (p 252) (AGS), PAD (claudication hx and assessment of pedal pulses) (p 67), sleep disorders (p 341), (ADA). Stress test screening for CAD is of no benefit in asymptomatic patients (p 45). In men, if symptoms of hypogonadism, consider screening with morning testosterone.

- Tx of comorbid conditions should be individualized based on life expectancy, patient preferences, and tx goals.
- Manage HTN (BP goal <140/80 mmHg [ADA] <130/80 [ACC]; also HTN, p 56) including an ACEI, ARB, dihydropyridine CCB, or thiazide diuretic (ACEI or ARB if albuminuria). If patient is black, CCB or thiazide diuretic is preferred as initial tx (JNC 8).
- Treat lipid disorders (p 53).
- ASA 75–162 mg/d if hx of heart disease but not for primary prevention[BC]; if allergic, clopidogrel 75 mg/d.
- Pneumococcal vaccination (PCV13 and PPSV23); revaccinate PPSV23 at age ≥65.
- Annual influenza vaccination
- Consider hepatitis B vaccination.

Goals of Glycemic Treatment (ADA, AGS) (Table 47)
- Older adults who are functional, cognitively intact, and have significant life expectancy should receive DM care with goals similar to those developed for younger adults (A1c <7.5%). Avoid using medications to achieve an A1c <7.5% in most older adults.[CW]
- If multiple coexisting chronic illnesses, cognitive impairment, or functional dependency, A1c goals should be 8.0–8.5%.

- In older persons and patients with cognitive dysfunction, individualize tx to avoid hypoglycemia.
- At end of life, focus should be to avoid symptoms and complications from glycemic management; most agents for type 2 DM, BP, and hyperlipidemia can be removed in dying patients.

Table 47. Goals of Treatment for Older Patients with Diabetes Mellitus

Patient Health	A1c goal	FPG or PPG, mg/dL	Bedtime glucose, mg/dL	BP goal, mmHg	Lipid Tx
Healthy	7.0–7.5%	90–130	90–150	<140/80	Statin
Complex/intermediate[1]	7.5–8.0%	90–150	100–180	<140/80	Statin
Very complex/poor health[2]	8.5–9.0%	100–180	110–200	<150/90	Consider statin

FPG = fasting plasma glucose; PPG = postprandial glucose.

[1] multiple (3+) coexisting chronic illness or 2+ IADL impairments or mild to moderate cognitive impairment

[2] LTC or end-stage chronic illnesses or moderate to severe cognitive impairment or 2+ ADL dependencies

Nonpharmacologic Interventions

- Patient and family education for self-management (reimbursed by Medicare)
- Individualize medical nutrition tx to achieve tx goals (diet plus exercise is more effective than diet alone)
  - Macronutrient (carbohydrate, protein, and fat) distribution based on individualized assessment of current eating patterns, preferences, and metabolic goals.
  - The amount of dietary saturated fat, cholesterol, and trans fat is the same as that recommended for the general population.
  - Carbohydrate intake from vegetables, fruits, whole grains, legumes, and dairy products— with an emphasis on foods higher in fiber and lower in glycemic load—should be advised over intake from other carbohydrate sources, especially those that contain added sugars.
  - Mediterranean diet high in monounsaturated fatty acids may be beneficial in glycemic control and cardiovascular risk reduction.
  - Limit alcohol intake to <1 drink/d in women and <2 drinks/d in men.
- Smoking cessation
- Exercise for ≥150 min/wk, resistance training 3×/wk if not contraindicated, balance and flexibility training
- Weight loss if overweight or obese. For younger and healthier older adults, consider bariatric surgery if DM with BMI ≥40, BMI 35–39 when hyperglycemia is inadequately controlled with lifestyle changes and medical tx, and BMI 30.0–34.9 if hyperglycemia is not controlled with oral or injectable medications.
- Psychosocial assessment and care

Pharmacologic Interventions for Type 2 DM (ADA)

- If diet and exercise have not achieved target A1c in 6 mo, begin drug tx.[1]
- *Monotherapy* (A1c<9): Metformin▲ (reduce dose in Stage 3 CKD; avoid in Stage 4 CKD) beginning 500 mg q12h or q24h; can titrate up q5–7d to max of 2000 mg/d if no AEs and blood glucose uncontrolled
- *Dual therapy* (A1c≥9): If A1c target is not achieved after 3 mo of monotx.
  - If established atherosclerotic CVD, empagliflozin, canagliflozin, or liraglutide are first choice.

- ○ If no atherosclerotic CVD, consider specific drug and patient factors in selecting drug (**Table 48**) in the following classes:
  - ▪ SGLT2 inhibitors: lower mortality compared to DPP-4 inhibitors
  - ▪ GLP-1 receptor agonists: lower mortality compared to DPP-4 inhibitors
  - ▪ Sulfonylurea (glipizide preferred)
  - ▪ DPP-4 enzyme inhibitors
  - ▪ Thiazolidinediones[BC]
- *Triple tx:* If fails to achieve target A1c after 3 mo dual therapy
- *Combination injectable tx:* If A1c≥10 %, BS >300 mg/dL, or markedly symptomatic. Insulin (basal and rapid acting) +/– GLP-1 receptor agonist

[1]Reinforce lifestyle modifications at every visit.

Table 48. Noninsulin Agents for Treating Diabetes Mellitus[1]

Medication	Dosage	Formulations	Comments (Metabolism)
Biguanide	Decrease hepatic glucose production; lower A1c by 1–2%; do not cause hypoglycemia		
Metformin▲	500–2550 mg divided	T: 500, 850, 1000	Contraindicated if eGFR <30 mL/min/1.73 m² and not recommended if 30–45 mL/min/1.73 m². If already taking and eGFR drops to 30–45 mL/min/1.73 m², consider risks and benefits. Do not administer for 48 h after iodinated contrast imaging if eGFR <60 mL/min/1.73 m². HF, COPD, ↑ LFTs; hold before contrast radiologic studies; may cause weight loss, B12 deficiency (K)
XR▲	1500–2000 mg/d	T: ER 500, 750	
2nd-Generation Sulfonylureas	Increase insulin secretion; lower A1c by 1–2%; can cause hypoglycemia and weight gain; use of clarithromycin, levofloxacin, trimethoprim-sulfamethoxazole, metronidazole, and ciprofloxacin are associated with increased risk of hypoglycemia		
✓ Glimepiride▲BC	4–8 mg 1× (begin 1–2 mg)	T: 1, 2, 4	Numerous drug interactions, long-acting (L, K)
✓ Glipizide▲	2.5–40 mg 1× or divided	T: 5, 10	Short-acting (L, K)
XL	5–20 mg 1×	T: ER 2.5, 5, 10	Long-acting (L, K)
Glyburide[BC] (aka glibenclamide)▲	1.25–20 mg 1× or divided	T: 1.25, 2.5, 5	Long-acting, ↑ risk of hypoglycemia; not recommended for use in older adults (L, K)
Micronized glyburide[BC] (Glynase)	1.5–12 mg 1×	T: 1.5, 3, 4.5, 6	Long-acting, ↑ risk of hypoglycemia; not recommended for use in older adults (L, K)

(cont.)

Table 48. Noninsulin Agents for Treating Diabetes Mellitus[1] (cont.)

Medication	Dosage	Formulations	Comments (Metabolism)
α-*Glucosidase Inhibitors*	Delay glucose absorption; lower A1c by 0.5–1%; can cause hypoglycemia and weight gain		
Acarbose▲	50–100 mg q8h, just ac; start with 25 mg/d	T: 25, 50, 100	GI AEs common, avoid if Cr >2 mg/dL, monitor LFTs (gut, K)
Miglitol *(Glyset)*	25–100 mg q8h, with 1st bite of meal; start with 25 mg/d	T: 25, 50, 100	Same as acarbose but no need to monitor LFTs (L, K)
Thiazolidinediones	Insulin resistance reducers; lower A1c by 0.5–1.5%; ↑ risk of HF; avoid if NYHA Class III or IV cardiac status[BC]; D/C if any decline in cardiac status; weight gain		
	Check LFTs at start, q2mo during 1st year, then periodically; avoid if clinical evidence of liver disease or if serum ALT levels >2.5× upper limit of normal; may increase risk of fractures in women (L, K)		
Pioglitazone▲	15 or 30 mg/d; max 45 mg/d as monotx, 30 mg/d in combination tx	T: 15, 30, 45	
Rosiglitazone *(Avandia)*	4 mg q 12–24h	T: 2, 4, 8	Prescribing and dispensing restrictions were removed in 2014
DPP–4 Enzyme Inhibitors	Protect and enhance endogenous incretin hormones; lower A1c by 0.5–1%; do not cause hypoglycemia, weight neutral		
Alogliptin *(Nesina)*	25 mg 1×/d; 12.5 mg/d if; CrCl 31–50; 6.25 mg/d if CrCl 15–29	T: 25, 12.5, 6.25	(K)
Linagliptin *(Tradjenta)*	5 mg	T: 5	(L)
Sitagliptin *(Januvia)*	100 mg 1×/d as monotx or in combination with metformin or a thiazolidinedione; 50 mg/d if CrCl 31–50; 25 mg/d if CrCl <30	T: 25, 50, 100	
Saxagliptin *(Onglyza)*	5 mg; 2.5 mg if CrCl <50	T: 2.5, 5	K
Meglitinides	Increase insulin secretion; lower A1c by 1–2%; can cause hypoglycemia and weight gain		
Nateglinide▲	60–120 mg q8h	T: 60, 120	Give 30 min ac
Repaglinide *(Prandin)*	0.5 mg q6–12h if A1c <8% or previously untreated; 1–2 mg q6–12h if A1c ≥8% or previously treated	T: 0.5, 1, 2	Give 30 min ac, adjust dosage at weekly intervals, potential for drug interactions, caution in hepatic, renal insufficiency (L)

(cont.)

Table 48. Noninsulin Agents for Treating Diabetes Mellitus[1] (cont.)

Medication	Dosage	Formulations	Comments (Metabolism)
♥*SGLT2 Inhibitors*	Decreases glucose reabsorption from kidney; lowers A1c by 0.5–1.5%; may cause ketoacidosis, AKI, genital mycotic infections, UTIs, increased LDL and fracture risk		
♥Canagliflozin *(Invokana)*	100–300 mg/d	T: 100, 300	Initial dose 100 mg and no more than 100 mg if eGFR 45–59 mL/min/1.73 m²; may increase fracture risk (L)
Dapagliflozin *(Farxiga)*	5–10 mg/d	T: 5, 10	Should not be used if eGFR <60 mL/min/1.73 m² (L)
Empagliflozin *(Jardiance)*	10–25 mg/d	T: 10, 25	Should not be used if eGFR <45 mL/min/1.73 m² (L). May reduce HF hospitalizations, cardiovascular and all-cause mortality, and progression of renal disease in patients with established CVD.
Ertugliflozin *(Steglatro)*	5–15 mg/d	T: 5, 15	(L,K)
GLP–1 Receptor Agonists	Hypoglycemia common if combined with sulfonylurea or insulin. Lowers A1c by 0.7–1%; less likely to cause hypoglycemia than insulin or sulfonylureas; can cause weight loss. Risks include acute pancreatitis and possibly medullary thyroid cancer.		
Albiglutide *(Tanzeum)*	30 or 50 mg SC 1×/wk	30, 50 mg single-dose pen	
Dulaglutide *(Trulicity)*	0.75 or 1.5 mg SC 1×/wk	0.75 mg/0.5 mL, 1.5 mg/0.5 mL single-dose pen or syringe	
Exenatide *(Byetta)*	5–10 mcg SC 2×/d with meals	1.2-, 2.4-mL prefilled syringes	Avoid if CrCl <30 (K)
Extended release *(Bydureon)*	2 mg SC 1×/wk	2-mg prefilled syringes	Avoid if CrCl <30 (K)
♥Liraglutide *(Victoza)*	0.6–1.8 mg SC 1×/d	0.6, 1.2, 1.8 (6 mg/mL) in prefilled, multidose pen	Lowers rates of CVD and all-cause mortality and composite outcome (cardiovascular mortality, nonfatal MI, nonfatal stroke) (L); 3-mg dose used for weight loss does not provide additional glucose lowering beyond 1.8-mg dose
Semaglutide *(Ozempic)*	0.5 or 1 mg SC 1×/wk	1.34 mg/mL (1.5-mL prefilled pen)	Starting dose is 0.25 mg 1×/wk for 4 wk
Amylin analog			
Pramlintide *(Symlin)*	60 mcg SC immediately before meals	0.6 mg/mL in 5-mL vial	Lowers A1c by 0.4–0.7%; nausea common; reduce premeal dose of short-acting insulin by 50% (K)

(cont.)

Table 48. Noninsulin Agents for Treating Diabetes Mellitus[1] (cont.)

Medication	Dosage	Formulations	Comments (Metabolism)
Other			
Bromocriptine *(Cycloset)*	1.6–4.8 mg 1×	0.8	Start 0.8 and increase 0.8 weekly; lowers A1c by 0.5% (L)
Colesevelam *(Welchol)*	3750 mg 1× or 1875 mg 2×	T: 625, 1875 pwd pk: 3750	Give with meals; lowers A1c by 0.5%; not absorbed (GI)

[1] Many combination drugs are available.

- Insulin. D/C sulfonylureas and meglitinides when insulins are started. Insulin analogues are not more effective than regular or NPH insulin and are much more expensive.
  - Begin with basal insulin (intermediate at bedtime or long-acting at bedtime or morning) 10 U or 0.2 U/kg; can increase by 2–4 U q3d depending on fasting blood glucose. 30–50 U is often needed. When fasting blood glucose is at goal, recheck A1c in 2–3 mo. If hypoglycemia or fasting blood glucose <70 mg/dL, reduce dose by 4 U or 10%, whichever is greater. If above target A1c, check before lunch, dinner, and bedtime blood glucose concentrations and add rapid- or intermediate-acting insulin or GLP-1 receptor agonist (**Table 49**).

Table 49. Insulin Preparations

Preparation	Onset	Peak	Duration	Number of Injections/d
Rapid-acting				
Insulin glulisine *(Apidra)* 200 U/mL (3 mL)	20 min	0.5–1.5 h	3–4 h	3
Insulin lispro *(Humalog)* 100 U/mL (3 mL) 200 U/mL (3 mL)	15 min	0.5–1.5 h	3–4 h	3
Insulin aspart *(NovoLog, Fiasp)* 100 U/mL (3 mL, 10 mL)	25 min	1–3 h	3–5 h	3
(Fiasp)	4 min	1 h	5–8 h	3
Inhaled *(Afrezza)*[1] 4 U, 8 U, 12 U	15 min	1 h	3–4 h	3
Regular (eg, *Humulin, Novolin*)[2] 100 U/mL (3 mL, 10 mL) 500 U/mL (3 mL, 20 mL)	0.5–1 h	2–3 h	5–8 h	1–3
Intermediate or long-acting				
NPH (eg, *Humulin, Novolin*)[2] 100 U/mL (3 mL, 10 mL)	1–1.5 h	4–12 h	24 h	1–2
Insulin detemir *(Levemir)* 100 U/mL (3 mL, 10 mL)	3–4 h	6–8 h	6–24 h depending on dose	1–2
Insulin glargine *(Lantus, Toujeo, Basaglar)*[3] 100 U/mL (3 mL) *Lantus, Basaglar*	1–4 h	—	24 h	1
300 U/mL (1.5 mL) *Toujeo*	1–6 h		24–36 h	1
Insulin degludec *(Tresiba)* 100 U/mL (3 mL) 200 U/mL (3 mL)	1–9 h	—	42 h	1

(cont.)

Table 49. Insulin Preparations (cont.)				
Preparation	**Onset**	**Peak**	**Duration**	**Number of Injections/d**
Combinations				
Isophane insulin and regular insulin inj, premixed *(Novolin 70/30)* 100 U/mL (3 mL, 10 mL)	See individual drugs	2–12 h	24 h	1–2
Insulin lispro protamine suspension and insulin lispro *(Humalog Mix 50/50; 75/25)* 100 U/mL (3 mL, 10 mL)	See individual drugs			

[1] Available as 4-unit and 8-unit single-use cartridges administered by inhalation

[2] Also available as mixtures of NPH and regular in 50:50 proportions

[3] To convert from NPH dosing, give same number of units 1×/d. For patients taking NPH q12h, decrease the total daily units by 20%, and titrate on basis of response. Starting dosage in insulin-naive patients is 10 U 1×/d hs.

  ○ Timing for prandial insulin: if blood glucose is in the 100s, give 10 min before eating; if blood glucose is in the 200s, give 20 min before eating; if blood glucose is in the 300s, give 30 min before eating.
  ○ If using fixed daily insulin doses, carbohydrate intake on a day-to-day basis should be consistent with respect to time and amount.
    ▪ Use 4-mm, 32-gauge needle if BMI <40 kg/m^2 and 8-mm, 32-gauge needle if BMI >40 kg/m^2. Inject at 90° without a pinch.
    ▪ Injection sites for human insulin: fastest onset is abdomen and slowest onset is thigh.

Glucose Monitoring

- If multiple daily injections or using insulin pump, self-monitor blood glucose (SMBG) before meals and snacks, occasionally postprandially, at bedtime, before exercise, when patient suspects low blood glucose, after treating low blood glucose until patient is normoglycemic, and before critical tasks such as driving.
- SMBG in patients with type 2 DM who are not receiving insulin does not improve A1c or quality of life; do not recommend.**^{CW}**
- There is no consensus about the frequency of SMBG patients on insulin.

Hypoglycemia

- Tx-associated hypoglycemia (most common with insulin, sulfonylurea, α-glucosidase inhibitors, and meglitinides)
  ○ Severe hypoglycemia: associated with severe cognitive impairment with no specific glucose threshold. Treat with glucagon 0.5–1 mg SC or IM. In medical settings, 25–50 g of D50 IV restores glucose quicker.
    ▪ Clinically significant hypoglycemia: <54 mg/dL
    ▪ Hypoglycemia alert value: ≤70 mg/dL. Treat with fast-acting carbohydrate (eg, glucose tabs, hard candy, paste [*Insta-Glucose*]) or instant fruit that provides 15–20 g of glucose. Effects may last only 15 min, so need to eat and recheck blood glucose. Also will likely need dose adjustment.
- If hypoglycemia unawareness or >1 episodes of severe hypoglycemia, then reevaluate regimen.

Monitoring (abridged ADA)

Initial and Annually

- Screen for depression, anxiety, and disordered eating
- Assess for cognitive impairment if ≥65
- Height, weight, and BMI (and at every follow-up visit)
- BP (and at every follow-up visit)
- Foot exam including visual inspection (and at every visit), checking pedal pulses and asking about claudication, and annual monofilament testing plus determination of either temperature or pinprick sensation or vibration.
- Comprehensive dilated eye and visual examinations by an ophthalmologist or optometrist who is experienced in the management of diabetic retinopathy
- A1c if results are not available in past 3 mo
- If not performed within the past year: lipid profile, LFTs, spot urinary albumin:Cr ratio, serum Cr, and eGFR, vitamin B12 if on metformin, serum potassium if on ACEI, ARB, or diuretics
- If 2nd-generation antipsychotics are being used, changes in weight, glycemic control, and cholesterol levels should be carefully monitored.

ADRENAL INSUFFICIENCY

Common Causes

Secondary (more common; mineralocorticoid function is preserved, no hyperkalemia or hyperpigmentation, dehydration is less common)

- Abrupt discontinuation of chronic glucocorticoid administration
- Megestrol acetate
- Brain irradiation
- Traumatic brain injury
- Pituitary tumors

Primary (less common)

- Autoimmune
- Tuberculosis

Evaluation

- Basal (morning) plasma cortisol >18 mcg/dL excludes adrenal insufficiency, and <3 mcg/dL is diagnostic.
- ACTH stimulation test: tetracosactrin *(Synacthen Depot)* 250 mcg IV; best administered in the morning; peak value at 30–60 min >18 mcg/dL is normal, <15 mcg/dL is diagnostic.
- If adrenal insufficiency is diagnosed with high ACTH (eg, >100 pg/mL), then insufficiency is primary.

Pharmacotherapy

For corticosteroid dose equivalencies, see **Table 50**.

Medication	Approx Equivalent Dose (mg)	Relative Anti-inflammatory Potency	Relative Mineralo-corticoid Potency	Biologic Half-life (h)	Formulations
Betamethasone▲	0.6–0.75	20–30	0	36–54	T: 0.6 S: 0.6 mg/5 mL
Cortisone▲	25	0.8	2	8–12	T: 5 S: 50 mg/mL
Dexamethasone▲	0.75	20–30	0	36–54	T: 0.25, 0.5, 0.75, 1, 1.5, 2, 4; S: elixir 0.5 mg/5 mL; Inj
Fludrocortisone▲ [1]	NA	10	4	12–36	T: 0.1
Hydrocortisone▲	20	1	2	8–12	T: 5, 10, 20 S: 10 mg/5 mL Inj
Methylprednisolone▲	4	5	0	18–36	T: 2, 4, 8, 16, 24, 32; Inj
Prednisolone▲	5	4	1	18–36	S: 5 mg/5 mL syr 5, 15 mg/5 mL
Prednisone▲	5	4	1	18–36	T: 1, 2.5, 5, 10, 20, 50 S: 5 mg/5 mL
Triamcinolone	4	5	0	18–36	T: 1, 2, 4, 8 S: syr 4 mg/5 mL

Table 50. Corticosteroids that Provide Gastroprotection[BC]

NA = not available.

[1] Usually given for orthostatic hypotension at 0.1 mg q8–24h (max 1 mg/d) and at 0.05–0.2 mg/d for primary adrenal insufficiency.

- For chronic adrenal insufficiency, hydrocortisone in 2 or 3 divided doses (total dose of 15–25 mg/d). Alternatives are dexamethasone or prednisone. If primary adrenal insufficiency, add fludrocortisone▲ to glucocorticoids.
- Stress doses of corticosteroids for patients with severe illness, injury, or undergoing surgery: In emergency situations, do not wait for test results. Give hydrocortisone 100 mg IV bolus (or if patient has not been previously diagnosed, dexamethasone 4 mg IV bolus). Also treat with IV fluids (eg, saline). For less severe stress (eg, minor illness), double or triple usual oral replacement dosage for 3 d.
- For minor surgery (eg, hernia repair), hydrocortisone 25 mg/d on day of surgery and return to usual dosage on the following day.
- For moderate surgical stress (eg, cholecystectomy, joint replacement), total 50–75 mg/d on the day of surgery and the 1st postoperative day, then usual dosage on the 2nd postoperative day.
- For major surgical procedures (eg, cardiac bypass), total 100–150 mg/d given in divided doses for 2–3 d, then return to usual dosage.

VISUAL IMPAIRMENT

Definition

Visual acuity 20/40 or worse; severe visual impairment (legal blindness) 20/200 or worse in the better eye.

Evaluation

- Acuity testing
  - Near vision: check each eye independently with glasses using handheld Rosenbaum card at 14" or Lighthouse Near Acuity Test at 16". *Note:* Distance must be accurate.
  - Far vision: Snellen wall chart at 20′
- Visual fields (by confrontation)
- Ophthalmoscopy
- Emergent referral for acute change in vision
- Medication review for drugs associated with blurry vision (eg, amiodarone, minocycline, sildenafil, tamoxifen) and any agent with anticholinergic properties

Prevention

Biennial full eye examinations for people aged >65, at diagnosis and every 1–2 y for people with DM (see Diabetic Retinopathy below).

SPECIFIC CONDITIONS ASSOCIATED WITH VISUAL IMPAIRMENT

Refractive Error

The most common cause of visual impairment. Incorrect refraction may account for 20% of IADL dysfunction.

Cataracts

Lens opacity on ophthalmoscopic examination. Risk factors: age, sun exposure, smoking, corticosteroids, DM, alcohol, low vitamin intake, quetiapine. Smoking cessation reduces risk for cataract extraction.

Nonpharmacologic Treatment:

- Reduce UV light exposure.
- Surgery (American Academy of Ophthalmology criteria):
  - If visual function no longer meets the patient's needs and cataract surgery is likely to improve vision.
  - When cataract coexists with lens-induced disease (eg, glaucoma) or other eye disease requiring unrestricted monitoring (eg, diabetic retinopathy).
  - The risk of bleeding is small when antithrombotic agents are continued in the perioperative period (p 286).
  - Do not perform preoperative medical tests for eye surgery without specific indications. Reasonable indications include an ECG in patients with heart disease, serum K+ in patients on diuretics, and serum glucose in patients with DM.[CW]

Age-related Macular Degeneration (AMD)

Atrophy of cells in the central macular region of retinal pigmented epithelium; on ophthalmoscopic examination, white-yellow patches (drusen) or hemorrhage and scars in advanced stages. Risk factors: age, smoking, sun exposure, family hx, white race (14% of white Americans by age 80). AMD has "wet" and "dry" forms.

- Patients with AMD have double the rate of depression compared to peers; evaluate for depression annually and treat.
- Dry AMD: Accounts for 85–90% of cases, is characterized by abnormalities in the retinal pigment with focal drusen, and has a natural hx of slow gradual loss of vision; may convert to the wet form.
- Wet AMD or neovascular type: Often causes rapid visual loss; causes 90% of severe visual loss in AMD. Early intervention when the dry form converts to the wet form saves vision.

Nonpharmacologic Treatment

- Monitor daily for conversion from dry to wet form using Amsler grid.
- Patients with large drusen most at risk of conversion to wet AMD.
- Dietary modification reduces risk of progression to neovascular AMD: high intake of beta-carotene, vitamin C, zinc, n-3 long-chain polyunsaturated fatty acids, and fish.

Pharmacotherapy of Wet AMD

- Vascular endothelial growth factor (VEGF) inhibitors reduce neovascularization, eg, bevacizumab *(Avastin)* or ranibizumab *(Lucentis)*, pegaptanib *(Macugen)* or aflibercept *(Eylea, Zaltrap)* intravitreal (various dosing intervals); maintains vision in the majority and improves it in a significant minority. Complications of the intraocular injections include uveitis, cataract, increased IOP, retinal detachment or endophthalmitis, and visual loss in 1–2% of patients.
- Photodynamic tx in combination with VEGF inhibitors may improve outcomes in those who fail to respond to VEGF inhibitors monotx.
- Most patients can receive intraocular VEGF inhibitors while taking anticoagulants and antiplatelet agents, but tx must be individualized.
- Patients have serious problems with depression in spite of effective VEGF inhibitor tx. Patients with depression perceive greater vision-related disability.

Pharmacotherapy of Both Wet and Dry AMD

- In intermediate or more advanced stages of dry AMD and all stages of wet AMD, zinc oxide 80 mg, cupric oxide 2 mg, lutein 10 mg, zeaxanthin 2 mg, vitamin C 500 mg, and vitamin E 400 IU taken in divided doses q12h reduces risk of progression (AREDS2 preparation).

Diabetic Retinopathy

Microaneurysms, dot and blot hemorrhages on ophthalmoscopy with proliferative retinopathy ischemia and vitreous hemorrhage. Risk factors: chronic hyperglycemia, smoking. Screen all patients with type 2 DM at the time of diagnosis, and at least annually if any retinopathy is found; if none at baseline, rescreen every 2 y.

Treatment

- Annual ophthalmologic evaluation determines the level of retinopathy (ie, mild, moderate, severe), whether retinopathy is proliferative or nonproliferative, and whether macular edema is present.
- The combination of these features determines the follow-up interval of 1–12 mo.
- For severe or very severe diabetic retinopathy, treat with panretinal photocoagulation; mild to moderate cases do not require tx.
- VEGF inhibitors are approved for use in severe retinopathy.
- The VEGF inhibitors are 1st-line tx for macular edema.

Diabetic Management to Reduce Risk or Progression of Retinopathy

Tailor glycemic control based on comorbidities and life expectancy (Diabetes, p 104); BP control <140/80 mmHg; benefits of lipid control have not been established.

Glaucoma

Characteristic optic cupping and nerve damage, and loss of peripheral visual fields. Risk factors: black race, age, family hx, increased ocular pressures. Most common cause of blindness in black Americans. Most patients need 6-mo follow-up appointments.

- Primary open-angle glaucoma is more common and asymptomatic until severe visual loss occurs. Initial tx may be either pharmacologic or laser surgery.
- Angle-closure glaucoma, while a less common disease, has both acute and chronic variants and is painful if acute, requiring emergent management.
- Angle-closure glaucoma is a surgical disease, although topicals are used preoperatively to control IOP.
- Normal-tension glaucoma (normal pressures but with visual field loss) is treated with the goal of reducing pressures 30% below baseline.

Nonpharmacologic Treatments

- Open angle—laser trabeculoplasty is 1st-line nonpharmacologic tx. Surgical procedures (filtration, shunts, etc) have complications such as scarring and visual loss.
- Angle closure (both acute and chronic)—laser peripheral iridotomy

Pharmacotherapy

- Treat when there is optic nerve damage or visual field loss (**Table 51**); goal is reducing IOP. Some advocate tx if 2 readings >25 mmHg. Prostaglandin analogs or laser tx are 1st-line tx.
- Combining drugs from different classes reduces pressure more than monotx.
- Patients receiving oral β-blockers do not benefit from adding the topical. The combination increases risk of drug-related AEs.
- Patients receiving many years of tx may have tachyphylaxis to drug effects. Switching rather than adding drugs may be appropriate.
- There is an age-related decline in aqueous humor production. Reduction of drug tx may be needed.
- Patients must use proper technique both for benefit and to avoid systemic drug-related AEs, ie, instill 1 gtt under lower lid, close eye for at least 1 min to reduce systemic absorption; repeat if a 2nd drop is needed. Systemic absorption is further reduced by teaching the patient to compress the lacrimal sac for 15–30 sec after instilling a drop. Always wait 5 min before instilling a 2nd type of drop.

Table 51. Medications for Treating Glaucoma

Medication	Dosage	Comments (Metabolism)
α2-Agonist (bottles with purple caps)		*Class AEs:* low BP, fatigue, drowsiness, dry mouth, dry nose, nightmares, depression, palpitation, ocular AEs, hyperemia, burning, foreign-body sensation (unknown)
Brimonidine▲ 0.1%, 0.15%, 0.2%	1 gtt q8–12h	
α-β Agonist		
Dipivefrin▲ 0.1%	1 gtt q12h	HTN, headache, tachycardia, arrhythmia (eye, L)
β-Blockers (bottles with blue or yellow caps)		*Class AEs:* hypotension, bradycardia, HF, bronchospasm, anxiety, depression, confusion, hallucination, diarrhea, nausea, cramps, lethargy, weakness, masking of hypoglycemia, sexual dysfunction. Avoid in asthma, bradycardia, COPD, or when taking oral β-blockers. (L)
✓Betaxolol▲ 0.25%, 0.5%	1–2 gtt q12h	
✓Carteolol▲ 1%	1 gtt q12h	
✓Levobunolol▲ 0.25%, 0.5%	1 gtt q12h	
✓Metipranolol▲ 0.3%	1 gtt q12h	
✓Timolol drops▲ 0.25%, 0.5%	1 gtt q12h	Not all formulations available as generic
Cholinergic Agonists (bottles with green caps)		*Class AEs:* brow ache, corneal toxicity, red eye, retinal detachment. Systemic cholinergic effects are rare (tissues, K)
Pilocarpine gel 4%	1/2" qhs	
Pilocarpine▲ 0.5–6%	1 gtt q6h	
Miotic Cholinesterase Inhibitor (bottles with green caps)		*Class AEs:* sweating, tremor, headache, salivation, confusion, high or low BP, bradycardia, bronchoconstriction, urinary frequency, GI upset (tissues, K)
Echothiophate 0.125%	1 gtt q12h	
Carbonic Anhydrase Inhibitors (bottles with orange caps)		
Topical		Caution in kidney failure and after corneal transplant (K)
✓Brinzolamide 1%	1 gtt q8h	
✓Dorzolamide▲ 2%	1 gtt q8h	
Oral		
Acetazolamide▲ 125–500 mg, SR 500 mg	250–500 mg q6–12h, SR 500 mg q12h	*Class AEs:* fatigue, weight loss, bitter taste, paresthesias, depression, COPD exacerbation, cramps, nausea, diarrhea, kidney failure, blood dyscrasias, hypokalemia, myopia, renal calculi acidosis; not recommended in kidney failure (K), (L, K)
Methazolamide▲ 25–50 mg	50–100 mg q8–12h	
Prostaglandin Analogs (bottles with turquoise caps)		First-line tx *Class AEs:* change in eye color and periorbital tissues, hyperemia, itching
✓Bimatoprost▲ 0.03%	1 gtt qhs	(L, K, F)
✓Latanoprost▲ 0.005%	1 gtt qhs	(L)
Latanoprostene *(Vyzulta)* 0.24%	1 gtt qhs	
Tafluprost[1] 0.0015%	1 gtt qhs	(L)
✓Travoprost 0.004%	1 gtt qhs	(L)

(cont.)

Table 51. Medications for Treating Glaucoma (cont.)

Medication	Dosage	Comments (Metabolism)
Combinations (May improve adherence when both agents required)		
Dorzolamide/timolol▲ 0.5%/0.2%	1 gtt q12h	See individual agents (K, L)
Brimonidine/timolol 0.2%/0.5%	1 gtt q12h	See individual agents (K, L)
Brinzolamide/brimonidine 1%/0.2%	1 gtt 2×/d	See individual agents (unknown, L)
Rho Kinase Inhibitor		
Netarsudil (Rhopressa) 0.02%	1gtt qhs	Rho kinase inhibitor (eye) ADEs: hyperemia, corneal verticillata, conjunctival hemorrhage

✓ = preferred for treating older adults; ¹preservative-free

Note: Patients may not know names of drugs but instead refer to them by the color of the bottle cap. The usual colors are listed above.

ADDITIONAL CONSIDERATIONS IN MANAGEMENT OF EYE DISORDERS

Topical Steroid Treatment

Are prescribed for serious ocular inflammatory disorders and require monitoring by an ophthalmologist. Serious and potentially vision-threatening adverse effects can occur from chronic topical corticosteroid use. Indications for topical steroid use include:

- allergic marginal corneal ulcer
- anterior segment inflammation
- bacterial conjunctivitis
- chorioretinitis, choroiditis
- cyclitis
- endophthalmitis
- Graves ophthalmopathy
- herpes zoster ocular infection with appropriate antiviral tx
- iritis
- nonspecific keratitis
- superficial punctate keratitis
- postoperative ocular inflammation
- optic neuritis
- sympathetic ophthalmia
- diffuse posterior uveitis
- vernal keratoconjunctivitis

Topical steroids are also used for corneal injury from thermal, chemical, or radiation burns or penetration of foreign bodies.

Low-vision Services

- Address the full range of functional visual impairment from blindness to partial sight. Refer patients with uncompensated visual loss that reduces function. Participation may reduce depression.
- Recommend and provide training for optical aids:
  - Electronic video magnifiers
  - Spectacle-mounted telescopes for distance vision, including driving
  - Closed-circuit television to enlarge text
  - A variety of high-technology devices are available (lighthouse.org).
  - iPad and iPhone apps are an inexpensive substitute for text-to-speech conversion, lighted magnifiers, big clocks, etc.
  - *Spotlight Text* is an eBook reader app for readers with vision loss and has a book share with >250,000 books.

- Environmental modifications that improve function include color contrast, floor lamps to reduce glare, motion sensors to turn on lights, talking clocks, spoken medication reminders.
- Many states have "Services for the Visually Impaired" through the health department.

Dual Sensory Impairment (DSI)

- 9–21% of adults aged >70 have loss of both vision and hearing.
- Compared with single-sensory impairment, DSI is more often associated with depression, poor self-rated health, reduced social participation, IADL and cognitive impairment, and higher mortality (OR=1.6–2.2 at 10 y).
- Nursing home residents with DSI have higher risk of behavioral problems and faster cognitive decline (unless they remain socially engaged).
- Management currently limited to vibrating devices such as alarm clocks, door bells, smoke alarms, etc.
- Rehab should be designed by a team of providers from audiology and visual rehab.

RED EYE

The "red eye" is an eye with vascular congestion: some conditions that cause this pose a threat to vision and warrant prompt ophthalmologic referral (**Table 52**).

Initial evaluation: check visual acuity, pupil reactivity; note if painful, corneal ulcer, or exudate in the anterior chamber (**Table 52**).

- Acute conjunctivitis, allergic conjunctivitis, and foreign bodies are common causes of red eye. Diagnosis and tx of acute and allergic conjunctivitis are discussed below.

Table 52. Signs and Symptoms of Serious Conditions in Patients with Red Eye	
Red Flag Signs and Symptom	**Potentially Dangerous Condition(s)**
Lid or lacrimal sac swelling or proptosis	Orbital cellulitis, orbital tumor
Subnormal visual acuity, foreign-body sensation, severe pain, photophobia, or circumcorneal hyperemia (ciliary flush)	Keratitis, anterior uveitis; acute angle-closure glaucoma; endophthalmitis, episcleritis and scleritis
Proptosis, chemosis, visual loss, and ophthalmoplegia	Cavernous sinus arteriovenous fistula

Acute Conjunctivitis

Symptoms: Red eye, foreign-body sensation, discharge, photophobia

Signs: Conjunctival hyperemia and discharge

Etiology: Viral, bacterial, chlamydial

Viral Versus Bacterial:

Viral—profuse tearing, minimal exudate, preauricular adenopathy common, monocytes in stained scrapings and exudates; may be part of upper respiratory infection. Extremely contagious; wash hands frequently and use separate towels to avoid spread.

Bacterial—moderate tearing, profuse exudation, preauricular adenopathy uncommon, bacteria and polymorphonuclear cells in stained scrapings and exudates

Both—minimal itching, generalized hyperemia, occasional sore throat and fever

Treatment: Most are viral; do not treat viral infections with antibiotics; if diagnosis is uncertain, patients may be followed closely for worsening that would warrant antibiotics.[CW]
- Treat viral infections with artificial tears and cool compresses.

- If purulent discharge, suspect bacterial. Many cases resolve without antibiotics and without adverse effect on visual function. Antibiotics reduce duration of symptoms. Some recommend use of erythromycin or polymyxin/trimethoprim. Avoid quinolones, which are expensive and select resistant organisms (**Table 53**). If severe, obtain culture and Gram stain, then start tx.
- If signs and symptoms do not improve in 24–48 h on tx for bacterial conjunctivitis, refer to ophthalmologist.
- If severe purulence or if patient wears contact lenses, refer to ophthalmologist immediately.

Table 53. Treatment for Acute Bacterial Conjunctivitis[1]

Medication/Formulations[2]	Comments
First Line (inexpensive, narrow spectrum)	
Erythromycin▲ 5 mg/g oint	Good if staphylococcal blepharitis is present
Trimethoprim and polymyxin▲ 1 mg/mL, 10,000 IU/mL sol	Well tolerated but some gaps in coverage
Second Line (more expensive, broad spectrum); preferred in contact lens wearers	
Besifloxacin *(Besivance)* 0.6% sol	Very broad spectrum, a 1st choice in severe cases, well tolerated, expensive
Ciprofloxacin 0.3% sol▲, 0.3% oint	See besifloxacin
Gatifloxacin *(Tequin)* 0.3% sol	See besifloxacin
Moxifloxacin *(Avelox)* 0.5% sol	See besifloxacin
Ofloxacin▲ 0.3% sol, 0.3% oint	See besifloxacin
Tobramycin 3 mg/g oint, 3 mg/mL sol▲	Well tolerated but more corneal toxicity

[1] Do not use steroid or steroid-antibiotic preparations in initial tx.

[2] In mild cases, solution is applied q6h and gel or oint q12h for 5–7 d. In more severe cases, solution is applied q2–3h and oint q6h; as the eye improves, solution is applied q6h and oint q12h.

Allergic Conjunctivitis

Symptoms: Prominent itching, watery discharge accompanied by nasal stuffiness (see allergic rhinitis, p 309)

Signs: Bilateral eyelid edema, conjunctival bogginess, and hyperemia.

Etiology: IgE–mediated hypersensitivity to airborne allergen

Treatment:

Mild to Moderate Symptoms

- Dilute and clear allergen with liberal use of refrigerated artificial tears.
- Topical H$_1$ antihistamine with mast cell stabilizing properties are the most effective agents, compared to mast cell stabilizers or topical NSAIDs (**Table 54**); 2 wk of tx required for full effectiveness. If symptoms are seasonal, begin tx 2–3 wk before pollen season.
- Nasal steroids reduce ocular symptoms to some degree (**Table 114**).
- Oral antihistamines may aggravate symptoms if there is a concomitant dry eye.

Severe or Persistent Symptoms

- If symptoms persist after 3 wk of topical antihistamine/mast cell stabilizer, refer to an ophthalmologist to confirm diagnosis.

- Topical steroids (eg, loteprednol) may be necessary but should be prescribed only by an ophthalmologist.
- The OTC vasoconstrictor/antihistamines are for short-term use only (**Table 54**).
- Recurrent or severe symptoms may benefit from desensitization.

Table 54. Topical Therapy for Allergic Conjunctivitis		
Category/Medication	**Formulation and Dosing**	**Adverse Events[1]/Comments**
H₁ Antihistamine/Mast Cell Stabilizers		
Alcaftadine *(Lastacaft)*	0.25%, 1 gtt OU q24h	*Class effects*: Itching, erythema, headache, rhinitis, dysgeusia, cold syndrome, headache, keratitis
Azelastine▲	0.05%, 1 gtt OU q6h	
Bepotastine *(Bepreve)*	1.5%, 1 gtt OU q12h	
Emedastine *(Emadine)*	0.05%, 1 gtt OU q12h	May not have mast stabilizing effect
Epinastine *(Elestat)*	0.5%, 1 gtt OU q12h	
Ketotifen▲	0.025%, 1 gtt OU q8–12h	Inexpensive, generic, OTC
Olopatadine *(Patanol)*	0.1%, 1 gtt OU q12h	May be more effective than ketotifen
Olopatadine *(Pataday)*	0.2%, 1 gtt OU q24h	
NSAID		
Ketorolac▲	0.5%, 1 gtt OU q6h	Ocular irritation, burning
Mast cell stabilizers[2]		
Lodoxamide *(Alomide)*	0.1%, 1–2 gtt OU q6h	Ocular irritation, burning
Cromolyn sodium▲	4%, 1 gtt q4–6h	Ocular irritation, burning
Nedocromil *(Alocril)*	2%, 1–2 gtt OU q12h	Headache, ocular irritation, burning
Pemirolast *(Alamast)*	0.1%, 1–2 gtt OU q6h	Headache, rhinitis, flu-like symptoms, ocular irritation, burning
Vasoconstrictor/Antihistamine combinations (for short-term <2 wk use only)		
Naphazoline▲ (0.03%, 0.1%, 0.13%)	OTC; 1-2 gtt q3–4h as needed for no more than a few days	*Class effects:* Caution in heart disease, HTN, BPH, narrow angle glaucoma; chronic use can cause follicular reactions or contact dermatitis
Pheniramine maleate (0.3–0.315%)/naphazoline hydrochloride (0.025–0.027%)▲	OTC; 1–2 gtt up to q6h for no more than a few days	

[1] Any may cause stinging, which can be reduced by refrigerating drops.

[2] Not used in acute allergy; use when allergen exposure can be predicted, and use well in advance of exposure; have slower onset of action.

BLEPHARITIS

Inflammation of the eyelid margin that causes eye irritation; may affect inner portion of the eyelid (posterior blepharitis) or the base of the eyelashes (anterior blepharitis).

Inflammation causes instability of tear film and abnormal secretions that have a toxic effect on the ocular surface, promoting bacterial growth. Long-term inflammation leads to gland dysfunction, fibrosis, and damage to the eyelid and ocular surface.

Symptoms: generally chronic recurrent symptoms, which vary over time, involving both eyes. These include:

- Red, swollen, or itchy eyelids
- Crusting of eyelashes in the morning
- Gritty or burning sensation
- Excessive tearing
- Flaking/scaling of the eyelid skin

Diagnosis is clinical, based on findings of bilateral red and irritated eyelid margins with crusting or flakes on the lashes or lid margins. If the diagnosis is unclear, refer to ophthalmology.

Therapy: Good lid hygiene is the mainstay of tx.

- **Mild to moderate symptoms**: Tx is symptomatic with warm compresses (5–10 min, 2–4×/d), lid massage (gentle circular motion against the eye), lid washing (with very dilute baby shampoo, rinse thoroughly, or use commercial preparation), and artificial tears (for dryness).
- **Severe or refractory symptoms**: Patients who do not respond to the above measures or those with severe symptoms need topical or oral antibiotic tx and need referral to ophthalmology.

DRY EYE SYNDROME

Symptoms: Itchy or sandy eyes (foreign-body sensation), visual impairment, excess tearing.

Signs: Symmetrical conjunctival injection, blepharitis, entropion, ectropion, reduced blink

Etiology: Altered tear film composition, reduced tear production, poor lid function, environment, drug-induced causes (eg, anticholinergics, estrogens, SSRIs, diuretics), or diseases such as Sjögren syndrome; refer to ophthalmology for diagnostic assistance.

Therapy:

- Artificial tear formulations (eg, *HypoTears*) administer q1–6h prn. Preservatives may cause eye irritation. Preservative-free preparations should be recommended if frequency of use is more often than q6h. Ointment preparations can be used at night or also during the day in severe cases.
- Environmental strategies: room humidifiers, frequent blinking, and swim goggles or moisture chambers fit to eye glasses are all helpful.
- Cyclosporine ophthalmic emulsion 0.05% *(Restasis)* 1 gtt OU q12h. Indicated when tear production is suppressed by inflammation. May take 4–6 wk to achieve results. Patients should have a complete ophthalmologic examination before receiving a prescription.
- Lifitegrast 5% *(Xiidra)*, an integrin antagonist, improves symptoms in mild to severe cases. Dose: 1 gtt q12h, ADEs: eye irritation, bad taste in 25%.
- Temporary or permanent punctal occlusion; do not place punctal occlusion for mild dry eye before trying other medical tx.[CW]

DEFINITION

An event whereby an individual unexpectedly comes to rest on the ground or another lower level without known loss of consciousness (AGS/BGS Clinical Practice Guideline: Prevention of Falls in Older Persons, 2010). Excludes falls from major intrinsic event (eg, seizure, stroke, syncope), which should be evaluated and managed.

ETIOLOGY

Typically multifactorial. Composed of intrinsic (eg, poor balance, weakness, chronic illness, visual or cognitive impairment), extrinsic (eg, polypharmacy), and environmental (eg, poor lighting, no safety equipment, loose carpets) factors. Commonly a nonspecific sign for one of many acute illnesses in older adults.

RISK FACTORS

Table 55. Risk Factors and Medications Associated with Falls

Risk Factor	OR for all fallers (those who fell at least once during follow-up)	OR for recurrent fallers (those who fell at least twice during follow-up)
Falls		
Hx of falls	2.8	3.5
Fear of falling	1.6	2.5
Pain		
Number of chronic musculoskeletal pain sites	5.3	ND
Pain (yes/no)	2.2	2.0
Severe foot pain	1.4	3.5
Moderate foot pain	1.2	1.8
Medical Conditions		
Parkinson disease	2.7	2.8
Rheumatic disease	1.5	1.6
Urinary incontinence	1.4	1.7
Arthritis	1.4	ND
Depression/Anxiety	1.3	ND
Comorbidity	1.2	1.5
Activity/Balance		
Balance limits activities	2.4	ND
Homebound	2.4	ND
Walking aid use	2.2	3.1
Gait deficit	2.1	2.2
Many problems moving around	1.8	ND

(cont.)

Table 55. Risk Factors and Medications Associated with Falls (cont.)

Risk Factor	OR for all fallers (those who fell at least once during follow-up)	OR for recurrent fallers (those who fell at least twice during follow-up)
Sensory		
Vertigo	1.8	2.3
Visual deficit, particularly unilateral visual loss	1.4	1.6
Hearing impairment	1.2	1.5
Cognitive/Psychiatric		
Depression	1.6	1.9
Poor self-rated health	1.5	1.8
Cognitive impairment	1.4	1.6
Other Risk Factors that Have Not Been Studied		
Impaired ADLs, higher pain severity	ND	ND
Pain interference with activities	ND	ND
Medications Associated with Falls		
Two or more CNS-active agents (Avoid ≥3 CNS-active agents[BC])	2.4	ND
Non-TCA/non-SSRI[1] (SNRI[BC])	ND	2.9
TCA (Avoid[BC])/SSRI[1]	1.5	1.5
Benzodiazepines[BC]	1.7	ND
Other sedatives (Avoid[BC]), hypnotics	1.7	ND
Opioids	2.4	1.0
Anticonvulsants (Avoid[BC,2])	1.9	2.6
Antipsychotics (Avoid[BC])	1.5	ND
Antiarrhythmics (Class 1A)	1.6	ND
Antihypertensives	1.2	ND
Diuretics	1.1	ND
Other Medications Associated with Falls		
Skeletal muscle relaxants (Avoid[BC]), systemic glucocorticoids		

OR = Odds ratio; ND = no data on OR or unable to calculate

[1] In a study of frail older women

[2] Avoid unless safer alternatives are not available; avoid except if seizure disorder.[BC]

SCREENING

Fall risk screening is an important 1st step in fall prevention, but must be followed by a thorough assessment and the development of a plan that tailors person-centered interventions to address identified risk factors. Fall risk screening or assessment is a quality measure included in the CMS MACRA and Medicare Annual Wellness Visit. Tool kits available to guide screening and tailored intervention from AHRQ in nursing facilities (AHRQ reviewed December 2017; ahrq.gov/professionals/systems/long-term-care/resources/injuries/fallspx) and in hospitals (AHRQ reviewed April 2018; ahrq.gov/professionals/systems/hospital/fallpxtoolkit/index.html) and Stopping Elderly Accidents, Deaths and Injuries (STEADI; cdc.gov/Steadi/index.html; cdc.gov/steadi/training.html).

See **Figure 5** for recommended assessment strategies. USPSTF does not recommend multifactorial assessment, although small benefit (6% reduction in fall risk; 11% when risk factors managed).

Assessment Considerations

USPSTF recommends 2 factors to identify increased risk for falls in older adults: hx of falls and hx of impairments in mobility, gait, and balance. Use assessments of gait and mobility, such as the *Timed Up & Go* (TUG) test.

Assess risk of falling as part of routine primary healthcare visit (at least annually). Risk of falling significantly increases as the number of risk factors increases. Falling is more frequent in ambulatory residents in long-term care and in acute care settings.

- Screen for fall risk in nursing home (Morse Fall Scale, www.ahrq.gov/professionals/systems/hospital/fallpxtoolkit/fallpxtk-tool3h.html).
- Screen for fall risk in acute care setting (Hendrich II Fall Risk Model, consultgeri.org/try-this/general-assessment/issue-8).
- Assess for risk factors (**Table 55**) using a multidisciplinary approach, including PT and OT if problems with gait, balance, or lower extremity strength are identified.
- Assess fear of falling using 7-item Falls Efficacy Scale-International (FES-I). Measures levels of concern about falling during physical and social activities on a 1- to 4-point Likert scale. https://sites.manchester.ac.uk/fes-i/

Gait, Balance, and Mobility Assessment

- Functional gait: observe patient rising from chair, walking (stride length, base of gait, velocity, symmetry), turning, sitting (Timed Up and Go Test)
- Balance: semi-tandem, and full-tandem stance; Functional Reach test; Berg Balance Scale (especially retrieve object from floor); Short Physical Performance Battery (SPPB)

Figure 5. Assessment and Prevention of Falls

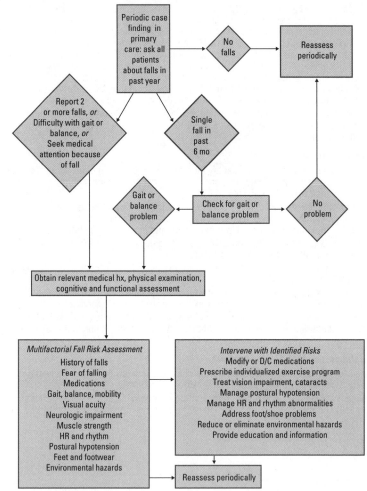

Adapted from American Geriatrics Society and British Geriatrics Society. *Clinical Practice Guideline for the Prevention of Falls in Older Persons*. New York: American Geriatrics Society; 2010; medcats.com/FALLS/frameset.htm; and Pighills AC et al. *J Am Geriatr Soc* 2011;59:26–33.

- Cognition: assess frontal-lobe cognitive function (eg, CLOCK or MiniCog) to identify impaired executive function and judgment that can impact fall risk.
- Mobility: observe patient's use and fit of assistive device (eg, cane, walker) or personal assistance, extent of ambulation, restraint use, footwear evaluation.
  - Cane fitting: top of the cane should be at the top of the greater trochanter or at the break of the wrist when patient stands with arms at side; when the patient holds the cane, there is approximately a 15-degree bend at the elbow. Canes are most often used to improve balance but can also be used to reduce weight-bearing on the opposite leg.
  - Walker fitting: walkers are prescribed when a cane does not offer sufficient stability. Front-wheeled walkers allow a more natural gait and are easier for cognitively impaired patients to use. Four-wheeled rolling walkers (ie, rollators) have the advantage for a smoother faster gait, but require more coordination because of the brakes; however, they are good for outside walking because the larger wheels move more easily over sidewalks.
- ADLs: complete ADL skill evaluation, including use of adaptive equipment and mobility aids as appropriate.
- Complete environmental assessment, including home safety, and mitigate identified hazards.

PREVENTION

See **Figure 5** for recommended prevention strategies.

Recommendations below are primarily based on studies of community-dwelling older adults with limited evidence from RCTs regarding single or multifactorial interventions in the long-term care setting and in cognitively impaired patients.

- Use strategies for lowering fall risk by targeting risk factors (**Table 56**).
  - Consider balance of benefits and harms of identified interventions, based on circumstances of prior falls, comorbid medical conditions, and patient values, in providing comprehensive intervention.
  - Multiple component interventions are most effective across care settings.
  - No evidence for hip protectors and medication review in long-term care facilities.
- Evidence-based programs advocated by the CDC and/or Administration for Community Living. Exercise: *Tai Chi: Moving for Better Balance* (or similar tai chi classes), *Otago Exercise Program, Stay Safe, Stay Active*. Multifactorial evidence-based educational programs: *Stepping On*, Prevention Of Falls in the Elderly Trial (PROFET), *A Matter of Balance*. Additional evidence-based programs at cdc.gov/homeandrecreationalsafety/Falls/compendium.html and community resources. Exercise videos for Otago home-based exercise available at med.unc.edu/aging/cgec/exercise-program/videos and for *Strategies to Reduce Injuries and Develop Confidence in Elders* (STRIDE).
- Additional CDC recommendations for visually impaired (eg, VIP trial home safety program) and for specific situations such as walking on ice and snow (eg, Yaktrax Walker). See cdc.gov/HomeandRecreationalSafety/Falls/compendium.html
- See Prevention (p 289) or Musculoskeletal Disorders (p 212) for details on exercise.

Table 56. Strategies for Lowering Fall Risk

Factors	Suggested Interventions (Outcome Reduction[1])
General Risk	Offer: exercise program to include exercises that address balance and stability, plus resistance (strength), flexibility, and endurance
	• medical assessment before starting • tailor to individual capabilities; consider strengths, weaknesses, and injury risk • initiate with caution in those with limited mobility not accustomed to physical activity • progress slowly, appropriate to ability and competence • maintain regular, comfortable, yet challenging plan • provide environment that builds self-efficacy • prescribed by qualified healthcare provider • regular review and progression
	(↓ risk 11% [USPSTF];
	↓ risk 15%; ↓ rate 29% [Cochrane];
	Tai Chi: ↓ risk 29%, ↓ rate 22% [Cochrane])
	Education and information, CBT intervention to decrease fear of falling and activity avoidance (limited evidence [Cochrane])
Medication-related Factors (Consider deprescribing [See Appropriate Prescribing, p 19])	
Use of benzodiazepines, sedative-hypnotics, antidepressants, or antipsychotics	Consider agents with less risk of falls
	Avoid if hx of falls or fracture[BC]
	Taper and D/C medications, as possible
	Address sleep problems with nonpharmacologic interventions (p 341)
	Educate regarding appropriate use of medications and monitoring for AEs
Recent change in dosage or number of prescription medications or use of ≥4 prescription medications or use of other medications associated with fall risk	Review medication profile and reduce number and dosage of all medications, as possible
	(Withdrawal of antipsychotics: no ↓ risk; ↓ rate 66% [Cochrane])
	Monitor response to medications and to dosage changes
Mobility-related Factors	
Environmental hazards (eg, improper bed height, cluttered walking surfaces, lack of railings, poor lighting)	Improve lighting, especially at night
	Remove floor barriers (eg, loose carpeting)
	Replace existing furniture with safer furniture (eg, correct height of beds/chairs, more stable)
	Install support structures, especially in bathroom (eg, railings, grab bars, elevated toilet seats)
	Use nonslip bathmats
	(↓ risk 12%; ↓ rate 19%; more effective delivered by OT [Cochrane])
Impaired gait, balance, or transfer skills	Provide exercise program resources (eg, NIA Exercise Booklet, Otago resources) or refer to local senior exercise program (↓ risk of fall 17%; ↓ risk of injurious falls 49%)
	Refer to PT for comprehensive evaluation and rehabilitation

(cont.)

Table 56. Strategies for Lowering Fall Risk (cont.)	
Factors	**Suggested Interventions (Outcome Reduction[1])**
	Refer to PT or OT for gait training, transfer skills, use of assistive devices, balancing, strengthening and resistance training, and evaluation for appropriate footwear
	Refer to podiatrist for evaluation and management of foot or ankle issues that affect mobility and balance
Impaired leg or arm strength or range of motion, or proprioception	Refer to PT or OT
Medical Factors	
Parkinson disease, osteoarthritis, depressive symptoms, impaired cognition, carotid sinus hypersensitivity, other conditions associated with increased falls	Optimize medical tx
	Monitor for disease progression and impact on mobility and impairments
	Address issues related to anxiety and impulsiveness, which may increase fall risk
	Determine need for assistive devices
	Use bedside commode if frequent nighttime urination cannot be managed by other methods
	Cardiac pacing in patients with carotid sinus hypersensitivity who experience falls due to syncope (See Syncope, p 68)
	($\downarrow$ rate 27%, but not risk [Cochrane])
Postural hypotension: drop in SBP $\geq$20 mmHg (or $\geq$20%) with or without symptoms, within 3 min of rising from lying to standing	See orthostatic postural hypotension, p 70
Visual (Eye Disorders, p 114)	Refer to ophthalmologist for evaluation and management of vision-related issues
	Cataract extraction (1st eye cataract removal, rate $\downarrow$ 34%, but not 2nd eye)
	Avoid wearing multifocal lenses while walking, particularly up stairs

[1] risk of falls = # people falling; rate of falling = # falls per person

EVALUATION OF FALL

Diagnose and treat underlying cause. Exclude acute illness or underlying systemic or metabolic process (eg, infection, electrolyte imbalance) as indicated by hx, examination, and laboratory studies. Determine if fall is syncopal or nonsyncopal (Syncope, p 68). Evaluate impact of cognition.

History

- Circumstances of fall (eg, activity at time of fall, location, time, footwear at time of fall, lighting)
- Associated symptoms (eg, lightheadedness, vertigo, syncope, weakness, confusion, palpitations, joint pain, joint stability, feelings of pitching [common in Parkinson disease], foot pain, ankle instability)
- Relevant comorbid conditions (eg, prior stroke, parkinsonism, cardiac disease, DM, seizure disorder, depression, anxiety, hyperplastic anemia, sensory deficit, osteoarthritis, osteoporosis, hyperthyroidism, glucocorticoid excess, GI or chronic renal disease, myeloma)
- Medication review, including OTC medications and alcohol use; note recent changes in medications (p 19)

Physical Examination

Look for:

- Vital signs: postural pulse and BP lying and 3 min after standing, temperature
- Head and neck: visual impairment (especially poor acuity, reduced contrast sensitivity, decreased visual fields, cataracts), motion-induced nystagmus (Dix-Hallpike test), bruit, nystagmus
- Musculoskeletal: arthritic changes, motion or joint limitations (especially lower extremity joint function), postural instability, skeletal deformities, podiatric problems, muscle strength
- Neurologic: slower reflexes, altered proprioception, altered mental status (focus on frontal-lobe impairment and impact on making poor choices), focal deficits, peripheral neuropathy, gait or balance disorders, hip flexor weakness, instability, tremor, rigidity
- Cardiovascular: heart arrhythmias, cardiac valve dysfunction (peripheral vascular changes, pedal pulses)

Diagnostic Tests

- Laboratory tests for people at risk include CBC, serum electrolytes, BUN, Cr, glucose, B_{12}, thyroid function
- Bone densitometry in all women aged >65 except those on osteoporosis tx or those who have osteopenic fragility fractures. Although bone density is not a risk factor for falls, it does affect serious fall-related outcomes (See Osteoporosis, p 247).
- Cardiac workup if symptoms of syncope or presyncope (Syncope Evaluation, p 68)
- Imaging: neuroimaging if head injury or new, focal neurologic findings on examination or if a CNS process is suspected; spinal imaging to exclude cervical spondylosis or lumbar stenosis in patients with abnormal gait, neurologic examination, or lower extremity spasticity or hyperreflexia

MANAGEMENT

- Use strategies to prevent future falls by addressing risk factors (**Table 56**)
- Treat osteoporosis. Recommend daily supplementation of vitamin D (at least 800 IU; See Osteoporosis)
- Maintain anticoagulation. Assess risk of anticoagulation. In most cases, benefits of anticoagulation tx outweigh risks. (See Antithrombotic Therapy and Thromboembolic Disease, [p 30])

DYSPHAGIA

See also p 279.

Types/Presentation/Patient Complaints

Table 57. Dysphagia Complaints

Classification	Presentation and Signs	Common Causes
Oral	Inability to move food or medication from mouth to pharynx. Food deposits in cheeks	Dementia
Pharyngeal	Impaired involuntary food transport pharynx to esophagus with airway protection. Coughing, choking, or nasal regurgitation	Stroke, Parkinson disease, CNS tumor, ALS, local strictures, Zenker diverticulum
Esophageal	Sensation that food is stuck in the throat	Impaired esophageal motility, obstruction, medication

Evaluation

Physical examination and history

- Oral cavity, head, neck, and supraclavicular region
- All cranial nerves with emphasis on nerves V, VII, IX, X, XI, XII
- Review medications for those that can decrease saliva production (eg, anticholinergics)
- Referral to speech-language pathologists

Diagnostic tests (as indicated)

- Modified barium swallow or videofluoroscopy to assess swallowing mechanism; may document aspiration; usual initial test before upper endoscopy (oral-pharyngeal)
- Upper endoscopy in patients with esophageal dysphagia (esophageal)
- Fiberoptic endoscopic evaluations of swallowing (FEES) provides detailed evaluation of lesions in oropharynx, hypopharynx, larynx, and proximal esophagus; also visualizes pooled secretions or food
- Esophageal manometry in combination with barium radiography; more useful for assessment of esophageal dysphagia and usually when a motility disorder is suspected or upper endoscopy is inconclusive (esophageal)

Treatment

- Identify and treat underlying cause (eg, endoscopic dilation, cricopharyngeal myotomy, botulinum toxin injection in cricopharyngeal muscle)

Oral-Pharyngeal

- Dietary modifications based on recommendation of speech pathologist or dietitian that are consistent with the patients and families wishes and quality of life
- Swallowing rehabilitation, eg, multiple swallows, tilt head back and place bolus on strong side, or chin tuck
- Avoid rushed or forced feeding
- Sit upright at 90 degrees
- Elevate head of the bed at least 30 degrees

- Review medications and administration for unsafe practices, eg, crushing enteric-coated or ER formulations (See Appropriate Prescribing, p 19)

Esophageal
- Symptomatic presbyesophagus responds to esophageal dilatation
- Neuromuscular electrical stimulation (NMES)

Food Consistencies
- Pureed: thick, homogenous textures; pudding-like
- Ground/minced: easily chewed without coarse texture; excludes most raw foods except mashed bananas
- Soft or easy to chew: soft foods prepared without a blender; tender meats cut to ≤1-cm pieces; excludes nuts, tough skins, and raw, crispy, or stringy foods
- Modified general: soft textures that do not require grinding or chopping

Fluid Consistencies and Thickening Agents
- Thin: regular fluids
- Nectar-like: thin enough to be sipped through a straw or from a cup, but still spillable (eg, eggnog, buttermilk); 2–3 tsp (10–15 mL) of thickening powder to ½ cup (120 mL) of liquid
- Honey-like: thick enough to be eaten with a spoon, too thick for a straw, not able to independently hold its shape (eg, yogurt, tomato sauce, honey); 3–5 tsp (15–25 mL) of thickening powder to ½ cup (120 mL) of liquid
- Spoon-thick: pudding-like, must be eaten with a spoon (eg, thick milk pudding, thickened applesauce); 5–6 tsp (25–30 mL) of thickening powder to ½ cup (120 mL) of liquid
- Thickening agents are starch- or gum-based. Liquids thickened with modified starch continue to thicken or over-thicken over time. The thicker the product, the less consumed and the greater risk for dehydration, UTI, and fever.

Note: In patients with dementia, the evidence is conflicting whether nectar- or honey-like thickened liquids reduce the risk for aspiration pneumonia compared to chin-down posture alone.

GASTROESOPHAGEAL REFLUX DISEASE (GERD)
Evaluation and Assessment
Empiric tx is appropriate when hx is typical for uncomplicated GERD.
- Upper GI endoscopy (if symptoms are chronic or persist despite initial management, atypical presentation)
- Ambulatory pH testing: confirm diagnostic when symptoms persist despite normal endoscopy and to monitor adequacy of pH suppressive tx
- Esophageal manometry when normal upper GI endoscopy and esophageal dysphagia

Risk Factors
- Obesity
- Hiatal hernia
- Use of estrogen, nitroglycerin, tobacco

Symptoms Suggesting Complicated GERD and Need for Evaluation
- Dysphagia
- Bleeding
- Weight loss
- Anemia
- Choking, cough, shortness of breath, hoarseness
- Chest pain
- Pain with swallowing
- Vomiting

Management

Universal Lifestyle and Dietary Interventions

- Avoid alcohol and fatty foods
- Avoid lying down for 3 h after eating
- Avoid tight-fitting clothes
- Change diet (avoid pepper, spearmint, chocolate, spicy or acidic foods, carbonated beverages)
- Drink 6–8 oz water with all medications
- Chew gum or use oral lozenges to stimulate salivation, which neutralizes gastric acid
- Elevate head of the bed (6–8 in)
- Lose weight (if overweight)
- Stop drugs that may promote reflux or that can induce esophagitis
- Stop smoking

Other Interventions

- Acid suppression with a PPI or H₂ antagonist (**Table 58**)
- Antacids
- Consider surgery (not recommended for PPI nonresponders)

Management of Treatment-Naïve Patients with Mild, Intermittent Symptoms

- Universal lifestyle and dietary interventions
- As needed H2RA
- As needed antacids

Treatment with PPIs: reserve for severe or frequent symptoms or erosive esophagitis

- Initial tx: 8 wk with 1×/d PPI with morning meal
- Maintenance tx if symptoms remain after stopping or if complicated by erosive esophagitis or Barrett esophagus
- Long-term use is associated with bone loss and fractures, community-acquired pneumonia, hypomagnesemia, and vitamin B12 deficiency.
- Lowering dose, frequency, or both (eg, 2×/d to 1×/d or every other day) for a short period may help prevent symptom rebound.
- See deprescribing.org for an algorithm for deprescribing PPIs (open-pharmacy-research.ca/evidence-based-ppi-deprescribing-algorithm/)

Table 58. Pharmacologic Management of GERD[1,CW]

Medication	Initial Oral Dosage	Formulations (mg) (Metabolism, Excretion)
PPIs[2, BC]		
Dexlansoprazole *(Dexilant)*	30 mg/d × 4 wk	C: ER 30, 60 (L)
✓Esomeprazole magnesium▲ᴼᵀᶜ	20 mg/d × 4 wk	C: ER 20, 40; T: ER 20; Inj (L)
Esomeprazole strontium▲	24.6 mg/d × 4 wk	C: ER 24.65, 49.3 (L)
✓Lansoprazole▲ᴼᵀᶜ	15 mg/d × 8 wk	C: ER 15, 30; T: 15, 30 (L)
✓Omeprazole▲ᴼᵀᶜ	20 mg/d × 4–8 wk	C: ER 10, 20,[3] 40; T: ER 20 (L); susp 2 mg/mL
✓Pantoprazole▲	40 mg/d × 8 wk	T: enteric-coated 20, 40; Inj (L)
✓Rabeprazole	20 mg/d × 4–8 wk; 20 mg/d maintenance, if needed	T: ER enteric-coated 20▲; C: 5, 10 (L)

(cont.)

Table 58. Pharmacologic Management of GERD[1,CW] (cont.)

Medication	Initial Oral Dosage	Formulations (mg) (Metabolism, Excretion)
H₂ Antagonists (for less severe GERD)(Avoid[BC] in patients with delirium)		
Cimetidine▲OTC,4	400 q6h or 800 mg q12h; reduce if CrCl <50	S: 300 mg/5 mL; T: 200,[3] 300, 400, 800; Inj (K, L)
✓Famotidine▲OTC	20 mg q12h × 6 wk; reduce if CrCl <50	S: oral sus 40 mg/5 mL; T: 10,[3] 20, 40; Inj (K)
✓Nizatidine▲	150 mg q12h × 6–12 wk; reduce if CrCl <50	C:150, 300; sol 15 mg/mL (K)
Ranitidine▲OTC	150 mg q12h; reduce if CrCl <50	C: 150, 300; T: 75, 150, 300; Syr: 15 mg/mL; Inj (K, F)
Prokinetic Agents [5]		
✓Domperidone[6]	10 mg 15–30 min ac (3×/d)	T: 10 mg (L)
Metoclopramide▲ 7, BC	5–15 mg q6h, ac, and hs × 4–12 wk	S: 5 mg/5 mL; T: 5, 10; inj (K, F)

✓ = preferred for treating older adults   CrCl unit = mL/min/1.73 m²

[CW]Use lowest dose needed to achieve symptom control.

[1] PPIs more effective than H₂ antagonists for tx and maintenance

[2] Associated with osteopenia/osteoporosis; can inhibit CYP2C19 (omeprazole and esomeprazole strongest, pantoprazole weakest); prolonged exposure may increase risk of fractures, community-acquired pneumonia, *Clostridium difficile* diarrhea, hypomagnesemia; reduce vitamins C and B₁₂ concentrations, kidney disease and gastric atrophy. Monitor magnesium if taken long-term or with digoxin.

[3] OTC strength

[4] Inhibits CYP1A2, –2D6, –3A4

[5] No role in absence of gastroparesis.

[6] Available in the United States only through an Investigational New Drug application for compassionate use in patients refractory to other tx (fda.gov); domperidone is approved in Canada as a tx for upper GI motility disorders associated with gastritis and diabetic gastroparesis, and for prevention of GI symptoms associated with use of dopamine-agonist anti-Parkinson agents.

[7] Risk of EPS high in people aged >65[BC] unless for gastroparesis.

PEPTIC ULCER DISEASE
Causes
Helicobacter pylori is the major cause. NSAIDs are the 2nd most common cause.

Diagnosis of *H pylori*
• Endoscopy with biopsy (definitive)

Noninvasive testing
• Urea breath test   • Fecal antigen test
• Definitive diagnostic evaluation by endoscopy with biopsy
• Serology: poor specificity and sensitivity; cannot differentiate between past and current infection
• PPIs, antibiotics, and bismuth-containing products interfere with testing (except serology). Hold PPIs and bismuth for ≥1–2 wk and antibiotics ≥4 wk before testing.

Who Should be Tested and Treated if Tested Positive

- Long-term, low dose ASA (consider)
- Before initiating long-term NSAID
- Unexplained iron deficiency anemia
- Idiopathic thrombocytopenia purpura
- Review patient's chronic medications for drug interactions before selecting regimen; many potential drug interactions and ADRs.

Table 59. Pharmacotherapeutic Management of *H pylori* Infection

Regimen	Duration	Comments
Bismuth Quadruple Therapy		Consider if penicillin allergy or previous macrolide exposure
PPI[1] q12h[2] *plus* Bismuth subsalicylate 525 mg q6h *plus* Metronidazole 250–500 mg q6h *plus* Tetracycline 500 mg q6h *(Helidac)*	10–14 d	Preferred 1st-line regimen Components prescribed separately Bismuth subsalicylate T: 262; C: 262, 527 mg/15 mL
Concomitant Quadruple Therapy		
PPI[1] q12h[2] *plus* Clarithromycin[3,BC] 500 mg q12h Amoxicillin 1000 mg q12h Metronidazole 500 mg q12h	10–14 d	Preferred 1st-line regimen
Clarithromycin Triple Therapy		Preferred if no previous macrolide exposure
PPI[1] q12h[2] *plus* Clarithromycin[3,BC] 500 mg q12h *plus* Amoxicillin 1000 mg q12h	14 d	Example: *PrevPac* (includes lansoprazole 30 mg); Omeclamox-Pak (includes omeprazole) Preferred when clarithromycin resistance is <15% and patients with no previous macrolide exposure
PPI[1] q12h[2] *plus* Clarithromycin[3,BC] 500 mg q12h *plus* Metronidazole 500 mg q12h	14 d	Preferred if penicillin allergy or unable to tolerate bismuth quadruple tx Preferred when clarithromycin resistance is <15% and patients with no previous macrolide exposure

[1] Associated with osteopenia/osteoporosis; can inhibit CYP2C19 and -3A4; prolonged exposure may increase risk of fractures, community-acquired pneumonia, hospital-acquired *C difficile* diarrhea; reduce vitamins C and B_{12} concentrations

[2] Esomeprazole is dosed 40 mg q24h.

[3] Clarithromycin may increase the risk of cardiac AEs and death in patients with CAD. Clarithromycin is a strong inhibitor of CYP3A4 and P-glycoprotein.

Source: Adapted from Chey WD et al. *Am J Gastroenterol.* 2017;112:212–238.

Medications

Bismuth subsalicylate▲ (for complete information, see **Table 62**)

Antibiotics: (for complete information, see **Table 77**)

PPIs: See **Table 58**.

STRESS-ULCER PREVENTION IN HOSPITALIZED OLDER ADULTS

Risk Factors (in order of prevalence in older adults)

- Hx of GI ulceration or bleed in past year[†]
- Sepsis
- Multiple organ failure
- Hypotension/shock

- Mechanical ventilation for >48 h (major risk factor)[†]
- Kidney failure
- Major trauma, shock, or head injury
- Glasgow Coma Scale <10
- Coagulopathy (platelets <50,000/µL, INR >1.5, or PTT >2 × control) (major risk factor)[†]
- Burns over >35% of BSA[†]
- Hepatic failure/partial hepatectomy
- Intracranial HTN
- Spinal cord injury[†]
- Organ transplant
- Quadriplegia

[†]Prophylaxis indicated; also if ≥2 of the following are present: sepsis, ICU stay >1 wk, occult GI bleeding × ≥6 d or glucocorticosteroid ≥250 mg hydrocortisone equivalents

Prophylaxis

- PPIs preferred (**Table 58**)
- H$_2$ antagonists (**Table 58**)
- Sucralfate▲ 1 g q6h
- Antacids 30–60 mL q1–2h
- Enteral feedings

Key Points

- Prophylaxis has not been shown to reduce mortality.
- No one regimen has shown superior efficacy.
- Choice of regimen depends on access to and function of GI tract and presence of nasogastric suction.
- D/C H$_2$ antagonists, PPIs, and other tx for stress-ulcer prevention when risk factors are eliminated, before transfer to skilled nursing facility or discharge from hospital.

IRRITABLE BOWEL SYNDROME (IBS)

Signs and Symptoms

Symptoms should be present ≥12 wk.

Consistent with IBS:

- Abdominal pain
- Bloating
- Constipation
- Diarrhea

Not Consistent with IBS:

- Weight loss
- First onset after age 50
- Nocturnal diarrhea
- Family hx of cancer or inflammatory bowel disease
- Rectal bleeding or obstruction
- Laboratory abnormalities
- Presence of fecal parasites

Diagnosis (of exclusion)

Exclude ischemia, diverticulosis, colon cancer, inflammatory bowel disease by physical examination and testing (colonoscopy, CT scan, or small-bowel series). Do not repeat CT unless major changes in clinical findings.[CW]

Treatment

Mild to moderate symptoms: reserve medications as adjunct to lifestyle and dietary changes
- Reassurance; not life threatening; focus on relief of physical and emotional symptoms
- Dietary modification
  ○ Avoid foods that trigger symptoms or produce excess gas or bloating
  ○ Consider a trial of a lactose-free diet

- Behavioral interventions: hypnosis, biofeedback, psychotherapy have been shown to be more effective than placebo. Other interventions: increase physical activity, trials of gluten-free diet.

Fiber supplements (Table 60)
- Synthetic: polycarbophil▲
- Natural: psyllium▲

Antispasmodics (short-term use only; avoid unless no other alternatives)
- Dicyclomine▲BC [C: 10▲; T: 20▲; syr: 10 mg/5 mL; inj] 10–20 mg po q6h prn (L)
- Hyoscyamine (Anaspaz, Levsin, Levsin/SL, others [T (sl): 0.125, 0.15; T ER, C: 0.375; inj: 125 sol]) 0.125–0.25 mg po/sl q6–8h prn (L, K)

Antidiarrheals: may be helpful for diarrhea but not for global IBS symptoms, abdominal pain, or constipation
- Loperamide▲ [C, T: 2; sol 1 mg/5 mL] 4 mg × 1, then 2 mg after each loose bowel movement; max 16 mg/24 h
- Eluxadoline (Viberzi) [T: 75, 100 mg] 100 mg q12h; 75 mg q12h if 100 mg not tolerated due to anticholinergic activity

Antidepressants
- TCAs and SSRIs may be beneficial for patients with diarrhea or pain. See Depression, p 86, for dosing.

Laxative for IBS constipation
- Polyethylene glycol (PEG)
- Linaclotide (Linzess [C:145, 290 mcg]): 290 mcg q24h on empty stomach
- Lubiprostone (women only) 8 mg q12h

Serotonin antagonist
- Alosetron (Lotronex [T: 0.5, 1 mg]): serotonin 3 antagonist; tx of women with severe diarrhea-predominant IBS who have not responded to conventional tx (restricted distribution in the US); 0.5 mg po q12h × 4 wk, increase to 1 mg q12h × 4 wk, stop if no response (K, L)

CONSTIPATION

Definition
Frequency of bowel movements <2–3×/wk, straining at defecation, hard feces, or feeling of incomplete evacuation. Clinically, large amount of feces in rectum on digital examination and/or colonic fecal loading on abdominal radiograph.

Medications That Constipate
- Analgesics—opioids
- Antacids with aluminum or calcium
- Anticholinergic drugs
- Antidepressants, lithium
- Antihypertensives
- Antipsychotics
- Barium sulfate
- Bismuth
- CCBs
- Diuretics
- Iron

Conditions That Constipate
- Colon tumor or mechanical obstruction
- Dehydration
- Depression
- DM
- Hypercalcemia
- Hypokalemia
- Hypothyroidism
- Immobility
- Low intake of fiber

- Panhypopituitarism
- Parkinson disease
- Spinal cord injury
- Stroke
- Uremia

Management of Non–opioid-related Chronic Constipation

Step 1: Stop all constipating medications, when possible.

Step 2: Increase dietary fiber to 6–25 g/d, increase fluid intake to ≥1500 mL/d, and increase physical activity; or add bulk laxative (**Table 60**), provided fluid intake is ≥1500 mL/d. If fiber exacerbates symptoms or is not tolerated, or patient has limited mobility, go to Step 3.

Step 3: Add an osmotic (eg, 70% sorbitol sol, polyethylene glycol *[MiraLAX]*).

Step 4: Add stimulant laxative (eg, senna, bisacodyl), 2–3×/wk. (Alternative: saline laxative, but avoid if CrCl <30 mL/min/1.73 m^2.)

Step 5: Use tap water enema or saline enema 2×/wk.

Step 6: Use oil-retention enema for refractory constipation.

Management of Opioid-induced Constipation

Avoid bulk-forming laxatives if insufficient oral intake.

Step 1: Stimulants (eg, bisacodyl, senna)

Step 2: Lubiprostone, linaclotide, or plecanatide if idiopathic constipation

Alvimopan, methylnaltrexone, naldemedine, or naloxegol if OIC

Medication	Onset of Action	Starting Dosage	Site and Mechanism of Action
Table 60. Medications That May Relieve Constipation			
Bulk laxatives—not useful in managing opioid-induced constipation			
Methylcellulose[▲OTC]	12–24 h (up to 72 h)	2–4 caplets or 1 heaping tbsp with 8 oz water q8–24h	Small and large intestine; holds water in feces; mechanical distention
Psyllium[▲OTC,1]	12–24 h (up to 72 h)	1–2 capsules, pk, or tsp with 8 oz water or juice q8–24h	Small and large intestine; holds water in feces; mechanical distention
Polycarbophil[▲1]	12–24 h (up to 72 h)	1250 mg q6–24h	Small and large intestine; holds water in feces; mechanical distention
Wheat dextrin[OTC]	24–28 h		Small and large intestine; holds water in feces; mechanical distention
Chronic secretagogues			
Lubiprostone (*Amitiza*)	24–28 h	24 mcg q12h with food C: 8, 24 mcg	Enhances chloride-ion intestinal fluid secretion; does not affect serum Na+ or K+ concentrations. For idiopathic chronic constipation.
Linaclotide (*Linzess*)		Chronic idiopathic constipation: 145 mcg q24h without food IBS-C: 290 mg/24h without food C: 145, 290 mcg	Guanylate cyclase-C agonist, which increases intracellular cGMP, which stimulates intraluminal secretion of chloride and bicarbonate increasing intestinal fluid and transit
Plecanatide (*Trulance*)	NA	T: 3 mg q24h for chronic idiopathic constipation; F	

(cont.)

Table 60. Medications That May Relieve Constipation (cont.)

Medication	Onset of Action	Starting Dosage	Site and Mechanism of Action
Opioid antagonists			
Alvimopan *(Entereg)*	NA	Initial: 12 mg po 30 min to 5 h before surgery Maintenance: 12 mg po q12h the day after surgery × 7 d max C: 12 mg	Hospital use only; for accelerating time to recovery after partial large- or small-bowel resection with primary anastomosis; contraindicated if >7 consecutive d of tx opioids (L, K, F)
Methylnaltrexone *(Relistor)*	30–60 min	SC: Weight-based dosing: <38 kg: 0.15 mg/kg 38 to <62 kg: 8 mg 62–114 kg: 12 mg >114 kg: 0.15 mg/kg (all SC q48h); if CrCl <30, decrease dosage 50% OIC with chronic noncancer pain: po: 450 mg 1×/d If CrCl <60, 150 mg 1×/d T: 150 mg; SC: 8 mg/0.4 mL, 12 mg/0.6 mL	Peripheral-acting opioid antagonist for the tx of OIC in palliative-care patients who have not responded to conventional laxatives (L, K, F)
Naloxegol *(Movantik)*		25 mg qam on an empty stomach; 12.5 mg qam initially if CrCl <60; 12.5 qam if taking mild or moderate CYP3A4 inhibitor. Avoid if taking strong CYP3A4 inhibitor T: 12.5, 25 mg	μ-opioid receptor antagonist. Composed of naloxone conjugated with a polyethylene glycol polymer, limits its ability to cross the blood-brain barrier. Functions peripherally in tissues such as the GI tract at recommended doses. (L, F, K)
Naldemedine *(Symproic)*		T: 0.2 mg 1×/d Avoid if taking a strong CYP3A4 inducer	Peripheral-acting opioid antagonist for the tx of OIC in adults with chronic noncancer pain
Osmotic laxatives			
Lactulose▲	24–48 h	10–20 g (15–30 mL) q12–24h S: 10 g/15 mL	Colon; osmotic effect
Polyethylene glycol▲OTC	48–96 h	17 g pwd q24h (~1 tbsp) dissolved in 8 oz water	GI tract; osmotic effect
Sorbitol 70%▲OTC	24–48 h	15–30 mL q12–24h; max 150 mL/d	Colon; delivers osmotically active molecules to colon
Glycerin suppOTC	15–30 min		Colon; local irritation; hyperosmotic
Sodium, potassium, and magnesium sulfate *(Suprep bowel prep kit)*	24 h		Small and large intestine; hyperosmotic

(cont.)

Table 60. Medications That May Relieve Constipation (cont.)

Medication	Onset of Action	Starting Dosage	Site and Mechanism of Action
Saline laxatives			
Magnesium citrate▲OTC	30 min–3 h	120–240 mL × 1; 10 oz q24h or 5 oz q12h followed by 8 oz water × ≤5 d	Small and large intestine; attracts, retains water in intestinal lumen; potential hypermagnesemia in patients with renal insufficiency or a low-salt diet
Magnesium hydroxide▲OTC	30 min–3 h	30 mL q12–24h 311-mg tab (130 mg magnesium); 400, 800 mg/5 mL sus	Osmotic effect and increased peristalsis in colon; potential hypermagnesemia in patients with renal insufficiency
Sodium phosphate/ biphosphate emollient enema▲OTC	2–15 min	14.5-oz enema × 1 per 24 h	Colon; osmotic effect; potential hypermagnesemia in patients with renal insufficiency
Stimulant laxatives			
Bisacodyl tablet▲OTC	6–10 h	5–15 mg × 1	Colon; increases peristalsis
Bisacodyl suppository▲OTC	15 min–1 h	10 mg × 1	Colon; increases peristalsis
Senna▲OTC	6–10 h	1–2 tabs or 1 tsp qhs	Colon; direct action on intestine; stimulates myenteric plexus; alters water and electrolyte secretion
Surfactant laxative (fecal softener)			
Docusate▲OTC	24–72 h	100 mg q12–24h	Small and large intestine; detergent activity; facilitates admixture of fat and water to soften feces (effectiveness questionable); does not increase frequency of bowel movements

CrCl unit = mL/min/1.73 m^2

[1] Psyllium caplets and packets contain ≥3 g dietary fiber and 2–3 g soluble fiber each. A teaspoonful contains ~3.8 g dietary fiber and 3 g soluble fiber.

NAUSEA AND VOMITING

Causes

- CNS disorders (eg, motion sickness, intracranial lesions)
- Drugs (eg, chemotherapy, NSAIDs, opioid analgesics, antibiotics, digoxin)
- GI disorders (eg, mechanical obstruction; inflammation of stomach, intestine, acute pancreatitis, or gallbladder; pseudo-obstruction; motility disorders; dyspepsia; gastroparesis)
- Infections (eg, viral or bacterial gastroenteritis, hepatitis, otitis, meningitis)
- Metabolic conditions (eg, uremia, acidosis, hyperparathyroidism, adrenal insufficiency)
- Psychiatric disorders

Evaluation

- If patient is not seriously ill or dehydrated, can probably wait 24–48 h to see if symptoms resolve spontaneously.
- If patient is seriously ill, dehydrated, or has other signs of acute illness, hospitalize for further evaluation.
- If symptoms persist, evaluate on the basis of the most likely causes.

Pharmacologic Management

- If analgesic drug is suspected, decrease dosage, consider adding antiemetic until tolerance develops, or change to a different analgesic drug.
- Drugs that are useful in the management of non–chemotherapy induced nausea and vomiting are listed in **Table 61**.

Table 61. Antiemetic Therapy		
Class/Site of Action	**Dosage (Metabolism)**	**Formulation**
Dopamine antagonists/CTZ vomiting center		
Haloperidol▲BC	IM, po: 0.5–1 mg q6h (L, K)	p 304
Metoclopramide▲BC	PONV: 5–10 mg IM, IV near the end of surgery Chemotherapy (IV): 1–2 mg/kg 30 min before and q2–4h or q4–6h (K)	T: 5, 10 S: 5 mg/mL, 10 mg/mL Inj: 5 mg/mL
Prochlorperazine▲BC	IM, po: 5–10 mg q6–8 h, usual max 40 mg/d IV: 2.5–10 mg, max 10 mg/dose or 40 mg/d; may repeat q3–4h prn (L)	T: 5, 10 mg Inj: 5 mg/mL Sp: 25
Serotonin (5-HT3) antagonists/CTZ, gut		
✓Ondansetron▲	PONV: ODT 8 mg po 1 h before anesthesia IM, IV: 4 mg immediately before end of anesthesia; repeat if needed (L) Radiation tx: 8 mg po 1–2 h before, then 8 mg po q8h × 1–2 d	T: 4, 8, 24 mg ODT: 4, 8 mg S: 4 mg/5 mL Inj: 2 mg/mL
Granisetron	PONV: 0.35–3 mg IV before end of anesthesia or anesthesia reversal Chemotherapy: 2 mg/d po (L, K) Radiation tx: 2 mg po 1 h before radiation tx	T:1 mg▲ S: 2 mg/10 mL▲ Inj: 1 mg/mL▲ Pch: 3.1 mg/24 h
Dolasetron *(Anzemet)*	PONV: 12.5 mg IV 15 min before stopping anesthesia; repeat as soon as nausea and vomiting are present (L)	T: 50, 100 mg Inj: 20 mg/mL
Antimuscarinic/H1 antagonist/vestibular apparatus^BC		
Dimenhydrinate▲OTC,1	IM, IV, po: 50–100 mg q4–6h; max 400 mg/d (L) Motion sickness: 50–100 mg q4–6h; max 400 mg/d	T, ChT: 50 mg Inj: 50 mg/mL
Meclizine▲OTC,1	Motion sickness: 12.5–50 mg 1 h before travel, repeat dose q24h if needed Vertigo: 25–100 mg/d in divided doses (L)	T: 12.5, 25 mg ChT: 25 mg
Scopolamine▲1	Motion sickness: apply 1 pch behind ear ≥4 h before travel/exposure; change q3d (L)	Pch: 1.5 mg

✓ = preferred for treating older adults

[1] Avoid unless no other alternatives.^BC

CTZ = chemoreceptor trigger zone; ODT = ondansetron disintegrating tablets; PONV = postoperative nausea and vomiting. All have potential CNS toxicity. Metoclopramide associated with EPS and TD.

DIARRHEA
Definition
- Passage of loose or watery stools ≥3× in 24 h
- Acute: ≤14 d
- Persistent: >14 d and <30 d
- Chronic: >30 d

Causes
- Drugs (eg, antibiotics [**Table 77** and below], laxatives, colchicine, metformin, cholinesterase inhibitors)
- Fecal impaction
- GI disorders (eg, IBS, malabsorption, inflammatory bowel disease)
- Infections (eg, viral, bacterial, parasitic)
- Lactose intolerance

Evaluation
- Obtain a stool culture from patients who are at high risk for complications (eg, aged ≥70, inflammatory bowel disease, or CVD exacerbated by hypovolemia)
- If patient is not seriously ill or dehydrated and there is no blood in the feces, can probably wait 48 h to see if symptoms resolve spontaneously.
- If patient is seriously ill, dehydrated, or has other signs of acute illness, hospitalize for further evaluation.
- If diarrhea persists, evaluate on the basis of the most likely causes.

Pharmacologic Management
Drugs that are useful in the management of diarrhea are listed in **Table 62**.

Probiotics containing *Saccharomyces boulardii* may be effective in decreasing the duration of *C difficile* infection.

Table 62. Antidiarrheals		
Drug	**Dosage (Metabolism)**	**Formulations**
✓ Bismuth subsalicylate▲OTC	2 tabs or 30 mL q30–60 min prn up to 8 doses/24 h (L, K) Duration: diarrhea/dyspepsia 48 h	S: 262 mg/15 mL, 525 mg/15 mL ChT: 262
Diphenoxylate with atropineBC▲OTC,1	15–20 mg/d of diphenoxylate in 3–4 divided doses; maintenance 5–15 mg/d in 2–3 divided doses (L) Duration: acute symptoms 48 h; chronic 10 d	S: oral, diphenoxylate hydrochloride 2.5 mg + atropine sulfate 0.025 mg/5 mL T: diphenoxylate hydrochloride 2.5 mg + atropine sulfate 0.025 mg
✓ Loperamide▲OTC	Initial: 4 mg followed by 2 mg after each loose bowel movement, up to 16 mg/d (L) Duration: acute use 48 h	Caplet: 2; C: 2; T: 2; S: oral, 1 mg/5 mL, 1 mg/1.75 mL
Rifaximin *(Xifaxan)*	Traveler's diarrhea: 200 mg 3×/d × 3 d IBS diarrhea: 550 mg q8h × 14 d; repeat × 2 if needed	T: 200, 550

✓ = preferred for treating older adults

[1] Anticholinergic, potential CNS toxicity

ANTIBIOTIC-ASSOCIATED DIARRHEA (AAD)

Antibiotic-associated pseudomembranous colitis (AAPMC)

Definition

A specific form of *C difficile* pseudomembranous colitis

Risk Factors

- Almost any oral or parenteral antibiotic and several antineoplastic agents, including cyclophosphamide, doxorubicin, fluorouracil, methotrexate
- Advanced age
- Duration of hospitalization
- PPI

Prevention

The use of probiotic products to prevent primary infection remains controversial. Two systematic reviews and meta-analyses found that they significantly reduce the risk of AAD and *C difficile* diarrhea. Since their publication, the largest trial, conducted in older inpatients, found the combination lactobacilli and bifidobacteria did not reduce the risk of AAD or *C difficile* diarrhea. The Infectious Diseases Society of America (IDSA)/ Society for Healthcare Epidemiology of America (SHEA) guidance cites insufficient data to recommend probiotics to prevent *C difficile*. Probiotics should be used with caution by immunocompromised patients.

Presentation

- Abdominal pain, cramping
- Dehydration
- Diarrhea (can be bloody)
- Fecal leukocytes
- Fever (100–105°F)
- Hypoalbuminemia
- Hypovolemia
- Leukocytosis

Symptoms appear a few days after starting to 10 wk after discontinuing the offending agent.

Evaluation, Empiric Management, and Diagnosis

- D/C unnecessary antibiotics, and agents that can slow gastric motility, such as opioids and antidiarrheal agents.
- Symptomatic patients who have had ≥3 liquid or soft stools (taking the shape of the container) in 24 h who have not taken a laxative in the past 48 h should be tested for *C difficile*.
- Test for *C difficile* with nucleic acid amplification tests (NAAT) alone or plus *C difficile* toxin, glutamate dehydrogenase (GDH) plus *C difficile* toxin, GDH plus *C difficile* toxin arbitrated by NAAT, or NAAT + *C difficile* toxin. NAAT is the most sensitive test.
- Place patient in contact isolation and observe infection control procedures. Hand washing is crucial and must be done with soap and water to remove spores. Hand sanitizers do not kill or remove spores.
- Provide adequate fluid and electrolyte replacement.
- Consider starting empiric tx when a delay in lab confirmation is anticipated or if fulminant infection (**Table 63** for dosing).
- Repeated testing within 7 d during the same episode of diarrhea is not recommended.
- Testing for a cure should not be performed.

Table 63. Treatment of Suspected or Confirmed *Clostridium difficile* Infection

Clinical Definition	Supportive Clinical Data	Treatment
Toxin negative on 2 specimens or NAAT negative		D/C contact isolation D/C metronidazole/vancomycin Begin antidiarrheal agent Evaluate other causes
Initial episode, mild or moderate	Leukocytosis (WBC ≤15,000 cells/µL), serum Cr <1.5× premorbid level	Vancomycin▲ 125 mg po q6h × 10–14 d *or* Fidaxomicin[1] 200 mg po q12h × 10 d Alternate: Metronidazole▲ 500 mg po q8h × 10 d
Initial episode, severe	Leukocytosis (WBC >15,000 cells/µL), which signifies colonic inflammation; serum Cr ≥1.5× premorbid level, which signifies dehydration	Vancomycin▲ 125 mg po q6h × 10 d or Fidaxomicin[1] 200 mg po q12h × 10 d Oral vancomycin is available as a cap (125, 250) or by reconstituting the pwd for injection for oral administration.
Initial episode, fulminant	Hypotension or shock, ileus, megacolon in the absence of abdominal distention	Vancomycin 500 mg po or nasogastric tube q6h plus metronidazole▲ IV 500 mg q8h; if complete ileus or toxic megacolon, add vancomycin 500 mg/500 mL pr is an option.
First recurrence		If metronidazole is used to treat initial episode: Vancomycin▲ 125 mg q6h po × 10 d if *or* If standard tx used initially: Vancomycin taper and pulsed (eg, 125 mg q6h po × 10–14 d, q12h × 7 d, q24h × 7 d, then q2–3d × 2–8 wk) *or* [1]Fidaxomicin 200 mg q12h po × 10 d, if vancomycin used initially
Second or subsequent recurrence		Vancomycin in a tapered and/or pulsed regimen *or* Vancomycin▲ 125 mg q6h po × 10 d followed by rifaximin 400 mg q8h po × 20 d *or* [1]Fidaxomicin 200 mg q12h po × 10 d *or* Fecal microbiota transplant

Source: Adapted from McDonald LC et al. *Clin Infect Dis* 2018;66:e1−e48.

[1] Fidaxomicin *(Dificid)* [T: 200 mg; 92% F, minimal systemic absorption]. Clinical trials did not include patients with life-threatening or fulminant *C difficile* infection, toxic megacolon, or with >1 *C difficile* infection in the previous 3 mo.

- Continue contact precautions for ≥48 h after diarrhea has resolved.
- Fecal microbiota transplant (FMT) is a promising alternative tx to antibiotics. It is not commercially available and meant for patients with recurrent infection after multiple courses of antibiotics.

Prevention of Recurrence

- Bezlotoxumab *(Zinplava)*, a human monoclonal antibody that binds to *C difficile* toxin B, indicated to reduce recurrence of *C difficile* infection (CDI) in patients aged ≥18 y who are receiving antibacterial drug tx of CDI and are at a high risk for CDI recurrence.

- Bezlotoxumab is not an antibacterial drug and is not indicated for the tx of CDI and should only be used in conjunction with antibacterial drug tx of CDI.
- Dose: single 10 mg/kg infusion over 60 min. Inj: 1000 mg/40 mL

HEMORRHOIDS

Contributing Factors

- Constipation
- Prolonged straining
- Exercise
- Gravity
- Low-fiber diet
- Pregnancy
- Increased intraabdominal pressure
- Irregular bowel habits
- Age

Classification

- External: distal to the dentate line and painful if thrombotic, itchy
- Internal: proximal to the dentate line without sensitivity to pain, touch, or temperature; mucous discharge; feeling of incomplete evacuation
  ○ *Grade*
    - First-degree: no prolapse, may bleed after defecation, only seen via anoscope
    - Second-degree: prolapse outside anal canal with defecation and retract spontaneously
    - Third-degree: prolapse and require manual reduction
    - Fourth-degree: prolapsed, nonreducible

Treatment

Diet and Lifestyle Changes

- High-fiber diet (20–35 g/d) or psyllium, methylcellulose, or calcium polycarbophil
- Increased fluid intake
- Avoid prolonged time on commode

Topical Treatments

- Sitz baths (40° C)
- Non–steroid-containing products: applied 4×/d
- Light shark liver oil plus phenylephrine oint[OTC] (*Preparation H*)
- Dibucaine 1% oint[OTC] (*Nupercainal*)
- Pramoxifen 1%[OTC] foam, gel (eg, *Proctofoam, PrameGel*)
- Witch hazel[OTC] liq, pads
- Steroid-containing products
- Light shark liver oil plus phenylephrine and hydrocortisone oint[OTC] (*Preparation H* [anti-itch formula])
- Hydrocortisone 1%[OTC] crm, enema
- Lidocaine 2% and hydrocortisone 2% crm (*AnaMantle HC, Ana-Lex*); rectal gel (*LidaMantle*)

Office-based Procedures

- Rubber band ligation: for first-, second-, or third-degree internal hemorrhoids
  ○ Contraindicated in patients who are anticoagulated
  ○ D/C antiplatelet drugs (including ASA) for 5–7 d before and after banding
- Sclerotherapy
- Bipolar diathermy
- Infrared photocoagulation

DEFINITION

The most common sensory impairment in old age; presbycusis affects 30–47% of the population older than 65. To quantify hearing ability, the necessary intensity (decibel = dB) and frequency (Hertz) of the perceived pure-tone signal must be described.

Importance: Hearing impairment is strongly correlated with depression, decreased quality of life, poorer memory and executive dysfunction, and incident dementia.

EVALUATION

Screening and Evaluation

- Note problems during conversation.
- Ask the question: Do you feel you have hearing loss? A "yes" response should prompt referral to audiology.
- Test with handheld audioscope or whisper test. Refer patients who screen positive for audiologic evaluation.
- Whisper test: stand behind patient at arm's length from ear, cover untested ear, fully exhale, whisper a combination of 3 numbers and letters (eg, 6-K-2) and ask patient to repeat the set; if patient unable to repeat all 3, whisper a 2nd set. Inability to repeat at least 3 of 6 is positive for impairment.

Audiometry

- Documents the dB loss across frequencies
- Determines the pattern of loss (see Classification, below)
- Determines if loss is unilateral or bilateral and assesses speech recognition.

CLASSIFICATION

See **Table 64**. Mixed hearing disorders are quite common, particularly involving features of age-related presbycusis and conductive loss. Central auditory processing disorders become clinically important when superimposed on other ear pathology.

Table 64. Classification of Hearing Disorders		
	Sensorineural Hearing Loss	**Conductive Hearing Loss**	**Central Auditory Processing Disorder**
Pathologic process	Cochlear or retrocochlear (cranial nerve VIII) pathology	Impaired transmission to inner ear from external or middle ear pathology	CNS change interfering with ability to discriminate speech, particularly when background noise is present
Weber test findings	Lateralizes away from impaired ear	Lateralizes toward impaired ear	Normal
Rinne test findings	Normal	Abnormal in impaired ear	Normal
Audiogram/ Audiometry findings	Air and bone-conduction thresholds equal	Air conduction thresholds greater than bone-conduction thresholds	Normal for pure-tone audiometry; impaired for speech discrimination

(cont.)

Table 64. Classification of Hearing Disorders (cont.)		
	Sensorineural Hearing Loss	**Conductive Hearing Loss**	**Central Auditory Processing Disorder**

	Sensorineural Hearing Loss	Conductive Hearing Loss	Central Auditory Processing Disorder
Common causes	Age-related presbycusis (high-frequency loss, problems with speech discrimination); most common cause	Cerumen impaction	Dementia
		Otosclerosis	Stroke
		RA	Presbycusis
		Paget disease	Possibly normal aging
	Excessive noise exposure	Psoriasis	
	Acoustic neuroma	Osteoma	
	Ménière disease (both high- and low-frequency loss)	Exostosis	
	Ototoxic drugs	Squamous cell cancer	

MANAGEMENT
Remove Ear Wax

Ear wax causes conductive loss and further reduces hearing. Soft wax can be flushed with a syringe, removed with a cerumen scoop, or suctioned. Dry wax should be softened before removal by doing the following:

Fill ear canal with 5–10 gtt water and cover with cotton q12h × ≥4 d. Liquid must stay in contact with ear for ≥15 min. Hearing may worsen as cerumen expands. Water is as effective as commercial preparations (eg, *Debrox, Cerumenex, Colace)*. Use of any of the commercial preparations for >4 d may cause ear irritation.

Table 65. Rehabilitation of Hearing Loss, by Level of Loss		
Level of Loss (dB)	**Difficulty Understanding**	**Need for Hearing Technology**
16–25 (slight)	None	None
26–40 (mild)	Normal speech	Hearing aid or MEI in specific situations
41–55 (moderate)	Loud speech	Hearing aid or MEI in many situations
56–69 (moderately severe)	Anything but amplified speech	Hearing aid, MEI, or EAS for all communication
70–90 (severe)	Even amplified speech	EAS or cochlear implant
≥91 (profound)	Even amplified speech	Cochlear implant and/or speech-reading, aural rehabilitation, sign language

EAS = electric acoustic stimulation; MEI = middle ear implant.

Hearing Technology

Hearing Aids: Digital devices enhance select frequencies for each ear.
- Amplification in both ears (binaural) provides best speech understanding; unilateral aid may be appropriate if hearing loss is asymmetrical, if hearing-aid care is challenging, or if cost is a factor.
- Features that enhance sound and speech quality include directional microphones, open-fit hearing aids, ear-to-ear wireless coordination, and in the canal extended-wear aids *(Lyric).*
- The mean cost of 2 hearing aids in the US is about $4700. Retailers such as Walmart and Costco sell brands at roughly half the price.

Personal Sound Amplification Products (PSAPs/OTC Hearing Aids): Some of these OTC devices are technologically comparable to hearing aids and may be suitable for persons with mild to moderate hearing loss at much lower cost (under $400/ear).

While data are presently limited, the following PSAPs have some evidence for accuracy in improving speech recognition to within 2% of what is achieved with a commonly sold hearing aid:

- Sound World Solutions CS50+ soundworldsolutions.com/store/personal-sound-amplifiers-psa/cs50
- Etymotic Bean https://www.etymotic.com/consumer/personal-sound-amplifiers/bean-qsa.html
- CAUTION: Very low-cost devices (under $50) amplify sound to a level that may cause injury to hearing.

These devices are not self-contained and all require interface with a computer, smart phone, tablet, or proprietary interface for fine-tuning or a hearing test (at an interface or by a hearing professional). They are sold in some audiology offices.

Cochlear Implants: Bypass the middle ear, directly innervate the cochlear nerve. Results after age 65 are comparable to those in younger people. Benefits are greater with bilateral implants. Early failure rate <1%, in the hands of experienced surgeons. Late complications of implants include vestibular problems (3.9%), device failure (3.4%), and taste problems (2.8%). Patient selection is important.

Selection criteria for cochlear implants:
- Moderate to profound bilateral sensorineural hearing loss
- **and** ≤60% sentence recognition in best aided ear
  or unilateral deafness with or without severe ipsilateral tinnitus
- **and** benefit from aids less than that expected from implant
- **and** no external or middle ear pathology causing hearing loss
- **and** no medical contraindication to general anesthesia
- **and** no contraindication to surgical placement of device
- **and** family support, motivation, appropriate expectations

Electric Acoustic Stimulation: Use of a cochlear implant and hearing aid in the same ear and also in the nonimplanted ear. Using both maximizes the range of sounds audible in both ears, aids in localization of sound, and speech perception in both noise and reverberation. The hearing aid amplifies residual hearing at low frequencies, while the cochlear implant provides electric stimulation to the high frequencies. Users still perform well when using the implant without the hearing aid.

Middle Ear Implants: A fully implantable ossicular stimulator; all components (including battery) are implanted under the skin; for adults who cannot wear hearing aids for medical (eg, collapsed ear canal, inability to handle device) or personal (ie, cosmetic) reasons. FDA-approved implant for severe hearing loss *(Esteem)* has limited availability, is expensive, and the reoperation rate exceeds 20%. Currently reserved for patients with conductive and mixed hearing losses who may have few, if any, other options.

Bone-Anchored Hearing Aids: *BAHA* is small titanium implant inserted into the skull where it osteointegrates. A small portion of the implant protrudes through the skin to form a snap attachment point for a removable bone-conduction hearing aid. The device bypasses the external canal and middle ear. *Potential indications:* Congenital atresia of the ear canal, chronic infection of the middle or outer ear, allergic reactions to standard hearing aids, single-sided deafness (eg, after removal of an acoustic neuroma or from a viral or vascular insult). The limited evidence on benefits is through case series reports.

Hearing Assistive Technology

Each patient should be asked if his or her needs are being met. If the prescribed hearing aids and implants do not fully meet these needs, additional technologies may be indicated. These technologies are referred to as Hearing Assistive Technology (HAT) and are available at various price points.

HAT benefit people at all levels of hearing, from normal to profound impairment. Even patients with hearing aids or cochlear implants who have difficulty hearing in some or many situations will benefit.

People have 4 basic reception/communication needs: at home, at work, in the community, and in the world at large. These include:

- Face-to-face communication (eg, restaurants)
- Electronic media (TV, radio, movie theater, concerts)
- Telephone—both land lines and cell phones
- Warning sounds (doorbells, telephone, smoke alarm)

Face-to-Face Communication, Media, Telephone

- *Pocketalker*. A personal amplifier with microphone and earphones, this device is inexpensive and useful for talking to patients with hearing loss who do not yet have hearing aids or can be used as a hearing aid for those who are not ready for hearing aids or who have situational hearing difficulties.
- Hardwired body-style amplifiers and wireless technologies (loop, FM, infrared, and digital systems).The same devices also can be used for reception of media.
- Various auditory and visual devices are also available to facilitate telecommunication (amplifiers, FaceTime, Skype, etc).

Devices for Safety

- Alert patients to a door knock, a doorbell, a smoke alarm, or an appliance signal.
- Wireless doorbell systems allow the chimes to be placed on each floor.
- *Ring Video Doorbell*. When visitors press the doorbell or motion sensors are activated, the owner uses an app to view and speak to the visitor remotely; allows for speech-reading.
- Smoke alarm systems will shake a bed when they go off.

Apps

In addition, apps are available to convert a smart phone and a headset into a personal listening device without the use of a hearing aid.

- Jacoti *ListenApp*®, FDA registered for mild to moderate hearing loss; based on an audiogram; left and/or right programming; settings for natural sound, speech, music, and movies.
- *HearYouNow* adjusts volume per ear in 3 bands (high, medium, low frequencies); its focus feature allows honing in on a conversation.
- Other amplifier apps: *i-Hear, EarMachine, Hearing Aid*.

Tips for Communication with People with Hearing Difficulties

- Ask the person how best to communicate
- Stand or sit 2–3 ft away
- Have the person's attention
- Have the person seated in front of a wall, which helps reflect sound
- Speak toward the better ear
- Use lower-pitched voice
- Speak slowly and distinctly; don't shout and don't exaggerate mouth movements

- Rephrase rather than repeat
- Pause at the end of phrases or ideas
- Ask the person to repeat what was heard

Tips for Approaches to Patients Resistant to Acquiring/Using Hearing Aids

Set appropriate expectations, inform the patient, support and assist the patient during the period of adjustment.

- Hearing aids do not produce normal hearing; they are aids to hearing
- New hearing aids usually need adjustments; expect to see the audiologist a few times. A resource to empower patients to work with their audiologist efficiently and to achieve the best fitting can be found at hearingloss.org/wp-content/uploads/HLM_JulAug2015_ Compton-Conley.pdf?pdf=2015-hlm-jacconley.
- Report problems: hearing or understanding speech in specific situations (eg, noisy environments); difficulty operating the hearing aid; aid-associated discomfort
- Inquire how the patient feels about hearing-aid appearance
- Recommend group audiologic visits of newly fitted patients, if available
- Include caregivers in the process of fitting hearing aids
- Regularly examine ears for cerumen or other pathology

Tips for Treating Hearing Loss in Older Adults with Frailty or Multiple Morbidities

- Include hearing evaluation in team-based geriatric assessment
- Assess, and when possible, improve visual function
- Assess and treat physical, cognitive, and affective disorders
- For patients with hearing aids and problems with manual dexterity, consider easier-to-use hearing-aid models (eg, behind-the-ear or in-the-ear types)
- For hearing-impaired patients with advanced cognitive deficits
  ○ Prevent loss of hearing aid by attaching a metal loop to its body and tying a thin nylon line through the loop, fasten the other end of the line to the patient's clothing
  ○ Educate caregivers on proper use of hearing aids
  ○ Consider use of personal amplifier *(Pocketalker)* or other assistive listening device if patient is unable to use a hearing aid
- Assess for hearing deficits and correct them in patients presenting with geriatric syndromes

TINNITUS
Definition

The perception of sound in the absence of external acoustic stimulus. The patient's description of the sound helps in diagnosis of the cause. Some tinnitus is normal, typically last <5 min, <1×/wk. Pathologic tinnitus last >5 min, >weekly. Prevalence is 30% after age 55 y.

Evaluation

- Examine ear canals for cerumen, otitis externa or interna; treat and reassess.
- Check medications that cause or exacerbate tinnitus, eg, NSAIDs, ASA, antibiotics (especially erythromycin), loop diuretics (especially furosemide), chemotherapy, quinine.
- Assess the severity of tinnitus using the Tinnitus Handicap Inventory https://www.ata.org/ sites/default/files/Tinnitus_Handicap_Inventory.pdf
- Unless initial evaluation shows the likely cause to be presbycusis or a myofascial disorder, refer to otolaryngology.
- If the examiner can hear the tinnitus (objective tinnitus), refer the patient to otolaryngology.

Some of the More Common Causes of Tinnitus

- **Originating from the auditory system:** presbycusis, otosclerosis, vestibular schwannoma, Chiari malformations
- **Myofascial disorders:** temporomandibular joint (TMJ) dysfunction, whiplash injuries, craniocervical disease
- **Vascular disorders:** arterial bruits, arteriovenous shunts, paraganglioma, venous hums, high cardiac output states
- **Neurologic disorders:** tensor tympani and/or stapedius muscle spasm, palatal muscles myoclonus
- **Patulous eustachian tube**

Treatment

- The 1st and often the only thing needed when tinnitus has a benign cause is patient education on the natural hx (may remit) and coping strategies.
- Also treat the underlying disorder (eg, hearing aids for hearing impairment)
- If the patient still has tinnitus that produces distress, symptom-oriented tx includes:
  - CBT: improves quality of life, reduces depression, and has the best evidence supporting its use.
  - Acoustic stimulation at levels that masks tinnitus; combination hearing aids with sound generators may be superior to aids alone for those with significant hearing loss.
  - Cochlear implants for those with moderate or greater sensorineural hearing loss may improve tinnitus in up to 75% of patients.

ANEMIA

Significance

Lower hemoglobin and mild anemia is associated with more severe disability, poorer mobility and cognition, frailty, and falls.

Evaluation

- Hematopoietic reserve capacity declines with age (eg, slower return of Hb to normal after phlebotomy); don't perform serial blood counts in clinically stable patients.[CW]
- Evaluate people aged >65 when Hb <13 g/dL in men and <12 g/dL in women.
- Evaluate if Hb falls >1 g/dL in 1 y.
- Physical examination and laboratory tests: BUN, Cr, ESR, CRP.
- Check WBC and peripheral blood smear; pursue suspected causes as appropriate.
- Combined deficiencies are common in older adults; reasonable to check B_{12}, folate, and iron in all cases. MCV is not reliable in combined deficiency states.
- Check reticulocyte count and reticulocyte index.
  ∘ Reticulocyte count or index high: suspect blood loss or hemolytic anemia, p 156.
  ∘ Reticulocyte count or index normal or low: suggests deficiency (B12, folate [**Figure 6**], or iron [**Figure 7**]).

Figure 6. Evaluation of Hypoproliferative Anemia Due to Possible B12 or Folate Deficiency

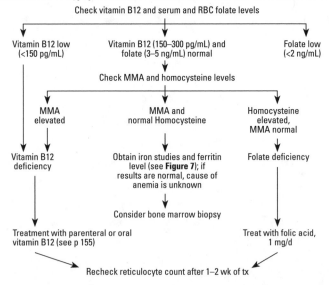

Source: Adapted from Balducci L. *J Amer Geriatr Soc* 2003; 51(3 Suppl):S2–9. Reprinted with permission.

Figure 7. Evaluation of Possible Iron Deficiency Anemia

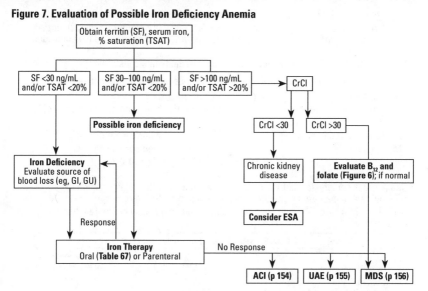

ACI = anemia of chronic inflammation; ESA = erythropoiesis-stimulating agent; MDS = myelodysplastic syndrome; UAE = undifferentiated anemia of the elderly.

Table 66. Differentiating Anemias of Chronic Inflammation, Chronic Kidney Disease, UAE, MDS, Iron Deficiency, and Mixed ACI/Iron Deficiency

Anemia Type	Ferritin, ng/mL	TSAT, %	ESR/CRP	Other Labs	% of All Late-Life Anemias
Anemia of chronic inflammation (ACI)	>100	>20	Elevated[1]	Hb not<10; CrCl >30	6–26
Anemia of CKD	>100	>20	WNL	CrCl <30	4–11
Unexplained Anemia of the Elderly (UAE)	WNL	WNL	WNL	B$_{12}$ and folate WNL; Hb not <10	25–40
Myelodysplastic Syndrome (MDS)	WNL	WNL	WNL	Hb <10, +/- other cytopenias	?
Iron Deficiency	<30	Low	WNL	TSAT <20	15–30
Mixed Iron Deficiency and ACI	30–100	Low	Elevated	TSAT <20	?

TSAT = transferrin saturation; WNL = within normal limits; CrCl unit = mL/min/1.73 m^2
[1]ESR >20 in men; >30 in women; or CRP >1.0 (10 mg/L)

Anemias of Later Life: Diagnosis and Treatment

Iron Deficiency Anemia (Figure 7)

- Serum iron and iron saturation (ie, transferrin saturation [TSAT]) are both low, transferrin is high, and ferritin ≤30 ng/mL (**Table 66**).
- Evaluate GI and GU source if iron deficient.

- Begin tx with oral iron using the steps outlined in **Table 67**.
- If oral iron replacement is inadequate or not tolerated, use parenteral replacement with iron sucrose *(Venofer)* ferumoxytol *(Feraheme)* or ferric carboxymaltose (see individual product information).
- Don't transfuse RBCs for iron deficiency without hemodynamic instability.^{CW}

Anemia of Chronic Inflammation (ACI; also known as anemia of chronic disease)

- Typically normocytic/normochromic and Hb about 10 g/dL
- Cause: hepcidin-induced alteration in GI iron absorption and iron trapping in macrophages.
- Most common causes in older adults:
  - Acute and chronic infection
  - Malignancy
  - Protein calorie malnutrition
  - Unidentified chronic disease
- Laboratory tests: usually low iron, low or normal TIBC, ferritin >100 ng/mL, and/or TSAT >20%; elevated ESR/CRP (**Table 66**).
- Check erythropoietin level; if <500 mU/mL may respond to the administration of recombinant human erythropoietin-stimulating agents (ESA); target level 10–11 g/dL.
- ADEs from ESA tx in ACI have not been well studied, and tx may not be reimbursed by Medicare.

Table 67. Steps in Oral Iron Replacement

	Hb, g/dL	Oral elemental iron total replacement dose, mg
Step 1: Estimate iron replacement dose based on Hb	>11 9–11 <9	5,000 10,000 15,000

	Preparation[1]	Number of tablets to achieve 5000-mg elemental iron replacement
Step 2: Select an oral iron preparation (only 10% of oral iron is absorbed)	Ferrous sulfate (Elixir 2.7 mg/15 mL, 324-mg tab, 65 mg elemental iron)	75
	Ferrous gluconate (300-mg tab, 36 mg elemental iron)	140
	Ferrous fumarate (100-mg tab, 33 mg elemental iron)	150
	Iron polysaccharide (150-mg tab, 150 mg elemental iron)	33
Step 3: Decide on dosing frequency	Many patients cannot tolerate more than a single tablet daily. Iron is best absorbed on an empty stomach. Assess tolerance after 1 wk (phone call); if not tolerating, adjust dose, interval, or preparation.	
Step 4: Recheck Hb and ferritin after each 5000-mg cycle	Give additional 5000-mg cycles prn.	

[1] Tolerance to GI side effects improves, however cost increases going down the list of preparations.

Note: 1 unit packed RBCs replaces 500 mg iron, or approximately the same as is absorbed from a 5000-mg cycle of oral iron. Reticulocytosis should occur in 7–10 d. Lack of correction with replacement suggests nonadherence, malabsorption, or ongoing blood loss. H$_2$-blockers, antacids, and PPIs reduce absorption, and some patients will need parenteral replacement. Enterically coated preparations are less well absorbed.

Combined Iron Deficiency and Anemia of Inflammation

- Iron, TIBC, and ferritin are less reliable in the presence of inflammatory conditions (**Figure 7**).
- Anemia is often more severe than in ACI alone.
- Suspect iron deficiency if ferritin 30–100 ng/mL and/or TSAT <20%. If ferritin ≤45 ng/mL, iron deficiency is confirmed. If 45–99 ng/mL, iron deficiency is possible; either treat presumed iron deficiency and evaluate response by reticulocyte count at 2 wk or check soluble transferrin receptor (sTfR). If sTfR/log (ferritin) >1.5, iron deficiency is confirmed.

Undifferentiated (or Unexplained) Anemia of the Elderly (UAE) and Idiopathic Cytopenias of Undetermined Significance (ICUS)

- UAE is the most common type of ICUS; and most ICUS develops in old age.
- Many patients with ICUS carry 1 or more of the 40 somatic mutations associated with myeloid malignancies and a portion of these evolve into a myelodysplastic syndrome.
- UAE is diagnosed when there is no evidence of B_{12} or folate deficiency, iron studies all normal, CrCl >30 mL/min/1.73 m²; hypocellular bone marrow; erythropoietin levels low for the degree of anemia; inflammatory markers (ESR/CRP) not elevated.

Anemia of Chronic Kidney Disease (suspect when CrCl <30 mL/min/1.73 m²)

- Caused by decreased erythropoietin production; check erythropoietin level, iron studies, B_{12}, and folate.
- Correct all correctable causes of anemia (iron deficiency, inflammation) before using ESAs. Keep transferrin saturation 20–50% and ferritin 100–500 ng/mL. Oral iron absorption is poor in CKD; parenteral replacement is often needed.
- Restoring Hb levels with ESAs decreases transfusions and fatigue but doubles stroke risk in people with DM, CKD, and anemia. Don't administer ESAs to CKD patients with Hb ≥10 g/dL without symptoms of anemia.**CW**
- Guidelines for ESAs (kdigo.org) recommend individualized tx.
  ○ Use ESAs with caution (if at all) in patients with malignancy, hx of stroke, or hx of malignancy.
  ○ For most patients, consider ESA and iron replacement when Hb is 9–10 g/dL with the goal of avoiding Hb <9 g/dL and the need for transfusion.
  ○ Some patients will have improved quality of life with Hb above 11.5 g/dL and will accept the risk; do not let Hb exceed 13 g/dL.
  ○ Patients who do not respond to usual dosages of ESAs may be at greater risk of cardiovascular events on high ESA dosages.
  ○ Evaluate for antibody-mediated pure red cell aplasia in patients using ESAs for >8 wk if Hb declines 0.5–1 g/wk.

Anemia of B_{12} and Folate Deficiency (Figure 6)

- Laboratory tests: anemia or pancytopenia, macrocytosis
- Serum B12 65–95% sensitivity for clinical deficiency if <200 pg/mL; deficiency is possible at <350 pg/mL; check serum methylmalonic acid level (MMA) to confirm deficiency.
  ○ **Treatment:** Expert panels recommend parenteral replacement for severe deficiency (neurologic complications, severe anemia). When adherence is not ensured, use:
    ▪ If neurologic impairment: B12 1000 mcg every other day for 2 wk, or until no further improvement, then 1000 mcg IM every 2 mo for life; if no neurologic impairment, every 3 mo.
    ▪ In cases of mild deficiency, randomized trials support the efficacy of oral replacement; ensure there will be adherence and malabsorption is not the cause, then use B12 1000–2000 mcg/d po.

- If using nonparenteral formulations, monitor MMA every 1–3 y to ensure replacement is adequate.
- Borderline folate levels 2–4 ng/mL should prompt homocysteine check. A few days of poor po intake lowers serum (but not body stores) of folate. RBC folate may be a more reliable test of deficiency.
  - **Treatment:** Folate 1 mg/d po for 1–4 mo or until complete hematologic recovery.

Hemolytic Anemia

- Hallmark is high reticulocyte count. About 2% of all anemias after age 65.
- The most common cause is autoimmune (low haptoglobin, positive direct antiglobulin) associated with chronic lymphocytic leukemia, medications, lymphoma, and collagen vascular disease; idiopathic.
- Causes if not autoimmune: mechanical heart valve, other intrinsic cause.

RBC Transfusion for Anemia

Acute Blood Loss

In general, withholding transfusion until Hb is 7–8 g/dL (restrictive) for people over age 65 results in equivalent outcomes (risk of bacterial infection, MI, mortality, rebleeding, pulmonary edema) compared to a more liberal transfusion for Hb <10 g/dL (liberal) transfusion policy. Exceptions are:

- Patients undergoing orthopedic procedures have better outcomes with restrictive transfusions.
- Patients with symptomatic CVD have better outcomes with liberal transfusions.

Avoid transfusions of RBC for arbitrary hemoglobin or hematocrit thresholds and in the absence of symptoms of active coronary disease, HF, or stroke.[CW]

Chronic Anemia

- Chronic anemia due to refractory aplastic anemia, myelodysplastic syndromes, etc, will require transfusion. For these patients, the transfusion threshold is based on symptoms to generally maintain Hb >9 g/dL in men and 8 g/dL in women.
- Don't transfuse more units of blood than absolutely necessary.[CW] Single-unit transfusions should be the standard in stable noncardiac patients.[CW]

PANCYTOPENIA

Unless due to B12 deficiency or drug-induced (eg, sulfonamides, carbamazepine, hydantoins, NSAIDs, antithyroid drugs, allopurinol, gold, etc), bone marrow aspirate is indicated; causes include cancer, fibrosis, myelodysplasia, and aplastic anemia.

Aplastic Anemia

- Hematopoietic stem cell failure; in 78%, cause is idiopathic but felt to be immune mediated.
- Diagnosis: hypocellular bone marrow
- Treatment: 75% respond to immunosuppressive tx.

Myelodysplastic Syndromes (MDS)

A group of stem cell disorders with decreased production of blood elements causing risk of symptomatic anemia, infection, and bleeding; risk of transformation to acute leukemia varies by syndrome. May be responsible for a proportion of unexplained anemias (ie, UAE) and ICUS in older patients (p 155).

Diagnosis

The diagnosis of MDS should be considered for any older patient with unexplained cytopenia(s) or monocytosis and for those who have had UAE when Hb falls below 10 g/dL. Inspection of the peripheral blood smear and bone marrow aspirate is a next step in diagnosis. Because these alone are not diagnostic of MDS, in vitro bone marrow progenitor cultures, trephine biopsies, flow cytometry, immunohistochemical studies, and chromosome analysis are routinely needed for diagnosis.

Staging and Prognosis

- Four different classification systems are available to help estimate prognosis, but none explain most of the variability in survival.
- Classification systems stratify patients from low- to high-risk groups based on various characteristics that differ by classification system.
- In general, poorer survival occurs with a higher proportion of blast cells, complex (>3 different) karyotypes or abnormal chromosome 7, and a greater number of cell lines with cytopenias (Hb <10 g/dL, absolute neutrophils <1800/µL, platelet count <100,000/µL).
- Median survival of high-risk patients is independent of age and is under 6 mo. However, among low-risk patients, survival is substantially affected by age with mean survival for those aged <60 is about 11.8 y, >60 about 4.8 y, and >70 about 3.9 y.
- The higher the blast count, the more likely the conversion to acute myelogenous leukemia (AML); but the most common causes of death are complications of the cytopenias, not acute leukemia.

Monitoring

- Should be under the direction of a hematologist and will vary by patient age, disease stage, prognosis, and tx status.
- Monitor all patients for the development of symptomatic cytopenias (anemia, infection, bleeding) and progression to AML.

Therapy (as directed by hematology; see subspecialty sources)

Supportive Care

- **Anemia** (usually present at diagnosis) is treated with ESAs if serum erythropoietin <500 mU/mL; if no response G-CSF may be added; RBC transfusion is an alternative; transfusion threshold generally Hb <8 g/dL.
- **Iron Overload**: risk increases with 20–30 U transfused; diagnosed when serum ferritin >1000 ng/mL; the use of chelating agents is controversial.
- **Infections**: are common and may be occult, respond poorly to antibiotics, and resolve slowly; bacterial skin infections are the most common; fungal disease is not uncommon.
  - In addition to influenza and pneumococcal, consider pertussis and haemophilus influenzae B vaccines.
  - Live vaccines (eg, live varicella vaccine or live-attenuated flu) should NOT be given.

PRIMARY MYELOPROLIFERATIVE DISORDERS

Polycythemia Vera

- Diagnosis: elevated RBC mass with normal arterial oxygen saturation and splenomegaly
- If no splenomegaly, 2 of the following: leukocytosis, increased leukocyte alkaline phosphatase, or increased B_{12}; or genetic testing showing JAK-2
- Treatment: phlebotomy to achieve iron deficiency and hematocrit ≤45% in men and <42% in women. Patients aged >60 are at higher risk for thrombosis and should receive hydroxyurea; if not tolerated, an alternate is ASA 81 mg/d.

Essential Thrombocytosis

- Platelet count >600,000/µL on 2 occasions ≥1 mo apart; Hb <13 mg/dL or normal RBC mass
- Normal iron marrow stores and no splenomegaly; exclude reactive thrombocytosis
- No Philadelphia or *bcr-abl* gene rearrangements or myelofibrosis in marrow
- Treatment: For patients at high risk (aged >60 or prior thrombohemorrhagic event), use ASA 81 mg and hydroxyurea. Anagrelide is less effective at preventing thrombosis.
- Target platelet count on tx: 100,000–400,000/mcL

Chronic Lymphocytic Leukemia (CLL)

- Progressive accumulation of functionally incompetent lymphocytes; only 30% of patients have an indolent 10- to 20-y course with the disease.
- Staging is based on CBC (anemia, thrombocytopenia) and physical exam (enlarged nodes, liver, or spleen); cytogenetic studies assist in prognosis.
- Monitoring and tx: 6- to 12-mo follow-up by hematology
- Treatment/prevention of complications:
  ◦ Infection: pneumococcal, influenza, and other inactivated adult vaccines; NOT live vaccines; neutrophil counts 500–1000 cells/µL with signs or symptoms of infection, treat with broad-spectrum antibiotics; neutrophil count >1000 cells/µL, treat as usual adult infection as indicated.
  ◦ Anemia in CLL is a result of hypersplenism, marrow infiltration, GI blood loss, chemotherapy, hemolytic anemia, or RBC aplasia. Tx should be directed at the underlying cause.
  ◦ Thrombocytopenia causes include extensive tumor burden, autoimmune destruction, and hypersplenism. Tx should be directed at the underlying cause.
  ◦ Malignancy: higher risk of other hematologic and solid malignancies. Patients should undergo age- and sex-appropriate screening.

Chronic Myelogenous Leukemia

- Leukocytosis with early myeloid forms evenly distributed in peripheral blood
- Philadelphia chromosome in >95% of cases
- Leukocyte alkaline phosphatase score low
- Treatment: Chronic phase, tyrosine kinase inhibitors (eg, imatinib); accelerated phase, initially a tyrosine kinase inhibitor then stem-cell transplant.

Myelofibrosis

- Pancytopenia, splenomegaly, and other extramedullary hematopoiesis
- Marrow fibrosis (dry tap) and peripheral blood: leukoerythroblastosis, tear-drop cells
- Acute leukemia develops in 5–20%.
- Treatment: Hematopoietic stem cell transplantation is the only tx with a potential for cure (may be an option for fit patients aged >65); ruxolitinib reduces symptoms and improves median survival for patients with high- or intermediate-risk disease; patients with low-risk disease are treated with danazol (for anemia), hydroxyurea, or both.

MONOCLONAL GAMMOPATHY AND MULTIPLE MYELOMA

Monoclonal Gammopathy of Undetermined Significance (MGUS)

- Definition: Premalignant clonal plasma cell disorder with the presence of monoclonal protein ≤3 g/dL, <10% clonal plasma cells in bone marrow; and the absence of multiple myeloma or other lymphoproliferative malignancy.
- Prevalence increases with age: 3.2% at age ≥50; 6.6% at age ≥80.

- Evaluation: CBC, calcium, comprehensive metabolic panel, LDH, spot urine protein, SPEP, serum immunofixation, and serum κ:λ light-chain ratio (if abnormal obtain urine electrophoresis and immunofixation).
  - If initial IgG MGUS is <1.5 g/dL or light-chain MGUS with κ:λ light chains ratio <8 and no other risk factors (see below), bone marrow may be deferred. Repeat laboratory testing at 6 mo and if stable; follow-up only with hx and physical exam (risk of progression 0.3–0.5%/y).
  - IgM MGUS has a higher risk for progression (1%/y) to Waldenstrom macroglobulinemia, amyloidosis, or rarely myeloma. Higher risk for peripheral neuropathy (bilateral sensory and demyelinating on nerve conduction study). Even if IgM MGUS <1.5 g/dL, if there are unexplained constitutional symptoms or signs (hepatosplenomegaly, lymphadenopathy), proceed to bone marrow biopsy, skeletal survey; echocardiography if unexplained heart disease (amyloidosis).
  - If MGUS ≥1.5 g/dL or any other of the risk factor (see below), obtain bone marrow biopsy and skeletal survey, and repeat laboratory testing at 6 mo and annually.
  - **Risk factors** for progression: MGUS ≥1.5 g/dL, IgM MGUS, abnormal serum-free light-chain ratio (κ:λ light chains) of <0.26 or >1.65. The greater the number of factors present, the greater the risk of progression.
  - Criteria for diagnosis of light-chain MGUS: abnormal κ:λ light chains ratio <0.26 or >1.65; increased κ if ratio >1.65 or λ if ratio <0.26; no heavy chains on immunofixation; no end-organ damage, clonal bone-marrow plasma cells <10%, urinary monoclonal protein <500 mg/24 h
- Increased risk of vertebral fracture; bone turnover markers are normalized with the use of bisphosphonates.

Multiple Myeloma

- Smoldering myeloma (asymptomatic stage) defined by presence of:
  - Serum monoclonal protein >3 g/dL and/or plasma cells >10% to <60%
  - No end-organ damage
  - A subset of high-risk patients may benefit from tx, but should enroll in clinical trials.
- Symptomatic multiple myeloma, defined by presence of:
  - Serum or urinary monoclonal protein >3 g/dL *and*
  - Clonal plasma cells in bone marrow >10% or plasmacytoma *and*
  - Presence of end-organ damage, hypercalcemia, lytic lesions, renal failure, anemia, *or* recurrent infections
  - Or >60% clonal plasma cells in bone marrow in the absence of end-organ damage
- Treat symptomatic patients. First, determine eligibility for stem cell transplant (for patients under age 70) and risk based on genetic abnormalities, comorbidities, functional status.
  - Transplant candidates 1st receive induction tx; exact agents selected based on risk.
  - Nontransplant candidates receive chemotherapy based on risk.
  - Frail older adults are generally treated with reduced doses of lenalidomide and dexamethasone; higher-risk patients may receive alternate agents.
  - Zoledronic acid (not all bisphosphonates) started at the time of diagnosis reduces skeletal events and improves overall survival independent of skeletal events. This effect was seen whether patients received transplant or oral agents.
  - Adverse effects of bisphosphonates include hypocalcemia, fever, osteonecrosis of the jaw in 1.3% in the 1st year (higher with denosumab). Risk of osteonecrosis of the jaw is reduced with good oral hygiene. Monitor for micro-albuminuria and stop tx if this develops.

- Performance status (ie, limitation in self-care ability: ≥50% of time in bed or chair), age >70, and albumin <3 g/dL have as much prognostic value as any of the disease factors.
- Patients at all stages are at risk of venous and possibly also arterial thrombosis related to both the disease and its tx (eg, thalidomide).
- Supportive care for all patients with advanced disease
  - Anemia may require transfusion. Erythropoietin is generally reserved for patients on chemotherapy with Hb <10 g/dL.
  - IV immunoglobulins monthly for recurrent bacterial infections and hypogammaglobulinemia; administer pneumococcal but NOT live vaccines (eg, live varicella vaccine or live-attenuated flu).
  - Surgical fixation and radiation tx for fractures and impending fractures.
  - Maintain hydration with at least 2 L/d and avoid NSAIDs and contrast because of renal dysfunction.
  - Provide adequate analgesia.

URINARY INCONTINENCE (UI)

UI is the complaint of involuntary leakage of urine. In older adults, it is most often multifactorial and results from some combination of lower urinary tract abnormalities, changes in neurologic control of voiding, multimorbidity, and functional impairment.

Like other geriatric syndromes, effective tx requires addressing more than one factor.

Classification of UI

Transient UI and Factors Contributing to UI: UI is caused or exacerbated by factors outside the lower urinary tract (eg, comorbidities, medications, mobility, see p 163). However, UI from these sources is transient only if they are recognized and addressed. These same factors are frequent contributors to UI in patients with urge, stress, and other causes of persistent UI.

Table 68. Types of Persistent Urinary Incontinence: Characteristics and Causes

Type	Characteristic	Causes
Urge	UI with compelling and often sudden need to void	Idiopathic or associated with CNS lesions or bladder irritation from infection, stones, or tumors
Stress	UI with increased intra-abdominal pressure (eg, cough or sneeze)	Due to failure of sphincter mechanisms to remain closed during bladder filling; insufficient pelvic support in women; prostate surgery in men
Mixed	UI with both urgency and increases in intra-abdominal pressure	Some of the above
Overflow (Detrusor Underactivity)	UI is continual, and postvoid residual urine is increased (typically >500 mL)	Impaired detrusor contractility from neuropathy, DM, vitamin B_{12} deficiency, tabes dorsalis, alcoholism, or spinal disease, or bladder outlet obstruction in men most often due to BPH, cancer, or stricture; in women due to prior incontinence surgery or a large cystocele
Detrusor Hyperactivity with Impaired Contractility (DHIC)	Characteristically UI with urge symptoms, but stress-related UI may occur; postvoid residual moderately elevated 200–300 mL	Detrusor does not contract sufficiently to empty but still has low-grade hyperactivity causing urgency. Underlying causes believed to stem from some of the same processes as urge and overflow UI.

Other (rare): Bladder-sphincter dyssynergia, fistulas, reduced detrusor compliance

Overactive Bladder: Frequency and urgency without UI; tx is the same as for urge UI.

Evaluation

History

- Determine type of UI (**Table 68**)
- Identify "red flag" symptoms including sudden onset of UI, pelvic pain (constant, worsened, or improved with voiding), or hematuria. These suggest neoplastic or neurologic disease and require prompt referral to a urologist if UTI is excluded.
- Lower urinary tract symptom review: frequency, nocturia, slow stream, hesitancy, interrupted voiding, terminal dribbling

- Medical condition status and medications used to treat them, reviewed in association with onset or worsening of UI
- Ask "How does UI affect your life?" and also ask about the presence of fecal incontinence (FI).

Physical Examination

- Functional status (eg, mobility, dexterity)
- Mental status (important for planning tx)
- Findings:
  - Bladder distention
  - Cord compression (interosseous muscle wasting, Hoffmann's or Babinski's signs)
  - Rectal mass or impaction
  - Sacral root integrity (anal sphincter tone, anal wink, perineal sensation)
  - Volume overload, edema

Male GU

Prostate consistency; symmetry; if uncircumcised, check phimosis, paraphimosis, balanitis

Female GU

Atrophic vaginitis (p 329); pelvic support (cystocele, rectocele, prolapse; p 361)

Testing

- **Bladder Diary:** Record time and volume of incontinent and continent voids, activities and time of sleep; knowing oral intake is sometimes helpful. Sample diary available at niddk.nih.gov/health-information/health-topics/urologic-disease/daily-bladder-diary/Pages/facts.aspx.
- **Postvoid Residual:** If available, bladder ultrasound after voiding is preferred to catheterization. If >200 mL, repeat; still >200 mL suggests detrusor weakness, neuropathy, medications, fecal impaction, outlet obstruction, or DHIC. Even if postvoid residual is not available, begin tx steps as shown in **Figure 8**.
- **Laboratory:** UA to check for hematuria or glycosuria; urine C&S if onset of UI or worsening of UI is acute; serum glucose and calcium if polyuric; renal function tests and B_{12} if urinary retention; urine cytology if hematuria or pain.

Figure 8. Stepwise Evaluation and Treatment of Common UI Conditions

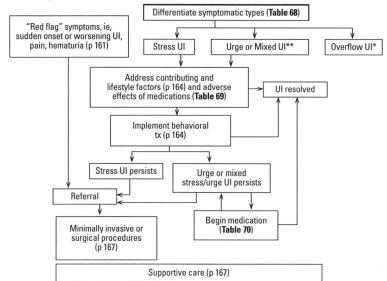

* Referral to differentiate neuropathy from obstruction (also **Table 68**)

** Treat both components of Mixed UI

- **Testing: Urodynamics** usually not needed; indicated before corrective surgery, when diagnosis is unclear, when empiric tx is ineffective, or if postvoid residual volume >200–300 mL (possibly lower in men).
- Don't perform cystoscopy, urodynamics or renal and bladder ultrasound in work-up of uncomplicated urge UI.**CW**
- Do not order upper tract imaging if there are only lower urinary tract symptoms.**CW**

Management in a Stepped Approach

Contributing Factors

- Environment: ensure adequate access
- Mentation: if the patient is cognitively impaired, recommend **Prompted toileting** (p 168).
- Manual dexterity: compensate for deficits, eg, by adapting clothing
- Medical conditions: optimize tx for HF, COPD, or chronic cough
- Medications: eliminate or minimize those with adverse effects (**Table 69**)
- Mobility: improve mobility or adapt environment

Lifestyle Factors

- Caffeine and diuretic (including carbonated) beverages produce rapid bladder filling and increase urgency
- Fluid intake: avoid extremes of fluid intake (<32 oz or >64 oz), reduce fluids after supper time to minimize nocturia
- Constipation: produces urethral obstruction or places pressure on bladder
- Weight loss: 60% UI reduction with large weight loss (≥16 kg); 30% decrease in odds for stress UI with 3.5 kg loss
- Smoking: produces chronic cough, encourage patient to quit

Behavioral Therapy

- Effective in urge, stress, and mixed UI
- Efficacy for behavioral tx: >35% reduction in UI; 50% greater patient perception of cure
- Two components of bladder training for urge UI:
  1) Voiding on schedule during the day (start q2h) to keep bladder volume low. When no incontinence for 2 d, increase voiding interval by 30–60 min until voiding q3–4h.
  2) Urge suppression (**Figure 9**), which retrains the CNS and pelvic mechanisms to inhibit contractions and leakage

Figure 9. Urge Suppression

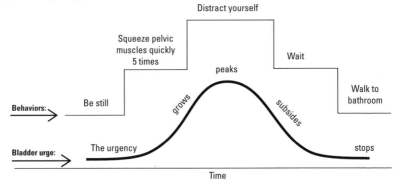

Note: Used with permission from Catherine E. DuBeau, MD

- Tx for stress UI involves timed toileting (as above) and also pelvic muscle (Kegel) exercises—isolate pelvic muscles (avoid thigh, rectal, buttocks contraction); perform slow velocity contraction, sustained for 6–8 sec. Perform 3 sets of 8–12 contractions in each set, on 3–4 d/wk (not daily) for at least 15–20 wk. An instructional booklet alone can reduce leakage by 50% (medlineplus.gov/ency/patientinstructions/000141.htm). Biofeedback can help with teaching; covered by Medicare if patient unsuccessful after 4 wk of conventional teaching (refer to continence specialist PT or APRN).
- Tx for postprostatectomy UI
  - Pelvic floor electrical stimulation and biofeedback begun soon after catheter removal in postprostatectomy patients improves early recovery of continence.
  - Even for those with UI ≥1 y after prostatectomy, pelvic floor exercises and urge control (**Figure 9**) reduces the number of incontinence episodes by more than half. Send patients to an experienced continence specialist for training (nurse practitioner or PT).

- Behavioral tx is at least as effective for overactive bladder symptoms in men on α-blocker tx as antimuscarinic tx. For benefit, patients should not have outlet obstruction (ie, postvoid residual urine <200 mL) (also Prostate, p 294).
- DHIC is first treated with behavioral methods; may add detrusor muscle-relaxing medications but follow postvoid residual; clean intermittent self-catheterization if needed.

Pharmacotherapy
- First eliminate medications causing/exacerbating UI if possible (**Table 69**).

Table 69. Medications Commonly Associated with UI

Medication/Class	Adverse Effects/Comments
ACEIs	Cough (stress UI) or cough-induced urge UI
Alcohol	Frequency, urgency, sedation, immobility
α-Adrenergic agonists	Outlet obstruction (men)
α-Adrenergic blockers (Avoid[BC])	Stress leakage (women)
Anticholinergics (Avoid[BC])	Impaired emptying, delirium, fecal impaction
Cholinesterase inhibitors	Increased uninhibited contractions and urgency
CCBs	Impaired detrusor contraction, edema with nocturnal diuresis
Estrogen (oral, transdermal)[BC]	Stress and mixed UI (women), avoid systemic estrogens in women with UI
GABA-ergics (gabapentin, pregabalin)	Edema, nocturnal diuresis
Loop diuretics	Polyuria, frequency, urgency
NSAIDs/thiazolidinediones	Edema, nocturnal diuresis
Sedative-hypnotics	Sedation, delirium, immobility
SGLT2 inhibitors	Diuresis, polyuria
Opioid analgesics	Constipation, sedation, delirium
TCAs and antipsychotics (Avoid[BC])	Anticholinergic effects, sedation, immobility

General Principles
- Data suggesting benefit of topical postmenopausal estrogen tx in urge and possibly stress UI are limited.
- See **Table 70** for pharmacotherapy for urge and mixed UI. All show efficacy in randomized controlled trials.
- Mirabegron has similar effectiveness to antimuscarinics; head-to-head trials are very limited.
- IR formulations are associated with greater side effects (ie, dry mouth, constipation, cognitive dysfunction).
- Special considerations in older people:
  - Longitudinal cohort studies suggest long-term use of antimuscarinics are associated with cognitive dysfunction, altered CNS metabolism, and brain atrophy.
  - Before using antimuscarinics, consider the total anticholinergic burden (eg, anticholinergic risk scale); mirabegron may be preferred to reduce cholinergic burden and is effective.
- Combining antimuscarinics and cholinesterase inhibitors should be avoided. Mirabegron is preferred tx for UI in patients who also take cholinesterase inhibitors.

- Select among alternative medications based on drug-related AEs (harms) (**Table 70**).
- >50% of patients stop tx by the end of 1 y.
- Chronic antimuscarinic use is associated with tooth loss and caries; routine dental care is important.
- Reevaluate use of these agents regularly after they are prescribed for lack of efficacy. D/C medication if not effective. Avoid use of anticholinergic agents.[BC]

Table 70. Pharmacotherapy for Urge or Mixed Urinary Incontinence

Medication	Dosage	Formulations	Adverse Events/Other RR for cure; NNT for cure
Antimuscarinics			*Class AEs:* dry mouth, blurry vision, dry eyes, delirium/confusion/dementia, constipation
Oxybutynin *(Ditropan*▲*, Ditropan XL*▲*, Gelnique)*	2.5–5 mg q8–12h 5–20 mg/d 1 g gel topically q24h	T: 5; S: 5 mg/5 mL SR: 5, 10, 15 10% gel, unit dose (1.14 mL)	Dry mouth and constipation less with XL and pch than immediate-release; doses above 10 mg/d not recommended. RR 1.7; NNT 9
(Oxytrol Women[OTC]*)*	3.9 mg/d (apply pch 2×/wk)	Transdermal pch 39 cm²	pch/gel: rotate sites to reduce skin irritation (L); OTC *Oxytrol* is less expensive
Tolterodine▲ *(Detrol*▲*, Detrol LA*▲*)*	2 mg q12h 4 mg/d	T: 1, 2 C: ER 2, 4	Withdrawal from tx trials for drug-related AEs not different from placebo; P450 interactions (L, CYP3A4 and CYP2D6) RR 1.2; NNT 12
Trospium *(Sanctura, Sanctura XR)*	20 mg q12–24h (on empty stomach) 60 mg/d (XR)	T: 20 C: ER 60	Dyspepsia, headache; caution in liver dysfunction; dose 1×/d at hs in patients aged ≥75 or with CrCl <30; XR formulation not recommended if CrCl <30 (L, K) RR 1.2; NNT 12
Darifenacin▲ *(Enablex)*	7.5–15 mg/d	T: 7.5, 15	Gastric retention; not recommended in severe liver impairment. Withdrawal from tx trials for drug-related AEs not different from placebo (L, CYP3A4 and CYP2D6) RR 1.3 NNT 9
Solifenacin▲ *(VESIcare)*	5–10 mg/d	T: 5, 10	Same as darifenacin; max dose 5 mg if CrCl <30 or moderate liver impairment. Women with urge UI who have taken other antimuscarinics that have failed may benefit from a trial dose of the 5-mg dose (no additional benefit at the 10-mg dose) (L, CYP3A4) RR 1.5; NNT 9
Fesoterodine *(TOVIAZ)*	4–8 mg/d	T: 4, 8	Max dose 4 mg if CrCl <30 (L, CYP3A4, CYP2D6) RR 1.3 ; NNT 8

(cont.)

Table 70. Pharmacotherapy for Urge or Mixed Urinary Incontinence (cont.)

Medication	Dosage	Formulations	Adverse Events/Other RR for cure; NNT for cure
β-3 agonist			
Mirabegron *(Myrbetriq)*	25–50 mg/d	T: 25, 50	Hypertension (monitor BP), nausea, headache, dizziness, tachycardia, AF; max dose 25 mg if CrCl <30; not recommended in severe kidney or severe liver impairment; raises digoxin and reduces metoprolol levels (L, CYP2D6). Combination with antimuscarinics should be done with caution while monitoring postvoid residual urine.

N/A = not available; RR = risk ratio for substantial improvement; NNT = number needed to treat for the effect according to 2017 guidelines of the European Urological Association; CrCl unit = mL/min/1.73 m^2

Note: For prostate obstruction UI, see Benign Prostatic Hyperplasia, p 294.

Procedures for Treatment of UI

- Electrical Modalities
  - Electrical stimulation with nonimplantable electrodes: electrical stimulation of bladder muscles through vaginal or anal probe or through a fine needle in the tibial nerve around the ankle:
    - More effective than antimuscarinics (OR=1.2), pelvic-floor muscle training (OR=1.6), or sham tx (OR=2.26) for achieving cure or improvement in symptoms of overactive bladder but not for cure of urge UI.
    - Less evidence that electrical stimulation is better for urge UI than pelvic-floor muscle exercises
  - Sacral nerve neuromodulation can be effective for refractory urge UI and urinary retention (both idiopathic and neurogenic). Electrode is implanted to stimulate S3; done as a trial before permanent device.
- Other Modalities
  - Pessaries benefit women with vaginal (p 361) or uterine prolapse who experience retention and stress or urge UI.
  - Botulinum toxin is also effective for refractory urge UI, but patients must be willing to perform self-catheterization because of the risk of retention and be willing to undergo serial intravesicular injections. Cure rates for overactive bladder and urge UI may be higher than with pharmacotherapy.

Surgical Therapy for Stress UI

- Consider for the 50% of women whose stress UI does not respond adequately to behavioral tx and exercise.
- Type of surgery depends on type of urethral function impairment, patient-related factors, and coexisting conditions (eg, prolapse).

Supportive Care

- Pads and protective garments should be chosen on the basis of gender and volume of urine loss. Medicaid (some states) covers pads; Medicare does not.
- Because of the expense, patients may not change pads frequently enough.
- Newer products (eg, Ultrasorbs® pads) contain large-volume UI and keep skin dry.

Causes of Nocturnal Frequency

Defined as greater than 2 voiding episodes/night

• Consider these more common causes first:

Cause	Characteristics	Therapy
Overactive bladder	Day- and nighttime frequency	**Table 70**
BPH	Elevated AUA symptom score (p 294)	Tx for BPH (p 295)
Sleep disorders	Complaints of poor sleep	p 341
Sleep apnea	Snoring or observed apnea	p 344
Stasis edema	Edema accumulates through the day	Compression stockings during the day
Uncontrolled DM	Elevated A1c	p 104–112
Excess PM fluid intake	Especially alcohol after supper	Restrict fluids 4 h before bedtime

• Then consider these causes of nocturnal polyuria defined as >1/3 of 24-h urine output between bedtime and waking; use bladder diary with measured voided volumes.

Heart failure	Consistent hx and exam	p 48–51
Autonomic dysfunction	Orthostatic hypotension; Parkinson disease and Parkinson plus syndromes; little voiding when upright, diuresis when supine; often hypotensive in the AM	Desmopressin[BC] 0.1–0.2 mg po hs; monitor for hyponatremia q7d after initiation and with dose increase; contraindicated if hyponatremic (or hx of hyponatremia) and with liver, renal, or heart failure
Reversal of diurnal fluid excretion	Patient often describes putting out more urine through the night than during the day	Trial short-acting potent diuretic after supper (eg, bumetanide 0.5–1.5 mg) to induce a brisk diuresis; if no response consider a trial of desmopressin[BC] or desmopressin acetate[BC] (as above)

UI in Special Populations

Nursing-home Residents and People with Cognitive Impairment

• Rather than bladder diaries, observe voiding patterns and UI episodes over several days.
• Trial of prompted voiding in patients who are able to state their name and transfer with assist of no more than one. Continue prompted schedule; if able to void at least 75% of the time during a 3-d trial which is considered a success.
• **Prompted voiding** consists of:
   ○ Asking if patient needs to void, and taking him or her to toilet starting at 2- to 3-h intervals during day; encourage patients to report continence status; praise patient when continent and responds to toileting.
   ○ Simply asking the patient if they need to void will NOT improve UI.
• Consider use of antimuscarinics in patients with urge UI who succeed with prompted voiding and still have UI episodes.
• Do not neglect evaluation for stress UI and outlet obstruction.

UI in Patients with Heart Failure

• 50% of HF patients have lower urinary tract symptoms
• If complaint is stress UI due to cough, check to see if patient is taking an ACEI; if so switch to ARB
• If complaint is urge UI or nocturia:
   ○ Rule out HF exacerbation and treat if needed

- If pedal edema is present, reduce or eliminate CCBs and other edema-causing drugs **(Table 69)**; use compression stockings if HF is stable and elevate legs at the level of the heart in late afternoon or evening
- Reduce/taper diuretics with careful follow-up of patient; avoid hs dosing
- Keep fluid intake at about 1.5 L/d and <2 L/d
- See Lifestyle and Behavioral Therapy p 164
- Caution in the use of antimuscarinics, which can cause dry mouth, increase fluid intake, and exacerbate HF

Catheter Care

- Use catheter **only** for chronic urinary retention, to protect pressure ulcers, and when requested by patients or families to promote comfort (eg, at end of life).[CW]
- Clean intermittent catheterization is a safe and effective alternative for many patients.
- Leakage around catheter can be caused by large Foley balloon, too large catheter diameter, constipation, impaction.
- Bacteriuria is universal; treat only if symptoms (eg, fever, inanition, anorexia, delirium) or if bacteriuria persists after catheter removal.
- Suprapubic catheters reduce meatal and penile trauma but not infection. Condom catheters are less painful and have a somewhat lower complication rate.
- Replace catheter if symptomatic bacteriuria develops, then culture urine from new catheter.
- Nursing-facility patients with catheters should reside in separate rooms.
- For acute retention, catheterize for 7–10 d, then do voiding trial after catheter removal.

Replacing Catheters: Routine replacement is not necessary. Changing q4–6wk is reasonable to prevent blockage. Patients with recurrent blockage need increased fluid intake, possibly acidification of urine, or change of catheter q7–10d.

FECAL INCONTINENCE (FI)

Definition

"Involuntary loss of liquid or solid stool that is a social or hygienic problem" (International Continence Society)

Prevalence

After age 65: 6–10% of men and 15% of community-dwelling women, 14% of hospitalized, 45% of nursing-home residents

Risk Factors

Constipation, diarrhea, age >80, female sex, UI, impaired mobility, dementia, neurologic disease

Age-related Factors

Decreased strength of external sphincter and weak anal squeeze, increased rectal compliance, decreased resting tone in internal sphincter, and impaired anal sensation

Causes: FI is commonly multifactorial.
- Overflow: from colonic distention by excessive feces, causing continuous soiling
- Loose feces: caused by medications, neoplasia, colitis, lactose intolerance
- Functional incontinence: associated with poor mobility
- Dementia related: uninhibited rectal contraction, often have UI
- Anorectal incontinence: weak external sphincter (surgery, multiparity, etc)
- Comorbidity: stroke, DM (autonomic neuropathy), sacral cord dysfunction

Evaluation

History

- Ask about "red flag" symptoms/signs that signal serious disease and require prompt referral to a gastroenterologist (ie, hematochezia, anemia, unexplained weight loss, refractory constipation, new-onset constipation or diarrhea, and positive family hx of colon cancer or inflammatory bowel disease)
- Description of FI (eg, diarrhea, hard feces), including usual bowel habit, change in habit, usual fecal consistency
- Frequency, urgency, ability to delay, difficulty wiping, postdefecation soiling, ability to distinguish feces and flatus
- Evacuation difficulties: straining, incomplete emptying, rectal prolapse or pain
- Functional: communication of needs, need for assistance, toilet access
- Other: bowel medications, other medications, UI, prior tx (eg, pads)

Examination

- Examine/palpate abdomen for colonic distention, and visually inspect anus for fissures and hemorrhoids.
- Check for rectal prolapse while patient seated on commode; check for rectocele in women.
- Perform rectal examination for sphincter tone, volume and consistency of feces; heme test.
- Observe gait, mobility, dressing, hygiene, mental status.

Laboratory

- TSH, electrolytes, calcium

Bowel investigations

- Abdominal radiograph: may identify colonic distention by excessive feces
- Colonoscopy: only when pathology suspected (unexplained loose feces, bleeding)
- Anorectal manometry and endorectal ultrasound: not generally needed for tx and are reserved for patients who do not respond to usual tx. Defecography not indicated unless surgery is planned.

Treatment: Multiple interventions may be required. Tx approaches based on symptoms and condition are effective, and significant improvement is maintained for up to 12 mo.

Main approach is to simulate the patient's usual bowel pattern.

- Use rectal evacuants to stimulate evacuation and to establish a bowel pattern.
- Use evacuants in the following order: glycerine Sp, bisacodyl Sp, microenemas (eg, *Enemeez*, docusate 5 mL), phosphate or tap water enemas; digital stimulation.
- Use antidiarrheals to slow an overactive bowel or to enable planned evacuation with rectal preparations.

Constipation (p 137): often plays a role; evaluate (if needed) and treat

Modify fecal consistency to achieve soft, formed feces.

- Loose feces: use fiber or loperamide titrated to effect, sometimes as little as q48h.
- Hard feces: modify diet; add stimulant (eg, *Senokot*) or osmotic (eg, polyethylene glycol) at low dosages. In poorly mobile people, bran and fiber may exacerbate constipation.

Patient education

- Respond promptly on urge to defecate.
- Take loperamide 2–4 mg 45 min before meal or social event to prevent evacuation.
- Use coffee to stimulate the gut.

- Position on toilet with back support, foot stool to achieve squat position.
- Exercise to improve bowel motility.

Rectal evacuation and toilet training: basic approach for most patients
- Following a routine improves bowel control.
- When no spontaneous bowel action, stimulate with suppositories or enemas (**Table 60**); those with incompetent sphincters may need microenemas.
- Bedpans should not be used; bedside commodes are not as good as toilets.

Exercise and other therapy
- Those who are able may be taught rectal sphincter exercises (tighten rectal sphincter for 10 sec 50× 2–3 d/wk) or may train using biofeedback (refer to PT).
- Biofeedback improves FI by strengthening pelvic floor muscles, improving the ability to sense rectal distension, and improving coordination of sensory and strength components.
- Eclipse System: an inflatable balloon inserted into the vagina places pressure on the rectum and reduces episodes of FI.
- Anal electrical stimulation of the anal sphincter a few minutes/d over 8–12 wk has modest benefit.
- Sacral nerve stimulation for patients with both intact and defective rectal sphincters is FDA approved for chronic FI in patients who cannot tolerate more conservative tx or in whom such tx has not been effective. Patients must show appropriate response to a trial of stimulation and must be able to operate the device.
- A perianal bulking agent *(Solesta)* is available for patients in whom other tx has failed. Gel is injected into the tissue below the anal lining to promote tissue growth. In turn, the anal opening narrows, and patients may have better bowel control. Tx is contraindicated in active inflammatory bowel disease, immunodeficiency disorders, previous pelvic radiation, and significant rectal prolapse.

Nursing-home residents and very disabled older adults: FI is most often due to colonic loading and overflow. Treat as follows:
- Daily enemas until no more results.
- Add a daily osmotic laxative (**Table 60**) and follow bowel training (above).
- Fecal transit can be stimulated with abdominal massage in the direction of colonic transit.

Other therapies
- Manual evacuation may be appropriate in some patients.
- Skin care: Wet wipes better than dry; commercial preparations better than soap and water; toilet tongs and bottom wipers help those with shoulder disease.
- Surgery:
  - Full-thickness rectal prolapse usually requires surgery using a transanal or intra-abdominal approach.
  - When FI is the result of sphincter injury (eg, obstetrical or fistula repair), surgical repair is often successful.
  - Sphincter dysfunction without an identifiable cause has a lower surgical cure rate, but may approach 50%.
  - Division of the external anal sphincter or anal fissure can be repaired, but long-term results are less than satisfactory.
- Selected patients have improved quality of life through the creation of a stoma.

ANTIMICROBIAL STEWARDSHIP: PRINCIPLES FOR PRESCRIBERS

- Collaborate with local antimicrobial stewardship teams and efforts.
- Be familiar with formulary restrictions and preauthorization requirements.
- Participate in educational offerings on antimicrobials and antimicrobial stewardship.
- In long-term care facilities, review antibiotic prescriptions upon admission, return from the hospital, or emergency department started by the covering provider, during monthly medication review.
- Streamline or deescalate empirical antimicrobial tx based on C&S results.
- Optimize and individualize antimicrobial dose and duration of tx.
- Avoid duplicative, redundant, or overlaps in tx (eg, piperacillin/tazobactam with metronidazole or another beta-lactam).
- Switch eligible patients from IV to oral antimicrobials.
- Use AHRQ minimum criteria toolkits on whether to treat UTI, skin and soft-tissue infection, or URI: https://www.ahrq.gov/nhguide/toolkits/determine-whether-to-treat/index.html
- CMS mandates that long-term care facilities develop, promote, and implement an antibiotic stewardship program (F881): https://www.cms.gov/Medicare/Provider-Enrollment-and-Certification/GuidanceforLawsAndRegulations/Downloads/Appendix-PP-State-Operations-Manual.pdf

PNEUMONIA

Presentation

Can range from subtle signs such as lethargy, anorexia, dizziness, falls, and delirium to septic shock or acute respiratory distress syndrome. Pleuritic chest pain, dyspnea, productive cough, fever, chills, or rigors are not consistently present in older adults.

Evaluation and Assessment

- Physical examination: Respiratory rate >25 breaths/min; low BP; chest sounds may be minimal, absent, or consistent with HF; 20% are afebrile.
- Imaging: infiltrates may not be present on the initial on CXR if the patient is dehydrated. CT scan may be indicated when CXR is inconclusive or compromised by other lung pathology.
- Sputum: Gram stain and culture (optional per ATS guidelines)
- CBC with differential: Up to 50% of patients have a normal WBC count, but 95% have a left shift.
- BUN, Cr, electrolytes, glucose
- Blood culture × 2 in hospitalized patients
- Oxygenation: ABG or oximetry <90% suggestive of pneumonia
- CRP >61 mg/L is associated with pneumonia.
- Test for *Mycobacterium tuberculosis* with acid-fast bacilli stain and culture in selected patients.
- Urinary antigen test for *Streptococcus* pneumonia and *Legionella* pneumophila in hospitalized patients. Legionella pneumophila urinary antigen test may be appropriate in residents of long-term care facilities when outbreaks are suspected or setting is optimal. Urinary antigen testing is highly specific for serotype 1 but lacks specificity for other serotypes. Value and use vary by geographic region.
- Thoracentesis (if moderate to large effusion)

CURB-65 Pneumonia Severity Scale (recommendation based on mortality probability)

Score each of the follow as 1 = Present and 0 = Absent: Confusion, BUN ≥19 mg/dL, RR ≥30, SBP <90 mmHg or DBP <60 mmHg, and age ≥65.

Interpretation: 1 = outpatient tx, 2 = consider hospitalization or outpatient tx, 3 = hospitalize, 4–5 = hospitalize consider ICU assessment

Aggravating Factors ([†] indicates modifiable)

- Age-related changes in pulmonary reserve
- Alcoholism
- Altered mental status
- Aspiration
- Comorbid conditions that alter gag reflexes or ciliary transport
- COPD or other lung disease
- Heart disease
- Heavy sedation[†] or paralytic agents
- Hyperglycemia[†]
- Intubation, mechanical ventilation (orotracheal intubation and orogastric intubation preferred)
- Malnutrition
- Medications[†]: immunosuppressants, sedatives, antipsychotics, inhaled corticosteroids, anticholinergic or other agents that dry secretions, agents that increase gastric pH
- Nasogastric tubes
- Oral care[†] (manual brushing plus rinse with fluoride/chlorhexidine 0.12% × 30 sec/d)
- Poor compliance with infection control[†] (eg, hand disinfection)
- Supine positioning[†] (semirecumbent, 30–45 degrees preferred)
- Swallowing[†] (eat/feed upright at 90 degrees over 15–20 min)

Predominant Organisms by Setting

Community-acquired:
- *Streptococcus pneumoniae*
- *Haemophilus influenzae*
- Respiratory viruses
- Enterobacteriaceae and other Gram-negative bacteria
- *Legionella* spp
- *Staphylococcus aureus* (including MRSA)

(including MRSA) Nursing-home–acquired:
- *Streptococcus pneumoniae*
- *H influenzae*
- *Staphylococcus aureus* (including MRSA)
- *Moraxella catarrhalis*
- Gram-negative bacteria
- Respiratory viruses
- *Legionella* spp
- Pseudomonas spp
- Mycoplasma pneumonia
- *Chlamydia pneumoniae*

Hospital-acquired:
- Gram-negative bacteria
- Anaerobes
- Gram-positive bacteria
- Fungi

Supportive Management
- Inhaled β-adrenergic agonists
- Mechanical ventilation (if indicated)
- Oxygen as indicated
- Rehydration

Empiric Antibiotic Therapy (Table 77)

The antibiotic regimen should be narrowed if the causative organism has been identified. If antibiotic tx is initiated ≥4 h posthospitalization, increased mortality may result.

Table 71. Treatment of Community-acquired Pneumonia for Immunocompetent Patients by Clinical Circumstances or Setting[1]

Clinical Circumstances or Setting	Treatment Options
Outpatient, previously healthy and no antibiotic tx in past 3 mo	Azithromycin, clarithromycin, or erythromycin Alternative: doxycycline
Outpatient, with comorbidities[2] or antibiotic tx in past 3 mo[4]	A fluoroquinolone[3] alone **or** Azithromycin, clarithromycin, or erythromycin *plus* amoxicillin (high dose) or amoxicillin-clavulanate Alternative β-lactams: ceftriaxone, cefpodoxime, or cefuroxime Alternative to a macrolide: doxycycline
Hospitalized patient	A fluoroquinolone[3] alone **or** Azithromycin or clarithromycin *plus* cefotaxime, ceftriaxone, or ampicillin Alternative β-lactam: ertapenem Alternative to a macrolide: doxycycline
Hospitalized patient, intensive care unit	
No concern about *Pseudomonas*	Cefotaxime, ceftriaxone, or ampicillin-sulbactam *plus* azithromycin or fluoroquinolone[3]
No concern about *Pseudomonas* but β-lactam allergy	Fluoroquinolone[3] *plus* aztreonam
Concern about *Pseudomonas*	Piperacillin-tazobactam, imipenem, meropenem, or cefepime *plus* ciprofloxacin or levofloxacin; **or** Piperacillin-tazobactam, imipenem, meropenem, or cefepime *plus* an aminoglycoside *and* azithromycin, ciprofloxacin, or levofloxacin
Concern about *Pseudomonas* and β-lactam allergy	Aztreonam *plus* ciprofloxacin or levofloxacin *plus* an aminoglycoside
Nursing-home patient[5,6]	Fluoroquinolone[3,4] alone **or** Azithromycin, clarithromycin, or erythromycin *plus* amoxicillin (high dose) or amoxicillin-clavulanate

[1] Because of the geographical variability in antimicrobial resistance patterns, refer to local tx recommendations.

[2] Comorbidities: chronic heart, lung, liver, or kidney disease; DM; alcoholism; malignancies; asplenia; immunosuppressing conditions or drugs

[3] Fluoroquinolones (respiratory): moxifloxacin, levofloxacin, or gemifloxacin

[4] Avoid fluoroquinolones in patients with a history of existing aortic aneurysm or increased risk of developing an aortic aneurysm.

[5] Patients being treated in the nursing home; for tx of nursing-home patients who are hospitalized, see hospitalized patient or intensive care unit.

[6] Because of the incidence of Gram-negative and atypical bacterial pneumonia in nursing-home patients, experts in geriatric infectious disease often recommend expanded Gram-negative antibiotic coverage.

Nursing-home or Hospital-acquired Pneumonia Requiring Parenteral Treatment: Alternative Recommendations

Antibiotics are indicated if:
- Temperature ≥102° F (38.9° C) + RR >25 or productive cough
- Temperature ≥100° F (37.8° C) + <102° F (38.9° C) + RR >25, pulse >100, rigors or new-onset delirium
- Afebrile with COPD + new or increased cough with purulent sputum
- Afebrile without COPD + new or increased cough + RR >25 or new-onset delirium

Empiric Treatment of Hospital- or Nursing-Home–Acquired Pneumonia (non–ventilator-dependent)

Antipseudomonal cephalosporin (cefepime or ceftazidime) *or*

Antipseudomonal carbapenem (imipenem or meropenem) *or*

β-lactam/β-lactamase inhibitor (piperacillin-tazobactam) *or*

Aztreonam *or*

Antipseudomonal fluoroquinolone (ciprofloxacin or levofloxacin) *or*
Aminoglycoside (amikacin, gentamicin, or tobramycin)—only if high risk of mortality and in combination with one of the above

Use 2 of the above (avoiding 2 beta lactams) if previous antibiotic tx within 90 days

plus

Linezolid or vancomycin (if risk factors for MRSA are present or if local incidence is high; until MRSA is excluded)

For both sets of empiric tx guidelines, the choice of combination depends on local bacteriologic patterns.

Duration of Treatment

Community-acquired pneumonia (CAP)
- Community setting: 5 days
- Hospital setting: A minimum of 5 d **plus** temperature <100°F (37.8°C) for 48 h **and** >1 CAP–associated sign of clinical instability:
  - Temp >37.8°C
  - HR >100 bpm
  - Respiratory rate ≥25/min
  - SBP <90 mmHg
  - O_2 saturation <90% or PaO_2 <60 mmHg

  Switch from parenteral to oral antibiotics when patient is hemodynamically stable, shows clinical improvement, is afebrile for 16 h, and can tolerate oral medications; total duration of tx 7–14 d depending on clinical response. Tx courses of 7–8 d are recommended for clinically improving hospital-acquired pneumonia not caused by *Pseudomonas* spp or other nonfermenting Gram-negative bacilli.
- Long-term care facility: usually 5–7 d is sufficient if stable ≥48–72 h before stopping antibiotics.

Note: The empiric use of vancomycin should be reserved for patients with a serious allergy to β-lactam antibiotics or for patients from environments in which MRSA is known to be a problem pathogen. For all cases, antimicrobial tx should be individualized after Gram stain or culture results are known.

URINARY TRACT INFECTION OR UROSEPSIS

See Prostate Disorders for prostatitis.

Definition

Bacteriuria is the presence of a significant number of bacteria in the urine without reference to symptoms.

- **Symptomatic bacteriuria** usually has signs of dysuria and increased frequency of urination; fever, chills, nausea may be present; $>10^5$ cfu/mL of the same organism from a single specimen supports the diagnosis of UTI, counts $\geq 10^3$ cfu/mL are diagnostic for specimens obtained by in and out catheterization.
- **Asymptomatic bacteriuria** is seen when there is an absence of symptoms, including absence of fever (<100.4°F [38°C]) plus:
  - the same organism(s) ($\geq 10^5$ cfu/mL) is found on 2 consecutive cultures in women
  - one bacterial species ($\geq 10^5$ cfu/mL) in a single clean-catch specimen in men
  - one bacterial species ($\geq 10^2$ cfu/mL) in a catheterized specimen in men and women
  - change in urine color, odor, or turbidity by themselves are not suggestive of UTI and do not warrant a urine culture
  - asymptomatic bacteria in the presence of delirium do not merit immediate antibiotic tx; first address hydration and other contributing factors and causes
- **Complicated UTI in women**—affecting the lower or upper urinary tract and associated with underlying condition that increases risk of infection and of tx failure (eg, obstruction, anatomical abnormality, resistant organisms, or urologic dysfunction)

Risk Factors

- Abnormalities in function or anatomy of the urinary tract
- Catheterization or recent instrumentation
- Comorbid conditions (eg, DM, BPH)
- Female sex
- Limited functional status

Assessment and Evaluation

- Screening and tx is recommended before a urologic procedure anticipated to result in mucosal bleeding, prosthesis implantation, and UTI symptoms. However, tx remains controversial for other than outright UTI. Tx of asymptomatic bacteriuria yields no difference in outcomes.
- Choice is based on presenting symptoms and severity of illness.
  - UA with culture (do not obtain sample from catheter bag)
  - Blood culture × 2
  - BUN, Cr, electrolytes
  - CBC with differential

Expected Organisms

Noncatheterized Patients: Most common: *Escherichia coli, Proteus* spp, *Klebsiella* spp, *Providencia* spp, *Citrobacter* spp, *Enterobacter* spp, coagulase-negative staphylococci, *Gardnerella vaginalis*, group B streptococci, and *Pseudomonas aeruginosa* if recent antibiotic exposure, known colonization, or known institutional flora

Nursing-Home–Catheterized Patients: All of the above plus enterococci, staphylococcus aureus, and fungus (eg, candida)

Empiric Antibiotic Treatment

- Routine tx of asymptomatic bacteriuria is not recommended.[CW]
  - Asymptomatic bacteriuria has not been associated with adverse outcomes.
- Empiric regimens should be changed based on C&S results, patient factors (eg, previous microbiology), and tx costs.

- Tx duration should be at least 3–7 d for women with uncomplicated UTI; 7–12 d for complicated UTI; and >14 d and up to 6 wk for men if prostatitis present (See Prostate Disorders for prostatitis).

First-line Treatment of Uncomplicated UTI (outpatient, oral)

- Cephalosporin, eg, cephalexin, or amoxicillin/clavulanate × 7 d
- Nitrofurantoin[BC] 50–100 mg q6h if CrCl >30 mL/min/1.73 m^2 × 7 d
- Trimethoprim/Sulfamethoxazole[BC] 160/800 mg 2×/d (if local resistance rate <20%) × 3–5 d if female and no catheter, × 7 d if catheter or male

When used systemically, fluoroquinolones can cause disabling and potentially permanent serious ADRs in patients with sinusitis, bronchitis, and uncomplicated UTIs. The FDA is advising that the serious ADRs associated with fluoroquinolone antibacterial drugs generally outweigh the benefits for patients with these conditions. Fluoroquinolones should only be used in patients who do not have alternative tx options. Serious ADRs associated with fluoroquinolones include hypo- and hyperglycemia (in people with DM); delirium; agitation; disturbances in attention, memory, and orientation; tendonitis and tendon rupture; *C difficile* infection; and QTc-interval prolongation and torsades de pointes (except delafloxacin). Avoid fluoroquinolones in patients with a history of existing aortic aneurysm or increased risk of developing an aortic aneurysm.

Empiric Treatment of Complicated UTI (Inpatient)

Not septic: Low risk of extended-spectrum beta-lactamase (ESBL): ceftriaxone; moderate- to high-risk ESBL: piperacillin/tazobactam, cefepime, or carbapenem

Suspected urosepsis (IV route): Low risk of carbapenem-resistant enterobacteriaceae (CRE): carbapenem ± vancomycin or piperacillin/tazobactam or 3rd-generation cephalosporin if ESBL risk is low; moderate- to high-risk CRE: ceftazidime-avibactam or ceftolozane-tazobactam.

Vancomycin should be reserved for patients with a serious allergy to β-lactam antibiotics.

UTI Prophylaxis

- Leads to antibiotic resistance regardless of patient's catheter status or duration of catheterization; generally not recommended. Noncatheterized women with a hx of UTI, especially if caused by *E coli*, may benefit from prophylaxis with cranberry juice (250–300 mL/d). Time to benefit may be ≥2 mo.
- Vaginal atrophy due to estrogen depletion may predispose women to recurrent UTIs. Local topical estrogen replacement may be indicated (**Table 126**). May take 2 to 3 mo to take effect.

SEPSIS AND SYSTEMIC INFLAMMATORY RESPONSE SYNDROME (SIRS)

Definition

Life-threatening organ dysfunction due to sepsis, a consequence of a dysregulated inflammatory response to an infection

Septic shock: subset of sepsis
- Serum lactate >2 mmol/L plus fluid resuscitation
- Hypotension requiring vasopressors to maintain mean BP ≥65 mmHg

Diagnostic Criteria

Outside the ICU (quick Sequential Oxygen Failure Assessment [qSOFA], www.mdcalc.com/qsofa-quick-sofa-score-sepsis):

1 point for each; used to predict mortality risk; >2 high risk
- Glasgow Coma Scale ≥15
- SBP ≤100 mmHg
- RR ≥22/min

ICU (SOFA, www.mdcalc.com/sequential-organ-failure-assessment-sofa-score): estimates ICU mortality risk

- PaO_2/FiO_2 ratio <300
- Glasgow Coma Scale >15
- Mean arterial pressure (MAP) <70 mmHg
- Use of vasopressors (eg, dopamine)
- Serum Cr as marker of urine output
- Bilirubin >4 mg/dL
- Platelet count <100,000

Risk Factors

- Bacteremia
- Age ≥65
- Immunosuppression
- DM or cancer
- Community-acquired pneumonia
- Genetic factors

Management

Supportive Care

- Respiratory: Oxygen and ventilator assistance as needed
- Goal-directed tx (if needed)
  ○ Rapidly infused bolus IV fluids defined by volume status; assess before and after each bolus
  ○ Use pressors when IV fluids are not sufficient or lead to cardiogenic pulmonary edema
  ○ Reserve inotropics (eg, dobutamine) for refractory patients with decreased cardiac output
  ○ RBC transfusion if Hb <7 g/dL, hemorrhagic shock, or myocardial ischemia

Early Goals of Treatment

- MAP >65 mmHg
- Urine output >0.5 mL/kg/h
- Central venous pressure 8–12 mmHg
- Central venous oxygen saturation ($ScvO_2$) ≥70% or SvO_2 ≥65%

Infection

- Identify and remove (when possible) infection loci
- IV antibiotics within 6 h associated with decreased mortality
- Empiric: vancomycin (or daptomycin for nonpulmonary MRSA, linezolid, ceftaroline) plus 1 or 2 other antibiotics depending if *Pseudomonas sp* is suspected
- Glucocorticoids if SBP <90 mmHg (severe septic shock)

METHICILLIN-RESISTANT STAPHYLOCOCCUS AUREUS (MRSA)

Risk Factors

- Long-term-care residence
- Hemodialysis or peritoneal dialysis
- IV drug use
- DM
- Recent surgery
- Previous colonization
- Poor functional status
- Wounds
- Invasive devices, (eg, catheters, feeding tube)

Types

Community-acquired

Usually skin and soft tissue infection (SSTI) or severe necrotizing pneumonia

Usual tx: clindamycin, doxycycline, minocycline, or TMP-SMX[BC]

Hospital-acquired

Usual tx: vancomycin +/– aminoglycoside and/or rifampin; daptomycin; or linezolid

Alternative tx for complicated SSTI: ceftaroline, delafloxacin, or telavancin

Duration of Treatment

- SSTI or pneumonia: 7–10 d
- Bacteremia, (–) valve endocarditis: 4 wk after culture negative
- Osteomyelitis or infected prosthetics: >6 wk

Decolonization with mupirocin or other antiseptics should be restricted to MRSA outbreaks and recurrent infections.

HERPES ZOSTER ("SHINGLES")

Definition

Cutaneous vesicular eruptions followed by radicular pain secondary to the recrudescence of varicella zoster virus. Recurrence may occur but rare in immunocompetent older people.

Prevention

Two zoster vaccines are available.

- A recombinant, adjuvanted zoster vaccine *(Shingrix)* was approved in October 2017 for individuals aged ≥50. Vaccination requires 2 doses given 2–6 mo apart. ACIP recommended vaccination of immunocompetent persons ≥50, including those who previously received the live vaccine or who had a prior episode of herpes zoster. CDC adopted ACIP's position in January 2018. The vaccine is available through most Part D and Medicare Advantage plans.
- A live vaccine *(Zostavax)* was approved in 2006 for individuals aged ≥50 who are immunocompetent and without contraindication to the vaccine. The USPSTF and ACIP recommend vaccination in immunocompetent persons aged >60. Patients who have had shingles in the past can receive the vaccine to prevent future episodes. There is no specific period of time that needs to have elapsed, but the rash should have resolved before administering the vaccine (**Table 103**).

Clinical Manifestations

• Abrupt onset of pruritus or pain along a specific dermatome (**Figure 1**)
• Macular, erythematous rash that becomes vesicular and pustular (Tzanck cell test positive) after ~3 d, crusts over and clears in 10–14 d
• Complications: postherpetic neuralgia, visual loss or blindness if ophthalmic involvement

Pharmacologic Management

When started within 72 h of the rash's appearance, antiviral tx (**Table 72**) decreases the severity and duration of the acute illness and possibly shortens the duration and reduces the risk of postherpetic neuralgias. (See p 246 for tx of postherpetic neuralgia.)

Table 72. Antiviral Treatments for Herpes Zoster

Medication, Route	Dosage	Formulations	Reduce dosage when CrCl[1] is
Acyclovir▲			
Oral	800 mg 5 ×/d for 7–10 d	T: 400, 800; C: 200; S: 200 mg/5 mL	<25
IV[2]	10 mg/kg q8h for 7 d	500 mg/10 mL	<50
Famciclovir▲			
Oral	500 mg q8h for 7 d	T: 125, 250, 500	<60
Valacyclovir▲[3]			
Oral	1000 mg q8h for 7 d	C: 500, 1000	<50

[1] The CrCl listed is the threshold below which the dosage (amount or frequency) should be reduced. See package insert for detailed dosing guidelines. CrCl unit = mL/min/1.73 m².

[2] Use IV for serious illness, ophthalmic infection, or patients who cannot take oral medication.

[3] Preferred to po acyclovir; prodrug of acyclovir with serum concentrations equal to those achieved with IV administration.

INFLUENZA

Vaccine Prevention (ACIP Guidelines)

Yearly vaccination is recommended for all adults aged ≥65, all residents and staff of nursing homes or residential or long-term care facilities, and all healthcare providers. Nursing-home residents admitted during the winter months after the vaccination program has been completed should be vaccinated at admission if they have not already been vaccinated. The influenza vaccine is contraindicated in people who have an anaphylactic hypersensitivity to eggs or any other component of the vaccine. Dose: 0.5 mL IM 1× in the fall for those living in the northern hemisphere.

Table 73. Influenza Vaccines 2018–2019

Influenza Vaccine Types	Antigen	Adult Age Group, y
Inactivated		
Trivalent, standard dose *(Afluria)*	2 A + 1 B	All adults
Trivalent, recombinant (RIV3, *Flublok*)	2 A + 1 B	All adults
Trivalent, adjuvanted. standard dose ≥65 *(Fluad)*	2 A + 1 B	≥65
Trivalent, high dose[1] *(Fluzone High-Dose)*	2 A + 1 B	≥65
Quadrivalent, standard dose *(Afluria, Fluarix, Flucelvax, FluLaval & Fluzone Quadravalent)*	2 A + 2 B	All adults
Quadrivalent, recombinant[2] (RIV4) *(Flublok Quadrivalent)*	2 A + 2 B	All adults
Live-attenuated Avoid in patients immune- or hematologically compromised, or receiving biologic agents		
Quadrivalent, intranasal *(Flumist Quadravalent)*	2 A + 2 B	Not approved for persons ≥50 y

[1] 4× the standard dose of antigen

[2] 3× the standard dose of antigen

Table 74. Diagnostic Tests for Influenza[1]

Method	Test Time	Acceptable Specimens, Detection and Differentiation
Rapid influenza diagnostic tests	<30 min	NP swab (throat swab), nasal wash, nasal aspirate
		Antigen (EIA) detects and differentiates between A and B, and detection of Type B varies with EIA
Reverse-transcriptase-polymerase chain reaction (RT-PCR)	1–6 h	Detect and differentiate Types A and B, including subtypes NP swab, throat swab, NP or bronchial wash, nasal or endotracheal aspirate, sputum
		Detect and differentiate Types A and B, including H1N1 and avian H5N1 subtypes
Immunofluorescence, direct (DFA) or indirect (IFA) antibody staining	1–4 h	NP swab or wash, bronchial wash, nasal or endotracheal aspirate
		Detect and differentiate between Types A and B, between A/B, and other respiratory viruses
Viral cell culture (conventional)	3–10 d	NP swab, throat swab, NP or bronchial wash, nasal or endotracheal aspirate, sputum

[1] Testing indicated early in the season or during outbreaks

EIA = enzyme immunoassay; NP = nasopharyngeal.

Pharmacologic Prophylaxis and Treatment with Antiviral Agents

Indications:

- Prevention (during an influenza outbreak): people who are not vaccinated, are immunodeficient, or may spread the virus
- Prophylaxis: during 2 wk required to develop antibodies for people vaccinated after an outbreak of influenza A
- Reduction of symptoms, duration of illness when started within the 1st 48 h of symptoms
- During epidemic outbreaks in nursing homes

- Resistance to antivirals and the emergence of specific strains of influenza (eg, H1N1) have led to frequent updates of recommendations for prophylaxis and tx. Check the CDC Web site for the most current information and guidance (cdc.gov/flu/professionals/antivirals/).

Duration: Tx of symptoms: 3–5 d or for 24–48 h after symptoms resolve. Prophylaxis during outbreak: min 2 wk or until ~1 wk after outbreak ends.

Table 75. Antiviral Treatment of Influenza

Agent	Formulation	Dosage
✓ Oseltamivir[▲1]	C: 30, 75 mg S: 360 mg/6 mL	Tx: 75 mg po q12h × 5 d; 30 mg po q12h× 5 d if CrCl >30–60; 30 mg po q24h × 5 d if CrCl = 10–30; 30 mg q24h; Hemodialysis: 30 mg immediately and 30 mg after every hemodialysis cycle for ESRD patients on hemodialysis, not to exceed 5 d; ESRD patients on CAPD: a single 30-mg dose immediately.
		Prophylaxis of influenza: 75 mg po q24h for 7–10 d; Community outbreak: 75 mg po q24h for up to 6 wk for immunocompetent patients and 12 wk for immunocompromised patients; Institutional outbreak: Continue for ≥2 wk until >7 d after onset in last patient.
Baloxavir marboxil *(Xofluza)*	T: 20, 40 mg	Tx: 40 kg to <80 kg: 40 mg po × 1 within 48 h of symptom onset
		≥80 kg: 80 mg × 1 within 48 h of symptom onset
Zanamivir *(Relenza)* [1,2]	Inh: 5 mg/blister	Tx: 2 × 5-mg inhalations q12h × 5 d
		Give doses on 1st d ≥2 h apart
		Prophylaxis: 2 × 5-mg inhalations q24h; Household setting: start 36 h after onset of signs and symptoms of initial case, duration 10 d; Community: begin within 5 d of outbreak, duration 30 d. Duration: until ~7 d after onset in last patient.
Peramivir *(Rapivab)*	IV: 200 mg/20 mL	600 mg IV × 1 CrCl 30–49: 200 mg × 1 CrCl 10–29: 100 mg × 1 End-stage renal disease requiring intermittent hemodialysis: 100 mg × 1, administered after dialysis

✓ = preferred for treating older adults; CrCl unit = mL/min/1.73 m²

[1] Must be started within 2 d of symptom onset or of contact with an infected individual.

[2] Do not use in patients with COPD or asthma.

OTHER RESPIRATORY VIRUSES
Coronavirus

Seasonality: Primarily winter

Presentation: Respiratory symptoms; influenza-like illness, acute exacerbation of chronic bronchitis and pneumonia. Pneumonia in immunocompromised patients or patients with HIV.

Diagnosis: Nasopharyngeal sample; RT-PCR

Treatment: Supportive, no known antiviral agent

Human Metapneumovirus

Seasonality in the US: Late winter, early spring

Presentation: respiratory, especially wheezing; may exacerbate asthma, pneumonia

Diagnosis: Nasopharyngeal sample; RT-PCR

Treatment: Supportive; ribavirin is active in vitro but has not been tested.

Parainfluenza Virus (PIV)

Seasonality in the US:
   PIV-1: Fall of odd number years
   PIV-2: Fall, annual
   PIV-3: Spring, less predictable
   PIV-4: Not yet characterized

Presentation: mild upper respiratory tract infection to pneumonia (in immunocompromised patients)

Diagnosis: Viral culture of nasal washing preferred with PCR for PIV detection

Treatment: Supportive; reduce immunosuppression if possible (eg, lower dose of corticosteroids); no known antiviral agent

Respiratory Syncytial Virus (RSV)

Seasonality:
   Northern hemisphere: November–April
   Southern hemisphere: May–September

Risk factors: Immunocompromised, significant asthma, cardiopulmonary disease, functional disability, institutionalization, residence in altitude >2500 m

Diagnosis: Isolation of human epithelial type 2 (HEp-2) cells

Treatment:
- Supportive (oxygen, bronchodilators, corticosteroids)
- Ribavirin + passive immunotherapy or corticosteroids

TUBERCULOSIS (TB)

TB in older adults may be the reactivation of old disease or a new infection due to exposure to an infected individual. If a new infection is suspected or if the patient has risk factors for resistant organisms, bacterial sensitivities must be determined.

Risk or Reactivating Factors
- Chronic institutionalization
- Corticosteroid use
- DM
- Malignancy
- Malnutrition
- Kidney failure

Diagnosis
- Mantoux tuberculin skin test (TST): 0.1 mL of tuberculin PPD intradermal injection into the inner surface of the forearm
- Read 48–72 h after injection (**Table 76** for interpretation).
- Repeat ("booster") 1–2 wk after initial skin testing can be useful for nursing-home residents, healthcare workers, and others who are retested periodically to reduce the likelihood of misinterpreting a boosted reaction to subsequent TSTs.

Interferon-gamma release assays (IGRAs)
- QuantiFERON = TB Gold In-Tube test (QFT-GIT)
- T-SPOT
  (+) Patient has been infected; additional tests if latent TB or tubercular disease
  (–) Latent TB or tubercular disease not likely

Table 76. Identification of Patients at High Risk of Developing TB Who Would Benefit from Treatment of Latent Infection

Population	Minimum Induration Considered a Positive Test
Considered positive in any person, including those considered low risk	15 mm
Residents and employees of hospitals, nursing homes, and long-term facilities for older adults, residential facilities for patients with AIDS, and homeless shelters	10 mm
Recent immigrants (<5 y) from countries where TB prevalence is high	10 mm
Injectable-drug users	10 mm
People with silicosis; DM; chronic kidney failure; leukemia; lymphoma; carcinoma of the head, neck, or lung; weight loss of ≥10%; gastrectomy or jejunoileal bypass	10 mm
Recent contact with TB patients	5 mm
Fibrotic changes on CXR consistent with prior TB	5 mm
Immunosuppressed (receiving the equivalent of prednisone at ≥15 mg/d for ≥1 mo), organ transplant recipients, patients receiving TNF-α inhibitors	5 mm
HIV-positive patients	5 mm

Treatment of Latent and Active Infection

Refer to CDC guidelines at cdc.gov/mmwr/preview/mmwrhtml/rr5211a1.htm#tab2.

HUMAN IMMUNODEFICIENCY VIRUS (HIV)

Reasons for increase in HIV infection in adults aged ≥50:
• Increased survival of people with HIV
• Age-associated decrease in immune function with resultant increased susceptibility
• Tx for erectile dysfunction leading to more sexual activity
• Difficulty with condom use secondary to erectile dysfunction
• Less condom use by partners of postmenopausal women
• Older women with vaginal dryness and thinning
• Older adults think only the young are at risk
• Mortality old > young secondary to non-HIV-related causes

Presentation

Many symptoms that may delay diagnosis are common in older adults:
• Anorexia
• Arthralgias
• Earlier, more symptomatic menopause
• Fatigue
• Flu-like symptoms
• Forgetfulness
• Hypogonadism
• Insomnia
• Myalgias
• Pain in hands or feet (neuropathy)
• Recurrent pneumonia
• Sexual disorders
• Weight loss

Comorbidities common in older adults that can occur earlier in people with HIV:
• Cancers (eg, anal, liver, lung)
• Cirrhosis
• Cognitive deficits
• CAD
• DM
• Dyslipidemia
• HTN
• Obstructive lung disease
• Osteoporosis
• Vascular disease

Laboratory Abnormalities

- Anemia
- Leukopenia
- Persons aged ≥65 have a lower CD4 count at diagnosis
- Low cholesterol
- Transaminitis

Screening

Routine screening of adults aged ≥65 is not recommended.

Screening is recommended regardless of age if:

- Starting tx for TB
- Treating a sexually transmitted disease
- Other HIV risk factors are present: unprotected sex and multiple partners, hazardous alcohol or illicit drug use
- Unexplained anemia
- Peripheral neuropathy
- Oral candidiasis
- Herpes zoster (widespread infection)
- Recurrent bacterial pneumonia
- Unexplained weight loss or pronounced fatigue

Treatment

Antiretroviral tx is recommended in patients aged >50, regardless of CD4 count.

- Viral load suppression greatest in patients aged ≥60 after initiating antiretroviral tx
- HIV-1 RNA suppression old > young
- CD4 response to tx young > old

For complete guidelines on antiretroviral regimens, see https://aidsinfo.nih.gov/guidelines.

Tx-naive patients:

- Nonnucleoside reverse transcriptase inhibitor (NNRTI) + 2 nucleoside reverse transcriptase inhibitors (NRTIs) *or*
- Protease inhibitor with ritonavir (preferred) + 2 NRTIs, *or*
- Integrase strand transfer inhibitor + 2 NRTIs

Pre-exposure Prophylaxis

The combination of emtricitabine and tenofovir *(Truvada*; T 200 mg/300 mg; K<60 mL/min) in combination with safer sex practices is approved for pre-exposure prophylaxis to reduce the risk of sexually acquired HIV-1 in adults at high risk.

Complications of Pharmacotherapy

- Increased cholesterol (accelerated atherosclerosis)
- Glucose intolerance
- Drug-drug interactions
- Drug toxicity
- Little data on the effects of age on drug pharmacokinetics in HIV-positive patients
- Increased pill burden

Monitor

- BMD
- Kidney function
- Liver function

Table 77. Antibiotics

Antimicrobial Class, *Subclass*	Dosage	Adjust When CrCl[1] Is: (Elimination)	Formulations
β-Lactams Penicillins			
Amoxicillin▲	po: 250 mg–1 g q8h	<50 (K)	T: film-coated 500, 875 C: 250, 500 ChT: 125, 250 S: 125, 200, 250, 400 mg/5 mL
Ampicillin▲	po: 250–500 mg q6h IM/IV: 1–2 g q4–6h	<30 (K)	C: 250, 500 S: 125, 250, 500 mg/5 mL Inj
Penicillin G▲	IV: 3–5 × 10⁶ U q4–6h IM: 0.6–2.4 × 10⁶ U q6–12h	<30 (K, L)	Inj procaine for IM
Penicillin VK▲	po: 125–500 mg q6h	[2] (K, L)	T: 250, 500 S: 125, 250 mg/5 mL
Antistaphylococcal Penicillins			
Dicloxacillin▲	po: 125–500 mg q6h	NA (K)	C: 250, 500
Nafcillin▲	IM: 500 mg q4–6h IV: 500 mg–2 g q4–6h	NA (L)	Inj
Oxacillin▲	IM, IV: 250 mg–2 g q6–12h	<10 (K)	Inj
Monobactam (antipseudomonal)			
Aztreonam▲	IM: 500 mg–1 g q8–12h IV: 500 mg–2 g q6–12h	<30 (K)	Inj
Carbapenems			
Doripenem▲	IV: 500 mg q8h	<50 (K)	Inj
Ertapenem *(Invanz)*	IM, IV: 1 g q24h × 3–14 d IM × 7 d max IV × 14 d max	<30 (K, F)	Inj
Imipenem-cilastatin▲	IM: 500 mg–1 g q8–12h IV: 500 mg–2 g q6–12h	<70 (K)	Inj
Meropenem▲	IV: 1 g q8h	≤50 (K, L)	Inj
Meropenem-vaborbactam *(Vabomere)*	IV: 4 g (2 g each) q8h × 14 d	<50 (K)	Inj
Penicillinase-resistant Penicillins			
Amoxicillin-clavulanate▲	po: 250 mg q8h, 500 mg q12h, 875 mg q12h	<30 (K, L)	T: 250, 500, 875, 1000 ChT: 200, 400 S: 125, 200, 250, 400 mg/5 mL

(cont.)

Table 77. Antibiotics (cont.)

Antimicrobial Class, *Subclass*	Dosage	Adjust When CrCl[1] Is: (Elimination)	Formulations
Ampicillin-sulbactam▲	IM, IV: 1–2 g q6–8h	<30 (K)	Inj
Penicillinase-resistant and Antipseudomonal Penicillins			
Ceftazidime-avibactam *(Avycaz)*	IV: 2.5 g q8h	<50 (K)	Inj
Ceftolozane-tazobactam *(Zerbaxa)*	IV: 1.5 g q8h	<50 (K)	Inj
Piperacillin-tazobactam▲	IV: 3.375 g q6h	<40 (K, F)	Inj
First-generation Cephalosporins			
Cefadroxil▲	po: 500 mg–1 g q12h	<50 (K)	C: 500 T: 1 g S: 250, 500 mg/5 mL
Cefazolin▲	IM, IV: 500 mg–2 g q12h	<55 (K)	Inj
Cephalexin▲	po: 250 mg–1 g q6h	<40 (K)	C: 250, 500, 750 T: 250, 500 S: 125, 250 mg/5 mL
Second-generation Cephalosporins			
Cefaclor▲	po: 250–500 mg q8h	<50 (K)	C: 250, 500 S: 125, 187, 250, 375 mg/5 mL T: ER 375, 500
Cefotetan▲	IM, IV: 1–3 g q12h or 1–2 g q24h (UTI)	<30 (K)	Inj
Cefoxitin▲	IM, IV: 1–2 g q6–8h	<50 (K)	Inj
Cefprozil▲	po: 250–500 mg q12–24h	<30 (K)	T: 250, 500 S: 125, 250 mg/5 mL
Cefuroxime axetil▲	po: 125–500 mg q12h IM, IV: 750 mg–1.5 g q6h	<20 (K)	T: 250, 500▲ S: 125, 150 mg/5 mL Inj▲
Third-generation Cephalosporins			
Cefdinir▲	po: 300 mg q12h or 600 mg/d × 10 d	<30 (K)	C: 300 S: 125, 250/5 mL
Cefditoren▲	po: 400 mg q12h × 10 d (bronchitis) 400 mg q12h × 14 d (pneumonia) 200 mg q12h × 10 d (soft tissue or skin)	<50 (K)	T: 200, 400
Cefixime▲	po: 400 mg/d	<60 (K)	C, T: 400 CT: 100, 200 S: 100, 200 mg/5 mL
Cefotaxime▲	IM, IV: 1–2 g q6–12h	<20 (K)	Inj

(cont.)

Antibiotics – INFECTIOUS 187

Table 77. Antibiotics (cont.)			
Antimicrobial Class, *Subclass*	**Dosage**	**Adjust When CrCl[1] Is: (Elimination)**	**Formulations**
Cefpodoxime▲	po: 100–400 mg q12h	<30 (K)	T: 100, 200 S: 50, 100 mg/5 mL
Ceftazidime▲	IM, IV: 500 mg–2 g q8–12h UTI: 250–500 mg q12h	<50 (K)	Inj
Ceftibuten▲	po: 400 mg/d	<50 (K)	C: 400 S: 90, 180 mg/5 mL
Ceftriaxone▲	IM, IV: 1–2 g q12–24h	NA (K)	Inj
Fourth-generation Cephalosporins			
Cefepime▲	IV: 500 mg–2 g q12h	<60 (K)	Inj
Fifth-generation Cephalosporin			
Ceftaroline fosamil *(Tefloro)*	400–600 mg q12h	≤50 (K)	IV: 400, 600 mg
Aminoglycosides			
Amikacin▲	IM, IV: 15–20 mg/kg/d divided q12–24h; 15–20 mg/kg q24–48h	<60, TDM (K)	Inj
Gentamicin▲	IM, IV: 2–5 mg/kg/d divided q12–24h; 5–7 mg/kg q24–48h	<60, TDM (K)	Inj ophth sus, oint
Plazomicin *(Zemdri)*	IV: 15 mg/kg q24h CrCl 30–<60: 10 mg/kg q24h CrCl 15–<30: 10 mg/kg q48h CrCl <15: No recommendation	<60, TDM (K)	Inj
Streptomycin▲	IM, IV: 10 mg/kg/d not to exceed 750 mg/d	<50 (K)	Inj
Tobramycin▲	IM, IV: 2–5 mg/kg/d divided q12–24h; 5–7 mg/kg q24–48h	<60, TDM (K)	Inj ophth sus, oint
Macrolides			
Azithromycin▲	po: 500 mg on day 1, then 250 mg/d IV: 500 mg/d	NA (L)	S: 100, 200 mg/5 mL, 1 g (single-dose pk) T: 250, 500, 600 mg Inj
Clarithromycin▲BC	po: 250–500 mg q12h ER: 1000 mg/d	<30 (L, K)	S: 125, 250 mg/5 mL T: 250, 500 ER: 500
Erythromycin▲BC	po: Base: 333 mg q8h Stearate or base: 250–500 mg q6–12h Ethylsuccinate: 400–800 mg q6–12h IV: 15–20 mg/kg/d divided q6h	NA (L)	Base: C, T: 250, 333, 500 Stearate: T: 250 Ethylsuccinate: S: 100, 200, 400 mg/5 mL T: 400 Inj

(cont.)

Table 77. Antibiotics (cont.)			
Antimicrobial Class, *Subclass*	**Dosage**	**Adjust When CrCl[1] Is: (Elimination)**	**Formulations**
Fidaxomicin *(Dificid)*	po: 200 mg q12h	NA (F)	T: 200 mg
Ketolide			
Telithromycin *(Ketek)*	po: 800 mg/d × 5–10 d	<30 (L, K)	T: 300, 400
Quinolones			
Ciprofloxacin ▲BC ophth: **Table 53**	po: 250–750 mg q12h	po: <50 (L, K)	T: 100, 250, 500, 750▲ S: 250 mg/5 mL, 500 mg/5 mL
	IV: 200–400 mg q12h	IV: <30	3.5 mg/5 mL Inj
(Cipro XR)			XR▲: 500, 1000
Delafloxacin *(Baxdela)*	po: 450 mg q12h × 5–14 d IV: 300 mg q12h × 5–14 d	IV: <30 (K)	T: 450 Inj
Gemifloxacin *(Factive)*	po: 320 mg/d	≤40 (K, L, F)	T: 320 mg
Levofloxacin▲	po, IV: 250–500 mg/d	<50 (K)	T: 250, 500, 750 S: 125 mg/5 mL Inj
Moxifloxacin▲	po: 400 mg q12h	NA (L, F, K)	Inj T: 400
Norfloxacin *(Noroxin)*	po: 400 mg q12h	<30 (K, F)	T: 400
Ofloxacin▲ ophth: **Table 53**	po, IV: 200–400 mg q12–24h	<50 (K)	T: 200, 300, 400▲
Tetracyclines			
Doxycycline▲	po, IV: 100–200 mg/d q12–24h	NA (K)	C, T: 50, 75, 100, 150; XR 40 S: 25, 50 mg/5 mL Inj
Minocycline▲	po, IV: 200 mg 1×, then 100 mg q12h	NA (K)	C: 50, 75, 100 TXR: 45, 90, 135 Inj
Tetracycline▲	po, IV: 250–500 mg q6–12h	NA (K)	C: 250, 500
Glycycline			
Tigecycline▲	IV: 100 mg 1×, then 50 mg q12h × 5–14 d	NA (K, F, L)	Inj
Other Antibiotics			
Chloramphenicol▲	po, IV: 50 mg/kg/d q6h; max: 4 g/d	NA (L)	Inj
Clindamycin▲	po: 150–450 mg q6–8h; max: 1.8 g/d IM, IV: 1.2–1.8 g/d q8–12h; max: 3.6 g/d	NA (L)	C: 75, 150, 300 S: 75 mg/5 mL Inj

(cont.)

Table 77. Antibiotics (cont.)

Antimicrobial Class, *Subclass*	Dosage	Adjust When CrCl[1] Is: (Elimination)	Formulations
Trimethoprim-sulfamethoxazole▲BC	Doses based on the trimethoprim component: po: 1 double-strength tab q12h IV: sepsis: 20 TMP/kg/d given q6h	≤30 (K, L)	T: SMZ 400, TMP 80 double-strength: SMZ 800, TMP 160 S: SMZ 200, TMP 40 mg/5 mL Inj
Dalbavancin *(Dalvance)*	IV: 1000 mg × 1 dose, then 500 mg × 1 dose 1 wk later	<30	Inj
Daptomycin▲	IV: 4 mg/kg/d × 7–14 d	<30 (K, L)	Inj
Fosfomycin *(Monurol)*	Complicated UTI: Women—po: 3 g in 90–120 mL water × 1 dose Men—po: 3 g in 90–120 mL water q2–3d × 3 doses Prostatitis—po: 3 g in 90–120 mL water q3d × 21 d	(K, F)	pwd: 3 g/pk
Linezolid▲	po: 600 mg q12h IV: 600 mg q12h	NA	T: 600 S: 100 mg/5 mL Inj
Metronidazole▲	po: 250–750 mg q6–8h	≤10 (L, K, F)	T: 250, 500▲ ER: 750 C: 375▲ Susp: 50, 100/mL
	Topical: apply q12h		Topical gel: 0.75%▲ (30 g)
	Vaginal: 1 applicator full (375 mg) qhs or q12h		Vaginal gel: 0.75%▲ (70 g) Inj▲
Nitrofurantoin▲BC	po: 50–100 mg q6h	Do not use if <30 (L, K)	C: 25, 50, 100 S: 25 mg/5 mL
Oritavancin *(Orbactiv)*	IV: 1200 mg × 1 dose for ABSSI	(K, F)	Inj
Quinupristin-dalfopristin *(Synercid)*	Vancomycin-resistant *E faecium:* IV: 7.5 mg/kg q8h Complicated skin or skin structure infection: 7.5 mg/kg q12h	NA (L, B, F, K)	Inj
Tedizolid *(Sivextro)*	po, IV: 200 mg q24h × 6 d for BSSI	(L)	T, Inj: 200 mg
Telavancin *(Vibativ)*	IV: 10 mg/kg q24h × 1–2 wk	≤50 (K)	Inj
Vancomycin▲	po: *C difficile:* 125–500 mg q6–8h IV: 500 mg–1 g q8–24h Trough: 10–20 mcg/mL; 15–10 mcg/mL if complicated or MRSA suspected	<60 (K)	C: 125, 250 S: 25, 50 mg/mL Inj

(cont.)

Antimicrobial Class, *Subclass*	Dosage	Adjust When CrCl[1] Is: (Elimination)	Formulations
Antifungals (also **Table 45**)			
Amphotericin			
Amphotericin B▲	IV: test dose: 1 mg infused over 20–30 min; if tolerated, initial therapeutic dosage is 0.25 mg/kg; the daily dosage can be increased by 0.25-mg/kg increments on each subsequent day until the desired daily dosage is reached Maintenance dosage: IV: 0.25–1 mg/kg/d or 1.5 mg/kg q48h; do not exceed 1.5 mg/kg/d	[3] (K)	Inj
Amphotericin B Lipid Complex *(Abelcet)*	2.5–5 mg/kg/d as a single infusion	[3] (K)	Inj
Amphotericin B Liposomal *(AmBisome)*	3–6 mg/kg/d infused over 1–2 h	[3] (K)	Inj
Amphotericin B Cholesteryl Sulfate Complex *(Amphotec)*	3–4 mg/kg/d infused at 1 mg/kg/h; max dosage 7.5 mg/kg/d	[3] (K)	Inj
Azoles			
Fluconazole▲	po, IV: 1st dose 200–800 mg, then 100–400 mg q24h for 14 d–12 wk, depending on indication Vaginal candidiasis: 150 mg as a single dose	<50 (K)	T: 50, 100, 150, 200 S: 10, 40 mg/mL Inj
Itraconazole *(Sporanox)*	po: 200–400 mg/d; dosages >200 mg/d should be divided. Life-threatening infections: loading dose: 200 mg q8h should be given for the 1st 3 d of tx IV: 200 mg q12h × 4 d, then 200 mg/d	<30 (L)	C: 100▲ T: 200 S: 10 mg/mL Inj
Ketoconazole▲	po: 200–400 mg/d shp: 2/wk × 4 wk with ≥3 d between each shp Topical: apply q12–24h	NA (L, F)	T: 200 shp: 2% crm: 2%
Miconazole▲	IT: 20 mg q1–2d IV: initial: 200 mg, then 1.2–3.6 g/d divided q8h for up to 2 wk	NA (L, F)	Inj
Posaconazole *(Noxafil)*	Candida or aspergillosis, invasive: Prophylaxis: T: 300 mg × 1 d; Maintenance: T: 300 mg q24h; Sus: 200 mg q8h; IV: 300 mg × 2 on day 1, maintenance 300 mg q24h. Duration: recovery from neutropenia or immunosuppression. Oropharyngeal infection: Initial: 100 mg q12h × 1 d; maintenance: 100 mg q24h × 13 d.	NA	T: 100 Sus: 40 mg/mL Inj

(cont.)

Table 77. Antibiotics (cont.)

Antimicrobial Class, *Subclass*	Dosage	Adjust When CrCl[1] Is: (Elimination)	Formulations
	Refractory oropharyngeal infection: Sus: 400 mg q12h; duration based on underlying disease and clinical response.		
Voriconazole▲	IV: loading dose 6 mg/kg q12h for 2 doses, then 4 mg/kg q12h po: >40 kg: 200 mg q12h; ≤ 40 kg: 100 mg q12h If on phenytoin, IV: 5 mg/kg q12h, and po: >40 kg: 400 mg q12h; ≤40 kg: 200 mg q12h	<50 (IV only) (L)	Inj T: 50, 200 mg Sus: 40 mg/mL
Echinocandins			
Anidulafungin *(Eraxis)*	Esophageal candidiasis: 100 mg on day 1, then 50 mg/d × ≥13 d and 7 d after symptoms resolve	NA (L, F)	Inj
Caspofungin▲	Initial: 70 mg infused over 1 h; esophageal candidiasis: 50 mg/d; dosage with concurrent enzyme inducers: 70 mg/d	NA (L, F)	Inj
Micafungin *(Mycamine)*	Esophageal candidiasis: 150 mg/d; prophylaxis in stem cell transplant: 50 mg/d	NA (L, F, K)	Inj
Other Antifungals			
Flucytosine▲	po: 50–150 mg/kg/d divided q6h	<40 (K)	C: 250, 500
Griseofulvin▲	po: Microsize: 500–1000 mg/d in single or divided doses Ultramicrosize: 330–375 mg/d in single or divided doses Duration based on indication	NA (L)	Microsize: S: 125 mg/5 mL T: 125, 250, 500
Isavuconazium *(Cresemba)*	IV po: 372 mg q8h × 6 doses, then 372 mg q24h	NA (L)	C: 186 Inj
Terbinafine▲	po: 250 mg/d × 6–12 wk for superficial mycoses; 250–500 mg/d for up to 16 mo Topical: apply q12–24h for max of 4 wk	<50 (L, K)	T: 250 mg▲

ABSSI = acute bacterial skin and skin structure infection; BSSI = bacterial skin and skin structure infection; NA = not applicable; TDM = adjust dose on basis of therapeutic drug monitoring principles and institutional protocols.

[1] The CrCl (mL/min/1.73 m^2) listed is the threshold below which the dosage (amount or frequency) should be adjusted. See package insert for detailed dosing guidelines.

[2] Dosage should not exceed 250 mg q6h in kidney impairment.

[3] Adjust dosage if decreased kidney function is due to the medication, or give every other day.

[BC]Avoid.

HEMATURIA

Definition

Microscopic: ≥3 RBCs per high-power field; Gross: red or brown urine visible to the naked eye; may be transient.

Common causes in older persons

- Bladder cancer (more common in older persons)
- UTI
- Stones
- Acute kidney injury
- Glomerulonephritis
- Interstitial disease (eg, analgesic nephropathy)
- BPH or prostate cancer
- Vigorous exercise
- Excessive anticoagulant tx
- No cause identified (may be up to 60%)

Evaluation

- Dipstick and microscopic analysis
- If microscopic (≥ 3 RBC/high-power field) only, assess for other causes including UTI or recent urologic procedures and treat appropriately. Repeat UA. If negative, no further workup. If positive, renal function testing, cystoscopy, and imaging with either CT urography or ultrasound and selective CT. If proteinuria, RBC or WBC casts, worsened KFTs or edema, refer to nephrology for glomerular evaluation.
- If gross, and visible clots, CT and urgent urology referral. If no clots, renal function testing, cystoscopy, and imaging with either CT urography or ultrasound and selective CT. If proteinuria, RBC or WBC casts, worsened KFTs or edema, refer to nephrology for glomerular evaluation.
- If due to UTI, repeat UA 6 wk after completing tx.
- Women may need pelvic exam to exclude vaginal bleeding.

ACUTE KIDNEY INJURY

Definition

An acute deterioration in kidney function defined by increased values of kidney function tests (eg, increase in Cr of ≥0.3 mg/dL within 48 h or by >50% within 7 d, or decreased urine volume (<0.4 mL/kg/h for 6 h). Oliguria (<500 mL urine output/d) has worse prognosis.

Precipitating and Aggravating Factors *(Italicized type indicates most common.)*

- *Acute tubular necrosis* due to hypoperfusion or nephrotoxins
- Medications (eg, aminoglycosides, radiocontrast materials, NSAIDs, ACEIs), including those causing allergic interstitial nephritis (eg, NSAIDs, penicillins and cephalosporins, sulfonamides, fluoroquinolones, allopurinol, rifampin, PPIs)
- Multiple myeloma
- Obstruction (eg, BPH)
- Cardiovascular disease (cardiorenal syndrome, thromboembolic, atheroembolic)
- *Volume depletion* or redistribution of ECF (eg, cirrhosis, burns)

Evaluation

- Review medication list
- Catheterize bladder or determine postvoid residual by ultrasound
- UA (**Table 78** for likely diagnoses)
- Renal ultrasonography
- Renal biopsy in selected cases
- If patient is not on diuretics, determine fractional excretion of sodium (FENa):

$$FENa = \left[\frac{urine\ Na/plasma\ Na}{urine\ Cr/plasma\ Cr} \right] \times 100$$

FENa <1% indicates prerenal cause; FENa >2% generally indicates acute tubular necrosis; FENa 1–2% is nondiagnostic. Some older adults who have prerenal cause may have FENa ≥1% because of age-related changes in sodium excretion.

- If patient is receiving diuretics, determine fractional excretion of urea (FEUrea):

$$FEUrea = \left[\frac{urine\ urea\ nitrogen/BUN}{urine\ Cr/plasma\ Cr} \right] \times 100$$

FEUrea ≤35% indicates prerenal azotemia; FEUrea >50% indicates acute tubular necrosis; FEUrea 36–50% is nondiagnostic.

Table 78. Likely Diagnoses Based on UA Findings	
Findings	**Diagnoses**
Hematuria, RBC casts, heavy proteinuria	Glomerular disease or vasculitis
Granular and epithelial cell casts, free epithelial cells	Acute tubular necrosis
Pyuria, WBC casts, granular or waxy casts, little or no proteinuria	Acute interstitial nephritis, glomerulitis, vasculitis, obstruction, renal infarction
Normal UA	Prerenal disease, obstruction, hypercalcemia, myeloma, acute tubular necrosis

Urinary eosinophils are neither sensitive nor specific for acute interstitial nephritis but may be helpful in some cases.

Prevention of Radiocontrast-induced Acute Kidney Failure in High-Risk Patients

Persons at risk: *High risk:* GFR <30 mL/min/1.73 m^2 BSA and not receiving dialysis; *Increased risk:* GFR <60 mL/min/1.73 m^2 BSA proteinuria >500 mg/d, DM, HF, liver failure, or myeloma, or GFR <45 mL/min/1.73 m^2 BSA without comorbidities)

Indications for Use of Radiocontrast

- MRI radiocontrast is gadolinium given IV. Avoid if GFR <30 mL/min/1.73 m^2. Can cause nephrogenic systemic fibrosis.
- CT radiocontrast are iodinated agents give IV or po (diluted). Low osmolal or iso-osmolal contrast agents should be used in low doses.
- Brain CTs generally should be noncontrast unless evaluating for an abscess, malignancy, or if focal deficits.
- Cardiothoracic CT can be noncontrast for coronary calcium scoring and pulmonary parenchymal evaluation.
- Abdomen and pelvic CT scan be noncontrast when evaluating for ureteral calculi, acute bleeding, or retroperitoneal hematoma, or CT colonography. For all other indications, contrast is preferred, usually IV unless looking for perforation, fistula, or obstruction of bowel.

- Risk of nephrotoxicity is almost exclusively associated with IV contrast.

Reducing Risk

- Hold NSAIDs and diuretics for 24 h and metformin for 48 h before administration.
- Avoid closely spaced repeat studies (eg, <48 h apart).
- If inpatient, IV hydration with 0.9% saline 1 mL/kg/h for 24 h beginning 6–12 h before administration and continuing 6–12 h after procedure.
- If outpatient, 3 mL/kg over 1 h before procedure, and 1–1.5 mL/kg/h during and 4–6 h after procedure
- Repeat serum Cr 24–48 h after administration.

Treatment of Acute Kidney Injury

- D/C medications that are possible precipitants; avoid contrast dyes.
- Crystalloid (eg, Ringers solution or *PlasmaLyte*) rather than saline fluid replacement.
- If prerenal pattern, treat HF (p 48) if present. Otherwise, volume repletion. Begin with fluid challenge 500–1000 mL over 30–60 min. If urine output does not increase in response, give furosemide 100–400 mg IV.
- If obstructed, leave urinary catheter in place during evaluation and while specific tx is implemented.
- If acute tubular necrosis, monitor weight daily, record intake and output, and monitor electrolytes frequently. Fluid replacement should be equal to urinary output plus other drainage plus 500 mL/d for insensible losses.
- If acute interstitial nephritis (except if NSAID-induced) and does not resolve with 3–7 d, glucocorticoids (eg, prednisone 1 mg/kg/d) for a minimum 1–2 wk and gradual taper when Cr has returned near baseline for a total duration of 2–3 mo.
- Dialysis is indicated when severe hyperkalemia, acidosis, or volume overload cannot be managed with other tx or when uremic symptoms (eg, pericarditis, coagulopathy, or encephalopathy) are present.

CHRONIC KIDNEY DISEASE

Definition

Kidney damage as evidenced by urinary albumin excretion of >30 mg/d or eGFR <60 mL/min/1.73 m^2, for 3 mo or more irrespective of the cause.

Classification (Kidney Disease Outcomes Quality Initiative)

- *Stage G1:* GFR >90 mL/min/1.73 m^2 and persistent albuminuria
- *Stage G2:* GFR 60–89 mL/min/1.73 m^2 and persistent albuminuria
- *Stage G3a:* GFR 45–59 mL/min/1.73 m^2
- *Stage G3b:* GFR 30–44 mL/min/1.73 m^2
- *Stage G4:* GFR 15–29 mL/min/1.73 m^2
- *Stage G5:* GFR <15 mL/min/1.73 m^2 or end-stage renal disease

Albumin

A1: Daily albumin excretion rate <30 mg/dL

A2: Daily albumin excretion rate 30–300 mg/dL

A3: Daily albumin excretion rate >300 mg/dL

- Cause of CKD also has prognostic value for kidney outcomes and other complications.
- Refer to a nephrologist for co-management if stages G4 or G5, or CKD complications (see below).

Evaluation

- Hx and physical examination: assess for DM, HTN, vascular disease, HF, NSAIDs, contrast dye exposure, angiographic procedures with possible cholesterol embolization, glomerulonephritis, myeloma, BPH or obstructive cancers, current or previous tx with a nephrotoxic drug, hereditary kidney disease (eg, polycystic)
- Blood tests (CBC, comprehensive metabolic profile, phosphorus, cholesterol, ESR, serum protein immunoelectrophoresis)
- Progression to kidney failure can be predicted by age, sex, eGFR, urine albumin:Cr ratio, serum calcium, serum phosphate, serum bicarbonate, and serum albumin using equation: qxmd.com/calculate-online/nephrology/kidney-failure-risk-equation.
- Estimate CrCl or GFR (p 1). CrCl is usually about 20% higher than true GFR. eGFR based on the MDRD equation and true GFR are very close when the GFR is <60 mL/min/1.73 m^2, but true GFR exceeds eGFR by a small amount when GFR is >60 mL/min/1.73 m^2. Older people with eGFR 45–59 mL/min/1.73 m^2 may have normal kidney function for their age and are less likely to progress to kidney failure compared younger persons.
- If GFR 15–59 mL/min/1.73 m^2, measure iPTH; if iPTH >100 pg/mL, measure serum 25(OH)D.
- UA and quantitative urine protein (protein:Cr ratio or 24-h urine for protein and Cr); urine immunoelectrophoresis, if indicated; at all stages, heavier proteinuria is predictive of mortality, ESRD, and doubling of serum Cr.
- Renal ultrasound (large kidneys suggest tumors, infiltrating disease, cystic disease; small kidneys suggest CKD; can also identify cysts, stones, masses, and hydronephrosis)
- Exclude renal artery stenosis with MRI angiography, spiral CT with CT angiography, or duplex Doppler ultrasound if acute rise in Cr shortly after beginning tx with ACEI or ARB
- Renal biopsy in selected cases

Treatment

- Attempt to slow progression of kidney failure by:
  - Controlling BP *most important* (target <130/80 if stage 3 or higher, or stage 1 or 2 if albuminuria >300 mg/d [ACC])
  - If DM or proteinuria, begin ACEI or ARB (**Table 24**) regardless of whether or not patient has HTN. Moderate dietary protein restriction, 0.8–1 g/kg/d, especially if diabetic nephropathy; if stage G4 or G5 CKD, consider low-protein (0.6 g/kg/d) diet. Goal is reduction of proteinuria to <1 g/d, if possible and at least to <60% of baseline.
  - Smoking cessation
  - Diet: if eGFR <60 mL/min/1.73 m^2
    - Restrict dietary caloric intake to 30–34 kcal/kg/d, with <30% as fat with saturated fat <10%
    - Restrict dietary protein to 0.8 g/kg/d
    - Restrict dietary sodium to <2 g/d if hypertension, volume overload, or increased protein excretion, and to <2.3 g/d if none of these comorbidities
    - Restrict total dietary calcium to 1000–1500/d
    - If eGFR <30 mL/min/1.73 m2, restrict dietary potassium
  - Treat hyperlipidemia (p 53).
  - Treat chronic acidosis: Sodium bicarbonate (daily dosage of 0.5–1 mEq/kg) tx to maintain serum bicarbonate concentration >23 mEq/L
  - Control blood sugar if patient has type 2 DM. Consider SGLT-2 inhibitors (**Table 47**)
  - Avoid triamterene, spironolactone, and NSAIDs[CW] in stages 4 and 5 CKD.[BC]
- Prevent and treat symptoms and complications
  - Hyperkalemia: if present (p 201); low-potassium diet <40–70 mEq/d; avoid NSAIDs.

- Mineral and bone complications:
  - Avoid aluminum and magnesium phosphate binders.
  - Normalize serum calcium with calcium carbonate▲ (500 mg elemental calcium q6–24h) or calcium acetate *(Phoslo)* (3 or 4 tabs q8h with meals); if hypocalcemia is refractory, consider calcitriol *(Rocaltrol)* 0.25 mcg/d.
  - Normalize serum phosphate (2.7–4.6 g/dL) if not on dialysis and maintain between 3.5 and 5.5 mg/dL if on dialysis; restrict dairy products and cola to phosphate intake <900 mg/d. When hyperphosphatemia is refractory, begin:
    - If serum calcium is low, calcium carbonate▲ (1250–1500 mg q8h with meals) or calcium acetate *(Phoslo)* (3 or 4 tabs q8h with meals).
    - If serum calcium is normal or calcium supplementation is ineffective:
      - Sevelamer hydrochloride *(Renagel)* [T: 400, 800; C: 403] or sevelamer carbonate *(Renvela)* [0.8 g pk, T: 800], which does not lower bicarbonate, 800–1600 mg po q8h with each meal.
      - Lanthanum carbonate *(Fosrenol)* [ChT: 250, 500] at initial dosage of 250–500 mg po q8h with each meal, then titrate in increments of 750 mg/d at intervals of 2–3 wk to max of 3750 mg/d.
- Treating vitamin D insufficiency improves biochemical markers but the effect on clinical outcomes is uncertain. Use vitamin D_2 (ergocalciferol) 50,000 U/mo or oral vitamin D with calcitriol 25 mcg/d if 25(OH)D is <30 ng/mL. Stop if corrected serum calcium is >10.2 mg/dL.
- Patients on dialysis with secondary hyperparathyroidism should be treated with the phosphate binders and vitamin D tx above as well as calcimimetics that increase the sensitivity of the calcium-sensing receptor in the parathyroid gland, including cinacalcet *(Sensipar)* 30–180 mg orally 1×/d [T: 30, 60, 90] or etelcalcetide *(Parsabiv)* 5 mg IV 3×/wk at the end of hemodialysis.
- Anemia: Monitor Hb yearly if stage G3, q6mo if stages G4 or G5, and q3mo if on dialysis. Treat anemia with iron (if iron deficient) to maintain transferrin saturation >20% and serum ferritin >100 ng/L and, if necessary, erythropoietin-darbepoetin to maintain a target Hb goal of ≤11 g/dL. Don't administer erythropoiesis-stimulating agents to patients with CKD with Hb ≥10 g/dL without signs or symptoms.[CW]
- Cardiovascular (as noted above)
- Prevention: Immunize with *Pneumovax, Prevnar,* and, if stage G4 or G5 CKD, hepatitis B vaccines if hepatitis B surface antigen and antibody are negative.
- Elicit the patient's goals of care, including discussions with family. Educate patients regarding options of hemodialysis, peritoneal dialysis, kidney transplantation, conservative medical tx, and hospice.
- If preferred by patient, prepare for dialysis or transplant. If eGFR <25 mL/min/1.73 m², recommend referral for arteriovenous fistula access, which takes months before it is ready to be used.
- If eGFR <20 mL/min/1.73 m², patients can be listed for cadaveric kidney transplant. Patients aged >65 can be considered for transplantation if substantial life expectancy.
- Dialysis is medically indicated when severe hyperkalemia, acidosis, or volume overload cannot be managed with other tx or when uremic symptoms (eg, pericarditis or pleuritis, coagulopathy, persistent nausea and vomiting, severe malnutrition, or encephalopathy) are present.
- Other than transplantation, renal replacement can be by hemodialysis or peritoneal dialysis (continuous or automated, which uses short dwells and automated technology to operate at near maximum solute clearance rates). Although more older persons select

hemodialysis and few switch from hemodialysis to peritoneal dialysis, differences in survival between approaches have not been demonstrated.

- Don't perform routine cancer screening for dialysis patients with limited life expectancies without signs or symptoms.**[CW]**
- If quality of life on dialysis is unsatisfactory or medical conditions have progressed, discuss discontinuing dialysis.

VOLUME DEPLETION (DEHYDRATION)

Definition

Losses of sodium and water that may be isotonic (eg, loss of blood) or hypotonic (eg, nasogastric suctioning)

Precipitating Factors

- Blood loss
- Diuretics
- GI losses
- Kidney or adrenal disease (eg, renal sodium wasting)
- Sequestration of fluid (eg, ileus, burns, peritonitis)
- Age-related changes (impaired thirst, sodium wasting due to hyporeninemic hypoaldosteronism, and free water wasting due to renal insensitivity to antidiuretic hormone)

Evaluation

Clinical Symptoms

- Anorexia
- Nausea and vomiting
- Orthostatic lightheadedness
- Delirium
- Weakness
- Acute weight loss

Clinical Signs

- Dry tongue and axillae
- Oliguria
- Orthostatic hypotension
- Elevated HR
- Weight loss (most specific)

Laboratory Tests

- Serum electrolytes
- Urine sodium (usually <10 mEq/L) and FENa (usually <1% but may be higher because of age-related sodium wasting, diuretics, renal ischemia)
- Serum BUN and Cr (BUN:Cr ratio often >20)

Management

- Weigh daily; monitor fluid losses and serum electrolytes, BUN, Cr.
- If mild, oral rehydration of 2–4 L of water/d and 4–8 g Na diet; if poor oral intake, give IV D5W 1/2 NS with potassium as needed.
- If hemodynamically unstable, give IV Ringer's lactate or 0.9% saline 1–2 L as quickly as possible until SBP ≥100 mmHg and no longer orthostatic. Then switch to D5W 1/2 NS. Monitor closely in patients with a hx of HF. Avoid hyperoncotic starch solutions, which are associated with acute kidney injury and increased mortality.

HYPERNATREMIA

Causes

- Pure water loss
  - Insensible losses due to sweating and respiration

- Impaired thirst (eg, delirious or intubated) or access to water (eg, functionally dependent) may sustain hypernatremia
- Central (eg, posttraumatic, CNS tumors, meningitis) diabetes insipidus or nephrogenic (eg, hypercalcemia, lithium) diabetes insipidus
- Hypotonic sodium loss
  - Renal causes: osmotic diuresis (eg, due to hyperglycemia), postobstructive diuresis, polyuric phase of acute tubular necrosis
  - GI causes: vomiting and diarrhea, nasogastric drainage, osmotic cathartic agents (eg, lactulose)
- Hypertonic sodium gain (eg, tx with hypertonic saline)

Evaluation
- Measure intake and output.
- Obtain urine osmolality:
  - >800 mOsm/kg suggests extrarenal (if urine Na <25 mEq/L) or remote renal water loss or administration of hypertonic Na+ salt solutions (if urine Na >100 mEq/L).
  - <250 mOsm/kg and polyuria suggest diabetes insipidus.

Treatment
- Treat underlying causes.
- If acute (eg, developing over hours), correct using D5W at a rate of 3–6 mL/kg/h with a goal of correcting by no more than 1–2 mmol/L/h.
- If chronic (present for >48 h), correct over 48–72 h using oral (can use pure water), nasogastric (can use pure water), or IV (D5W, 1/2 or 1/4 NS) fluids at 1.35 mL/h × body weight in kg (approximately 70 mL/h for a 50-kg person and 100 mL/h for a 70-kg person) with correction goal of 6–10 mmol/L/d.
- Correct with NS only in cases of severe volume depletion with hemodynamic compromise; once stable, switch to hypotonic solution.

HYPONATREMIA

Classifications

Acuity: hyperacute (within hours), acute (within 24 h), chronic (at least 48 h or unknown)

Severity: mild (130–135 mEq/L), moderate (121–129 mEq/L), severe (≤120 mEq/L)

Symptoms: absent, mild to moderate (eg, headache, nausea, vomiting, fatigue, gait disturbances, confusion), severe (eg, seizures, obtundation, coma, respiratory arrest)

Causes
- With increased plasma osmolality: hyperglycemia (1.6 mEq/L decrement for each 100 mg/dL increase in plasma glucose)
- With normal plasma osmolality (pseudohyponatremia): severe hyperlipidemia, hyperproteinemia (eg, multiple myeloma)
- With decreased plasma osmolality:
  - With ECF excess: kidney failure, HF, hepatic cirrhosis, nephrotic syndrome
  - With decreased ECF volume: renal loss from salt-losing nephropathies, diuretics, cerebral salt wasting, osmotic diuresis; extrarenal loss due to vomiting, diarrhea, skin losses, and 3rd-spacing (usually urine Na <20 mEq/L, FENa <1%, and uric acid >4 mg/dL)
  - With normal ECF volume: primary polydipsia (urine osmolarity <100 mOsm/kg), hypothyroidism, adrenal insufficiency, SIADH (urine Na >40 mEq/L and uric acid <4 mg/dL)

Management

Treat underlying cause. Specific tx only if symptomatic (eg, altered mental status, seizures), severe acute hyponatremia (eg, <120 mEq/L), or hyperacute regardless of symptoms.

- If initial volume estimate is equivocal, give fluid challenge of 0.5–1 L of isotonic (0.9%) saline.
- If volume depletion, give saline IV (corrects ~1 mEq/L for every liter given) or oral salt tablets.
- If edematous states, SIADH, or chronic renal failure, fluid restriction to below the level of urine output is the primary tx.
- Hypovolemic hyponatremia is almost always chronic (except for cerebral salt wasting and after diuretic initiation), and hypertonic saline is seldom indicated.
- Emergent tx with hypertonic (3%) saline initially with 100 mL bolus over 10–15 min; correct 2–4 mEq/L (goal is 4–6 mEq/L) in 1st 2–4 h. Concurrent desmopressin (1–2 µg IV or SC q6–8h for 24–48 h) may help prevent overly rapid correction but is usually not used if HF or cirrhosis. Monitor sodium q2h. Indications include:
  - severe symptoms
  - acute hyponatremia (<24 h) even with mild symptoms
  - hyperacute due to self-induced water intoxication
  - symptomatic postoperative hyponatremia or associated with intracranial pathology
- Nonemergent tx for
  - asymptomatic acute or subacute hyponatremia or chronic severe hyponatremia with mild to moderate symptoms: 3% hypertonic saline 50 mL bolus or slow infusion 15–30 mL/h
  - chronic moderate hyponatremia with mild to moderate symptoms
  - If edematous states, SIADH, advanced CKD, or primary polydipsia, restrict fluids.
- Goal is <4–6 mEq/L Na rise during 1st 24 h and no more than 8 mEq/L in any 24 h (more rapid correction can result in central pontine myelinolysis).
- Monitor Na closely and taper tx when >120 mEq/L or symptoms resolve.
- Arginine vasopressin receptor antagonists
  - Conivaptan *(Vaprisol)* is effective in euvolemic hyponatremia in hospitalized patients; 20 mg IV over 30 min 1×, followed by continuous infusion of 20–40 mg over 24 h for 4 d max (L) (CYP3A4 interactions).
  - Tolvaptan *(Samsca)* 15–60 mg/d [T: 15, 30]: initiate in hospital and monitor blood sodium concentration closely. Not to be given to patients with liver disease and not to be used for ≥30 d.

SYNDROME OF INAPPROPRIATE SECRETION OF ANTIDIURETIC HORMONE (SIADH)

Definition

Hypotonic hyponatremia (<280 mOsm/kg) with:

- Less than maximally dilute urine (usually >100 mOsm/kg)
- Elevated urine sodium (usually >40 mEq/L)
- Normal volume status
- Normal kidney, adrenal, and thyroid function

Precipitating Factors, Causes

- Medications (eg, SSRIs and SNRIs, especially if borderline low Na; chlorpropamide; carbamazepine; oxcarbazepine; NSAIDs; barbiturates; antipsychotics; mirtazapine. Use with caution.[BC])
- Neuropsychiatric factors (eg, neoplasm, subarachnoid hemorrhage, psychosis, meningitis)
- Postoperative state, especially if pain or nausea
- Pulmonary disease (eg, pneumonia, tuberculosis, acute asthma)

- Tumors (eg, lung, pancreas, thymus)
- Reset osmostat (mild hyponatremia stable over days despite variations in Na and water intake)

Evaluation

- BUN, Cr, serum cortisol, TSH
- CXR
- Review of medications
- Neurologic tests as indicated
- Urine sodium and osmolality
- If osmostat reset is suspected, give water load (10–15 mL/kg po or IV); if reset osmostat, will excrete water load within 4 h.

Management

Acute Treatment: See euvolemic hyponatremia management, p 200.

Chronic Treatment:

- D/C offending medication or treat precipitating illness.
- No tx is needed for reset osmostat.
- Restrict water intake (unless due to subarachnoid hemorrhage) to <800 mL/d with goal of Na ≥130 mEq/L. Rate of correction should be <8 mEq/L/d.
- Liberalize salt intake or give salt tablets. Can also give IV saline but the electrolyte concentration of the fluid must be greater than the electrolyte concentration of urine. Usually, hypertonic saline, if given.
- If urinary osmolality is twice the plasma osmolality, loop diuretics (eg, furosemide 20 mg q12h) may help facilitate excess water excretion.
- Demeclocycline▲ 150–300 mg q12h [T: 150, 300] (may be nephrotoxic in patients with liver disease) only if symptomatic and above steps do not work.
- Tolvaptan *(Samsca)* 15–60 mg/d [T:15, 30]: initiate in hospital and monitor blood sodium concentration closely only if symptomatic and above steps do not work. Risk of hepatotoxicity. Do not use for >30 d and do not use in patients with chronic liver diseases.

HYPERKALEMIA

Causes

- Kidney failure
- Addison disease
- Hyporeninemic hypoaldosteronism
- Renal tubular acidosis
- Acidosis
- Diabetic hyperglycemia
- Hemolysis, tumor lysis, rhabdomyolysis
- Medications (potassium-sparing diuretics, ACEIs, trimethoprim-sulfamethoxazole, β-blockers, NSAIDs, cyclosporine, tacrolimus, pentamidine, calcineurin inhibitors, heparin, digoxin toxicity)
- Pseudohyperkalemia from extreme thrombocytosis or leukocytosis or improper blood drawing (betadine antiseptic, mechanical trauma, repeated fist clenching, prolonged tourniquet application) or handling (not centrifuged within 30 min of drawing)
- Transfusions of stored blood
- Constipation

Evaluation

- ECG; peaked T waves typically occur when K+ exceeds 6.5 mEq/L. ECG changes are more likely with acute increases of K+ than with chronic increases.

Treatment

- K+ <6 mEq/L without ECG changes:

- Low-potassium diet (restrict orange juice, bananas, potatoes, cantaloupe, honeydew, tomatoes)
- May be stable and not need medical tx
- Oral diuretics (eg, oral torsemide or bumetanide, combined oral loop and thiazide-like diuretics; metolazone is the most K+ wasting); avoid hypovolemia
- Oral sodium bicarbonate (650–1300 mg q12h); not recommended as a single agent
- Reduce or D/C medications that increase K+
- K+ 6–6.5 mEq/L without ECG changes: above tx plus
  - Sodium polystyrene sulfonate▲ 15–30 g po q6–24h, or prn as enema 30–50 g in 100 mL of dextrose; full effect takes 4–24 h and generally requires multiple doses over 1–5 d. Can expect approximately 1 mEq/L reduction. If taken orally, can bind to other drugs, and when given rectally, can cause intestinal necrosis if bowel dysfunction or recent GI surgery.
  - Patiromer *(Veltassa)* 8.4 g/d with food and may be titrated up each wk to max 25.2 g. If taking ciprofloxacin, levothyroxine, or metformin, separate administration of patiromer and other drug by 3 h.
- K+ 6.5 mEq/L with peaked T waves but no other ECG changes: hospitalization is decided case-by-case based on acuteness of onset, cause, and other patient factors.

Absolute indications for hospitalization

- K+ >8 mEq/L
- ECG changes other than peaked T waves (eg, prolonged PR, loss of P waves, widened QRS)
- Acute deterioration of kidney function

Inpatient Management of Hyperkalemia

- Antagonism of cardiac effects of hyperkalemia (most rapid-acting acute tx; use only for severe hyperkalemia with significant ECG changes when too dangerous to wait for redistribution tx to take effect)
  - 10% calcium gluconate IV infused over 2–3 min (20–30 min if on digoxin) with ECG monitoring; effect lasts 30–60 min, may repeat if needed
- Reduction of serum K+ by redistribution into cells (acute tx; can be used in combination with calcium gluconate, and different redistribution tx can be combined depending on severity of hyperkalemia)
  - Insulin (regular) 10 U in 500 mL of 10% dextrose over 30–60 min or bolus insulin (regular) 10 U IV followed by 50 mL of 50% dextrose
  - Albuterol 0.5 mg in 100 mL of 5% dextrose given over 10–15 min or nebulized 10–20 mg in 4 mL of NS over 10 min (should not be used as single agent)
  - Sodium bicarbonate if significant metabolic acidosis, but should not be used as single agent.
- Removal of potassium from body (definitive tx; work more slowly)
  - Diuretics (eg, oral torsemide or bumetanide, IV furosemide, combined oral loop and thiazide-like diuretics; metolazone is the most K+ wasting). Avoid hypovolemia.
  - Fludrocortisone▲ 0.1–0.3 mg/d
  - Sodium polystyrene sulfonate▲ 15–30 g po q6–24h or prn as enema 30–50 g in 100 mL of dextrose; full effect takes 4–24 h and typically requires multiple doses over 1–5 d. Can expect ~1 mEq/d reduction. Do not use in postoperative patients, patients with ileus, patients receiving opiates, or patients with ulcerative colitis, *C difficile* colitis, or bowel obstruction. If packaged in sorbitol to prevent fecal impaction, may cause intestinal necrosis.
  - Dialysis

REQUIREMENTS, DIET, AND SUPPLEMENTS

Calculating Basic Energy (Caloric), Protein, and Fluid Requirements

- WHO energy estimates for adults aged 60 and older:
  - Women (10.5) (weight in kg) + 596
  - Men (13.5) (weight in kg) + 487
- Harris-Benedict energy requirement equations:
  - Women: 655 + (9.6) (weight in kg) + (1.7) (height in cm) – (4.7) (age in y)
  - Men: 66 + (13.7) (weight in kg) + (5) (height in cm) – (6.8) (age in y)
  - Depending on activity and physiologic stress levels, these basic requirements may need to be increased (eg, 25% for sedentary or mild, 50% for moderate, and 100% for intense or severe activity or stress).
  - Based on observational data that associated lower protein intake with increased incident mobility limitation, protein intake of ≥1 g/kg body weight/d may be optimal.
- Fluid requirements for older adults without heart or kidney disease are ~30 mL/kg/d.

Mediterranean and Related Diets

- Observational data indicate improved health status and reductions in cardiovascular disease, cancer, and overall mortality, as well as lower incidences of Parkinson disease and Alzheimer disease (AD).
- Clinical trial data demonstrate reduction in major cardiovascular events and cognitive decline with Mediterranean diet supplemented by either extra-virgin olive oil or mixed nuts.
- In observational studies, DASH and Mediterranean-DASH Intervention for Neurodegenerative Delay (MIND) diets have also been associated with slowed cognitive decline and reduced incidence of AD.

Vitamins and Supplements

Vitamin D and Calcium

- All older adults should receive calcium 1200 mg/d and vitamin D 800–1000 IU/d. Each 8 oz glass of milk or fortified orange juice has approximately 100 IU. D_3 (cholecalciferol) is the preferred form of supplementation. The USPSTF concluded that there is insufficient evidence to recommend screening for vitamin D deficiency and recommends against vitamin D to prevent falls. Don't routinely measure 1,25(OH)2D or 25(OH)D unless the patient has hypercalcemia or decreased kidney function.[CW]
- Calcium supplements probably don't increase the risk of CVD. Data on risk of dementia and stroke-related dementia remain inconclusive. Risk of kidney stones is increased.

Multivitamins and Other Supplements

- Most older persons who eat a balanced diet do not need multivitamins.
- Observational data in postmenopausal women indicate no effect of multivitamins on breast, colorectal, endometrial, lung, or ovarian cancers, MI, stroke, VTE, or mortality.
- In clinical trials in middle-aged men, multivitamins have not been shown to decrease CVD or mortality, but there is a small reduction in total cancer risk.
- Clinical trial data show no benefit of multivitamins in reducing infections in outpatient and nursing-home settings.

- Clinical trial data show no benefit of fatty acids (docosahexaenoic acid [DHA]/ eicosapentaenoic acid [EPA]), antioxidants (lutein/zeaxanthin), or zinc supplements on cognitive decline.
- USPSTF recommends against use of beta carotene or vitamin E supplements to prevent CVD or cancer.
- Treat specific vitamin (eg, vitamin B12, folate) or micronutrient deficiencies if there are medical indications (See Hematologic Disorders, p 152, Neurologic Disorders, p 234). Don't routinely use vitamin B supplements for tx of polyneuropathy or neuropathic pain unless a deficiency exists.[CW]

UNDERNUTRITION
Definition
There is no uniformly accepted definition of undernutrition in older adults. Some commonly used definitions include those listed below.

Community-dwelling Older Adults
- American Society for Parenteral and Enteral Nutrition (ASPEN) criteria for adult malnutrition (2 of the following):
  - Insufficient energy intake
  - Loss of muscle mass
  - Fluid accumulation (eg, edema)
  - Weight loss
  - Loss of subcutaneous fat
  - Diminished function by hand-grip strength
- Involuntary weight loss (eg, ≥2% over 1 mo, >10 lb over 6 mo, ≥4% over 1 y)
- BMI <22 kg/m^2
- Hypoalbuminemia (eg, ≤3.8 g/dL)
- Hypocholesterolemia (eg, <160 mg/dL)
- Cancer-related anorexia/cachexia syndrome: a hypercatabolic state (increased resting energy expenditure) with high levels of tumor-activated or host-produced immune responses (eg, proinflammatory cytokines) to the tumor
- Sarcopenia age-related loss of muscle mass (eg, 2 SDs below mean for young healthy adults) with loss of strength and performance; contributors include decreased sex hormones, increased insulin resistance, increased inflammatory cytokines, decreased physical activity, inadequate protein intake, and spinal cord changes (decreased motor units)

Hospitalized Patients
- Dietary intake (eg, <50% of estimated needed caloric intake)
- Hypoalbuminemia (eg, <3.5 g/dL)
- Hypocholesterolemia (eg, <160 mg/dL)
- Refeeding syndrome caused by the glucose-induced acute transcellular shift of phosphate typically occurs in malnourished patients who have had poor oral intake and then receive either IV glucose-containing fluids or enteral or parenteral nutrition. Symptoms occur most commonly within 2–4 d of refeeding and include hypophosphatemia, hyperglycemia, and hyperinsulinemia, which may be accompanied by hypokalemia, hypomagnesemia, and fluid retention. Supplementing IV fluids with potassium phosphate or oral phosphate and potassium may help prevent this syndrome.

Nursing-home Patients (triggered by the CMS Minimum Data Set)
- Weight loss of ≥5% in past 30 d; ≥10% in 180 d
- Dietary intake <75% of most meals

Screening

Proposed screening instruments have not been adequately validated or do not demonstrate sufficient sensitivity and specificity to warrant use in clinical practice.

Multidimensional Assessment

In the absence of valid nutrition screening instruments, clinicians should focus on whether the following issues may be affecting nutritional status:
- Economic barriers to securing food
- Social isolation (eg, eating alone)
- Availability of sufficiently high-quality food
- Dental problems that preclude ingesting food
- Medical illnesses that:
  ◦ interfere with ingestion (eg, dysphagia), digestion, or absorption of food
  ◦ increase nutritional requirements or cause cachexia (especially cancer)
  ◦ require dietary restrictions (eg, low-sodium diet or npo)
  ◦ are treated with digoxin, cholinesterase inhibitors, SSRIs, amiodarone, topiramate
- Functional disability that interferes with shopping, preparing meals, or feeding
- Food preferences or cultural beliefs that interfere with adequate food intake
- Poor appetite
- Depressive symptoms (most common cause)

Anthropometrics

Weight on each visit and yearly height (p 1)

Evaluation for Comorbid Medical Conditions

- CBC, ESR, and comprehensive metabolic panel (if none abnormal, likelihood ratio for cancer is 0.2)
- CXR
- TSH

Biochemical Markers

Serum Proteins: All may drop precipitously because of trauma, sepsis, or major infection.
- Albumin (half-life 18–20 d) has prognostic value in all settings.
- Transferrin (half-life 7 d)
- Prealbumin (half-life 48 h) may be valuable in monitoring nutritional recovery.

Nonpharmacologic Treatment

- If possible, remove disease-specific (eg, for hypercholesterolemia) dietary restrictions.
- If needed, help arrange shopping, cooking, and feeding assistance, including home-delivered meals and between-meal snacks.
- Increase caloric density of foods.
- Posthospitalization home visits by a dietitian may be valuable.

Pharmacologic Treatment: Appetite Stimulants

- No medications are FDA approved to promote weight gain in older adults. Avoid using prescription appetite stimulants.[CW]
- Dronabinol and megestrol acetate (not covered by Medicare Part D) have been effective in promoting weight gain in younger adults with specific conditions (eg, AIDS, cancer). Avoid megestrol; may increase risk of thrombosis and death.[BC]

- A minority of patients receiving mirtazapine▲ report appetite stimulation and weight gain.
- All medications used for appetite have substantial potential AEs.

Nutritional Supplements

- Protein and energy supplements in older adults at risk of malnutrition appear to have beneficial effects on weight gain and mortality, and shorten length of stay in hospitalized patients. Among those who are well nourished at baseline, the benefit is less clear. Supplements should be given between rather than with meals.
- For ICU patients, enteral nutrition is preferred over parenteral nutrition and should be started within the 1st 24–48 h after admission. Absence of bowel sounds and evidence of bowel function (eg, passing flatus or feces) are not contraindications to beginning tube feeding.
- Many formulas are available (**Table 79** and **Table 80**). Read the content labels and choose on the basis of calories/mL, protein, fiber, lactose, and fluid load.
  ○ Oral: Many (eg, *Resource Health Shake*) are milk-based and provide ~1–1.5 calories/mL.
  ○ Enteral: Commercial preparations have between 0.5 and 2 calories/mL; most contain no milk (lactose) products. For patients who need fluid restriction, the higher concentrated formulas may be valuable, but they may cause diarrhea. Because of reduced kidney function with aging, some recommend that protein should contribute no more than 20% of the formula's total calories. If the formula is the sole source of nutrition, consider one that contains fiber (25 g/d is optimal).

Table 79. Examples of Lactose-free Oral Products

Product	Kcal/mL	mOsm	Protein (g/L)	Water (mL/L)	Na (mEq/L)	K (mEq/L)	Fiber (g/L)
Routine use formulations							
Boost Original[1]	1.01	780	42.3	890	27.5	49.9	12.7
Boost Plus	1.50	670	59.2	780	36.8	38.9	12.7
Ensure Original[2]	0.93	590	38.0	840	36.8	40.1	4.2
Ensure Plus	1.48	680	54.9	760	40.4	43.4	4.2
Low volume (packaged as 44-mL supplement; nutrients are provided per serving)							
Benecalorie[3]	330 kcal	NA	7.0	0	20 mg	0	0
Clear liquid							
Boost Breeze	1.06	750	38.0	830	14.8	0.0	0
Ensure Clear[4]	0.61	700	27.0	830	6.6	0.0	0
Diabetes formulations							
Boost Glucose Control	0.80	400	67.6	870	40.2	5.5	12.7
Glucerna shake	0.80	670	42.2	850	38.6	54.2	12.7

NA = not available.

[1] Also has pudding product that has 160 Kcal/5 oz and 1 g fiber/serving

[2] Also has pudding product that has 170 Kcal/4 oz and 3 g fiber/serving

[3] Per serving, not per mL

[4] Institutional formulation of *Ensure* differs slightly

Table 80. Examples of Lactose-free Enteral Products							
Product	**Kcal/mL**	**mOsm**	**Protein (g/L)**	**Water (mL/L)**	**Na (mEq/L)**	**K (mEq/L)**	**Fiber (g/L)**
Diabetes formulations							
Diabetisource AC	1.20	450	60.0	820	46.0	41.0	15.2
Glucerna 1.0 Cal [1]	1.00	355	41.8	850	40.4	40.1	14.4
Low residue							
Isosource HN [2]	1.20	510	54.0	810	49.0	49.0	0
Osmolite 1 Cal [1]	1.05	300	44.4	840	40.6	40.2	0
Nutren 1.0 [3]	1.00	330	40.0	850	38.0	41.0	0
Low volume							
Nutren 2.0	2.00	780	84.0	690	65.0	54.0	0
TwoCal HN	2.00	725	84.1	700	63.4	62.6	5.1
High fiber							
Jevity 1 Cal [1]	1.06	310	43.8	830	32.2	31.8	14.0
Fibersource HN	1.20	480	54.0	810	49.0	49.0	15.2
Nutren 1.0 FIBER	1.00	340	40.0	830	38.0	41.0	15.2

[1] Also has 1.2- and 1.5-calorie formulations

[2] Also has 1.5-calorie formulation with 15.2 g fiber/L

[3] Also has 1.5-calorie formulation

Important Drug-Enteral Interactions

- Soybean formulas increase fecal elimination of thyroxine; time the administration of thyroxine and enteral nutrition as far apart as possible.
- Enteral feedings reduce absorption of phenytoin, L-dopa, levofloxacin, and ciprofloxacin; administer these medications at least 2 h after a feeding and delay feeding at least 2 h after medication is administered; monitor levels (if taking phenytoin) and adjust dosages, as necessary.
- Check with pharmacy about suitability and best way to administer SR, enteric-coated, and microencapsulated products (eg, omeprazole, lansoprazole, diltiazem, fluoxetine, verapamil).

Gastrostomy/Jejunostomy Tube Feeding

- Chronic artificial nutrition and hydration is not a basic intervention and is associated with uncertain benefit and considerable risks and discomfort.
- Do not insert percutaneous feeding tubes if advanced dementia; instead offer oral assisted feedings.[cw]
- Artificial nutrition and hydration should be used only for specific medical indications, not to increase patient comfort.
- Some evidence supports the use of gastrostomy tubes in patients with head and neck cancer.
- For dysphagia and aspiration, the evidence for gastronomy tubes is conflicting and there are no randomized trials.

Tips for Successful Tube Feeding

- Tube feeding can begin 4 h after placement, though early feeding may result in increased gastric residual volumes.
- Bolster should be positioned to allow 1 to 2 cm movement.
- Gauze pads should be placed over, not underneath, the external bolster.
- Gastrostomy tube feeding may be either intermittent or continuous.
- Jejunostomy tube feedings must be continuous.
- Polyurethane tubes have less dysfunction than silicone tubes.
- Continuous tube feeding is associated with less frequent diarrhea but with higher rates of tube clogging.
- To prevent clogging and to provide additional free water, flushing with at least 30–60 mL of water q4–6h is recommended. Do not allow formula bags to run dry. Administer only liquid or crushed and dissolved medication through tubes.
- Do not give more than one medication at a time; flush with 20 mL of water before and after medication administration and with 5–10 mL between medications. Do not mix medications directly into the enteral feeding formula.
- Do not administer bulk-forming laxatives (eg, methylcellulose or psyllium) through feeding tubes.
- If clogged, begin with gentle flush with warm water with 30- to 60-mL syringe. Allow water to sit for 5 min and repeat. Pancrelipase *(Viokase)* mixed with a bicarbonate 324-mg tab or 1/8 tsp baking soda in warm water may be helpful. Papain and chymopapain are more effective at clearing clogged tubes than sugar-free carbonated beverages or cranberry juice. Commercial devices (eg, *Clog Zapper*) may be effective.
- Diarrhea, which develops in 5–30% of people receiving enteral feeding, may be related to the osmolality of the formula, the rate of delivery, high sorbitol content in liquid medications (eg, APAP, lithium, oxybutynin, furosemide), or other patient-related factors such as antibiotic use or impaired absorption.
- To help prevent aspiration, maintain a 30- to 45-degree elevation of the head of the bed during continuous feeding and for at least 2 h after bolus feedings.
- Check gastric residual volume before each bolus feeding. Gastric residual volumes in the range of 200–500 mL should raise concern and lead to the implementation of measures to reduce the risk of aspiration, but automatic cessation of feeding should not occur for gastric residual volumes <500 mL in the absence of other signs of intolerance. If needed, naloxone *(Narcan)* 8 mg q6h per nasogastric tube, metoclopramide▲ 10 mg, or erythromycin 250 mg IV [5 mg/5 mL] q6h may be useful for problems with high gastric residual volume after mechanical obstruction has been excluded.
- Tubes removed inadvertently during the 1st 4 wk should not be reinserted blindly. Rather, they should be endoscopically, radiologically, or surgically reinserted, which can usually occur through the same site.

Parenteral Nutrition

- Indicated in those with digestive dysfunction precluding enteral feeding.
- In ICU settings, if enteral nutrition is not feasible, should wait 8 d to begin parenteral nutrition.
- Delivers protein as amino acids, carbohydrate as dextrose (D5 = 170 kcal/L; D10 = 340 kcal/L), and fat as lipid emulsions (10% = 1100 kcal/L; 20% = 2200 kcal/L).
- Usually administered as total parenteral nutrition through a central catheter, which may be inserted peripherally.

OBESITY AND OVERWEIGHT

Definitions

- Overweight (BMI 25–29.9 kg/m^2); not associated with increased mortality if aged >70
- Obesity (BMI ≥30 kg/m^2)

Nonpharmacologic Treatment

- Overweight probably does not increase mortality risk; however, weight loss in obese older adults may decrease mortality risk.
- Combinations of weight management (eg, low-calorie diet with deficit of 500–750 calories/d) plus moderate exercise (90 min/3×/wk, preferably combined aerobic and resistance) has resulted in weight loss of 10% and improved functional status in younger (mean age 70) obese older persons.
- Various macronutrient composition low-calorie diets are equally effective.
- Very low–calorie programs with intake <800 calories/d (Health Management Resources, Medifast, and OPTIFAST) are no more effective than low-calorie diets and require medical supervision.
- Patients on diet tx tend to lose weight over initial 6 mo and regain it over next 2–3 y. Lower energy-density diet (fewer calories per volume of food) and high-protein, low-glycemic index may be more effective in reducing weight regain after loss. Behavioral interventions (up to 52 mo) may be helpful in maintaining weight loss.
- No commercial weight-loss programs have been evaluated in older persons. In younger patients:
  - Weight Watchers is more effective than education alone.
  - Jenny Craig is more effective than education or behavioral counseling but more expensive than Weight Watchers.
  - Self-directed programs (Atkins) are more effective than education or counseling. Internet-based (The Biggest Loser Club, eDiets, Lose IT!) appear more effective than education alone but are comparable to counseling.

Procedures (outcome is the percent of excess weight lost [excess weight is above BMI 25])

- Bariatric surgery: In younger patients (usually BMI ≥35), increased remissions from DM and lower incidence of micro- and macrovascular complications. Reduced cardiovascular and all-cause mortality. Guidelines for surgery include DM with BMI ≥40 or BMI ≥35 with comorbidities.
  - Adjustable gastric banding placed laparoscopically: 47% excess weight loss at 15 y; safest but least effective procedure
  - Sleeve gastrectomy with most of greater curvature removed: 59% excess weight loss; less effective than gastric bypass or Roux-en-Y but lower rate of complications
  - Roux-en-Y gastric bypass creating pouch of stomach anastomosing jejunum: 54–74% excess weight loss
  - Biliopancreatic diversion with duodenal switch: ≥70% excess weight loss
- Gastric balloon device endoscopically placed and left in place for up to 6 mo: 25–30% excess weight loss
- *Maestro* Rechargeable System uses high-frequency electric pulses to block vagus signals: 25% excess weight loss
- *AspireAssist* allows patients to partially drain (similar to PEG feeding tube) stomach contents after meal, reducing absorbed calories by 30%; 32% excess weight loss
- Biliopancreatic diversion with duodenal switch combines restrictive procedure similar to sleeve with bypass about 3/4 small intestine; more weight loss (70% of excess weight) but higher complications and mortality

Pharmacologic Treatment

- Drugs to treat obesity have not been studied extensively in older persons; the information below is based on studies of younger persons.
- Consider if BMI ≥30 or 27–29 if comorbidities, especially DM.
- When using pharmacologic management, weight loss of 10–15% is considered a good response and >15% is considered excellent. If ≥5% weight loss is not achieved in 12 wk, stop or taper depending on the specific drug.
- Based on a meta-analysis, 23% of placebo recipients achieved 5% weight loss; 5% loss rates for individual drugs are listed in **Table 81**.

Table 81. Drugs for Weight Loss in Older Persons

Drug	Dose	How supplied	Average weight loss, kg	Percentage losing ≥5%	Conditions for which drug is a preferred tx	Adverse Effects
Orlistat (Xenical)	120 mg q8h	C: 120 mg	2.5–3.4	35–73%	Type 2 DM, high BP, CAD, arrhythmia, CKD (mild or moderate), depression, anxiety, glaucoma, seizure disorder	Abdominal discomfort, flatus; may increase risk of calcium oxalate renal stones
(Alli)ᴼᵀᶜ	60 mg q8h	C: 60 mg				
Lorcaserin (Belviq)	10 mg q12h	T: 10 mg	2.9–3.6	38–48%	Type 2 DM, high BP, CAD, CKD (mild or moderate), glaucoma, seizure disorder	Hypoglycemia (if diabetic), bradycardia, nausea, vomiting, serotonin syndrome
Phentermine-topiramate ER (Qsymia)	Begin 3.75 mg/23 mg daily for 14 d, then increase; 7.5 mg/46 mg may be more effective but should not be used if CVD or HTN	ER T: 3.75 mg/23 mg, 7.5 mg/46 mg, 11.25 mg/69 mg, 15 mg/92 mg	4.1–10.7	45–70%	Type 2 DM, high BP (monitor HR), CKD (mild or moderate, lower max dose), depression, anxiety,[1] seizure disorder	Dry mouth, paresthesia, constipation, dysgeusia, cognitive changes
Naltrexone-bupropion (Contrave)	Titrate from 1 tab daily to 2 tab q12h over 4 wk (1 tab if moderate or severe renal impairment)	ER T: 8/90 mg	3.7–5.2	39–66%	Type 2 DM, CKD (mild or moderate, lower max dose), anxiety	Nausea, vomiting, headache, constipation, dizziness, dry mouth, lowered seizure threshold, abnormal LFTs

(cont.)

			Average weight loss, kg	Percentage losing ≥5%	Conditions for which drug is a preferred tx	Adverse Effects
Drug	**Dose**	**How supplied**				
Liraglutide (*Saxenda*)	Begin 0.6 mg daily × 7 d, then each wk increase dose by 0.6 mg/d to a total of 3 mg SC daily	inj: 18 mg/3 mL	3.7–5.8	44–62%	Type 2 DM, high BP (monitor HR), CAD, arrhythmia, CKD (mild or moderate), depression, anxiety, glaucoma, seizure disorder	Nausea, vomiting, constipation, diarrhea; contraindicated if medullary thyroid carcinoma (or family hx) or multiple endocrine neoplasia type 2

Table 81. Drugs for Weight Loss in Older Persons

[1] Avoid max dose.

Note: Other drugs have limited effectiveness or high potential for ADRs or abuse.

NECK PAIN: DIFFERENTIAL DIAGNOSIS AND TREATMENT
Cervical Stenosis/Radiculopathy

May present with weakness or atrophy in arms, legs, or both; sensory loss; neck or shoulder pain; gait disorder; bladder or rectal sphincter dysfunction

Noncompressive: Herpes zoster, Lyme disease, lymphoma, carcinomatosis, demyelination

Compressive: Cervical spondylosis, disc herniation; MRI abnormalities are common in asymptomatic older persons; must have correlation between findings and clinical symptoms.

Treatment: Most patients improve without specific tx. If radicular pain, paresthesias, numbness, or nonprogressive neurologic deficits, prescribe oral analgesics and avoidance of aggravating movements. If severe, short course of oral prednisone. PT when pain is tolerable. If severe or disabling persistent symptoms, epidural steroids. Surgery if symptoms and neurologic signs, documented nerve root compression by MRI or CT, and persistence of pain for 6–12 wk or progressive motor weakness. Acute deterioration or sudden presentation with myelopathy warrants IV corticosteroids and urgent surgical consultation.

SHOULDER PAIN: DIFFERENTIAL DIAGNOSIS AND TREATMENT

Rotator Cuff Tendonopathy, Subacromial Bursitis, or Rotator Tendon Impingement on Clavicle

Dull ache radiating to upper arm. Painful arc is characteristic. Also can be distinguished by applying resistance against active range of motion while immobilizing the neck with hand.

May cause shoulder impingement syndrome (insidious onset of anterolateral acromial pain frequently radiating to lateral midhumerus). Pain is worse at night, exacerbated by lying on the involved shoulder or sleeping with the arm overhead. Active and passive range of motion are normal. Lidocaine injection can be used to distinguish different shoulder pain syndromes. Insert a 1½-inch, 22-gauge needle 1½ inches below the midpoint of the acromion to a depth of 1 to 1½ inches. The angle of entry parallels the acromion. Inject 1 mL of lidocaine into the deltoid and 1–2 mL into the subacromial bursa. Dramatic relief of pain and improvement of function by injection into subacromial bursa effectively excludes glenohumeral joint process. Lidocaine injection will result in normal strength and temporary pain relief.

Most accurate bedside tests are (muscle being tested):
- Painful arc test: pain on abduction 60–120 degrees and external rotation suggests impingement or rotator cuff disorder due to compression
- Drop arm test (supraspinatus): inability to maintain the arm in an abducted 90-degree position indicates tear
- External rotation resistance test (infraspinatus): elbows flexed, thumbs up with examiner's hands outside patient's elbows; patient is asked to resist inward pressure; pain or weakness indicates tendonitis or tear
- External rotation lag test (supraspinatus and infraspinatus): elbow at 90-degree flexion and 20-degree abduction, examiner passively rotates patient's arm into full external rotation; inability to maintain this position indicates tear
- Internal rotation lag test (subscapularis): elbow at 90-degree flexion, dorsum of hand on back; hand is lifted off back by examiner; inability to maintain position indicates tear
- Imaging, if indicated, with ultrasound or MRI; plain x-ray of limited value

Treatment: Identify and eliminate provocative, repetitive injury (eg, avoid overhead reaching). A brief period of rest and immobilization with a sling may be helpful. Pain control with APAP or a short course of NSAIDs (**Table 82**), home exercises or PT (especially assisted range of motion and wall walking), and corticosteroid injections (p 222) may be useful.

Rotator Cuff Tears

Mild to complete; characterized by diminished shoulder movement. Chronic full-thickness tear may not have pain but have loss of range of active or passive motion. After lidocaine injection of shoulder (see above), weakness persists despite pain relief. Ultrasound (preferred test), MRI, or MR arthrography establishes diagnosis.

Treatment: If due to injury, a brief period of rest and immobilization with a sling may be helpful. Pain control with APAP or a short course of NSAIDs (**Table 82**), home exercises or PT (especially assisted range of motion and wall walking) may be useful. Subacromial glucocorticoid injections may provide short-term pain relief, but multiple injections may be deleterious to healthy tendons. If no improvement after 6–8 wk of conservative measures, consider surgical repair, which may improve long-term (5 y) pain but not function.

Bicipital Tendonitis

Pain felt on anterior lateral aspect of shoulder, tenderness in the groove between greater and lesser tuberosities of the humerus. Pain is elicited on resisted flexion of shoulder, flexion of the elbow, or supination (external rotation) of the hand and wrist with the elbow flexed at the side.

Treatment: Identify and eliminate provocative, repetitive activities (eg, avoid overhead reaching). A period of rest (at least 7 d with no lifting) and corticosteroid injections (p 222) are major components of tx. After rest period, PT should focus on stretching biceps tendon (eg, putting arm on doorframe and hyperextending shoulder, with some external rotation). Tendon sheath injection, often with ultrasound guidance, with corticosteroids may be helpful.

Frozen Shoulder (Adhesive Capsulitis)

Loss of passive external (lateral) rotation, abduction, and internal rotation of the shoulder to <90 degrees. Usually follows 3 phases: painful (freezing) phase lasting weeks to a few months; adhesive (stiffening) phase lasting 4–12 mo; resolution phase lasting 6–24 mo. Lidocaine injection (see above) does not restore range of motion.

Treatment: Avoid rest and begin with gentle home exercises for shoulder mobility including stretching the arm in flexion, horizontal adduction, and internal and external rotation. Transition to PT when patient begins to improve. Low-dose (eg, 20 mg triamcinolone) corticosteroid injections (p 222) given early reduces pain and improves range of motion but duration of effect is limited. Intra-articular injection of saline and anesthetic (hydrodilatation) may be of benefit. If no response after 6–12 mo, consider surgical manipulation under anesthesia or arthroscopic release.

BACK PAIN: DIFFERENTIAL DIAGNOSIS AND TREATMENT OF COMMON CAUSES IN OLDER PERSONS

Axial mechanical back pain is associated with osteoporotic fractures, metastatic bone lesions with or without fractures, internal disc disruption (typically in younger patients), and ligament tears.

Lateral mechanical pain can result from facet arthropathy, sacroiliac joint dysfunction, fascial strain or injury (myofascial pain), or ligament strain. These patients may present with different patterns of radiating pain, but typically the pain does not spread to below the knee. In contrast, pain from lumbar spinal stenosis typically radiates below the knee.

Acute (<4 wk) Back Pain

Do not perform imaging for lower back pain within the 1st 6 wk unless red flags are present (severe or progressive neurologic deficits or when serious underlying conditions are present).**CW**

Acute Lumbar Strain (Low-Back Pain Syndrome)

Acute pain frequently precipitated by heavy lifting or exercise. Pain may be central or more prominent on one side and may radiate to sacroiliac region and buttocks. Pain is aggravated by motion, standing, and prolonged sitting, and relieved by rest. Sciatic pain may be present even when neurologic examination is normal. In sciatica, pain radiating below the knee is more likely to represent true radiculopathy (usually L5 or S1) than proximal leg pain.

Treatment: Most can continue normal activities. If a patient obtains symptomatic relief from bed rest, generally 1–2 d lying in a semi-Fowler position or on side with the hips and knees flexed with pillow between legs will suffice. Do not recommend bedrest without completing an evaluation or for more than 2 days.**CW** Treat muscle spasm with the application of ice, preferably in a massage over the muscles in spasm. A short course of NSAIDs (**Table 82**) can be used to control pain. Spinal manipulation, including high-thrust osteopathic manipulation, is also effective for uncomplicated low-back pain. If severe refractory symptoms, consider systemic or epidural glucocorticoids. Do not prescribe opioids for acute disabling low-back pain before evaluation and trial of other alternatives is considered.**CW** As pain diminishes, encourage patient to begin isometric abdominal and lower-extremity exercises. Symptoms often recur. Education on back posture, lifting precautions, and abdominal muscle strengthening may help prevent recurrences.

Acute Disc Herniation

Over 90% of cases have herniation at L4–L5 or L5–S1 levels, resulting in unilateral impairment of ankle reflex, toe and ankle dorsiflexion, and pain (commonly sciatic) on straight leg raising (can be tested from sitting position by leg extension). Pain is acute in onset and varies considerably with changes in position. If progressive or severe motor deficit, suspected neoplasm or epidural abscess, urinary retention, saddle anesthesia, or bilateral symptoms, urgent MRI, CT, or CT myelography.

Treatment: Initially same as acute lumbar strain (above). The value of epidural injections and surgery for pain without neurologic signs is controversial. Epidural injection of a combination of a long-acting corticosteroid with an epidural anesthetic may provide modest, transient relief and results in less surgery at 1 y if symptoms unresponsive to conservative tx. Consider surgery if recurrence or neurologic signs persist beyond 6–8 wk after conservative tx. The value of epidural injections and surgery for pain without neurologic signs is controversial. Surgery for severe sciatica provides faster pain relief and perceived recovery rates but no difference in perceived recovery and disability at 1 y compared with conservative management.

Vertebral Compression Fracture

Immediate onset of severe pain; worse with sitting or standing; sometimes relieved by lying down. CT scan can help determine instability and MRI can determine acuity of fracture.

Treatment: See Osteoporosis, p 247. Bed rest, analgesia, and mobilization as tolerated. Bracing is unproved except for traumatic vertebral fractures. Nasal calcitonin (for no longer than 2–4 wk), teriparatide or pamidronate (30 mg/d IV for 3 consecutive d) may provide symptomatic improvement. May require hospitalization to control symptoms. Although evidence does not support the effectiveness of percutaneous vertebral augmentation (vertebroplasty and kyphoplasty), some groups recommend augmentation for severe ongoing pain from a known fracture (AAOS, NICE). Vertebroplasty is easier to perform and less expensive but has higher complication rates. Avoid muscle relaxants. Pain may persist for 1 y or longer. As pain diminishes, exercise program (eg, aquatic-based) should be initiated.

Subacute (4–12 wk) and Chronic (>12 wk) Low-Back Pain

Osteoarthritis and Chronic Disc Degeneration

Characterized by aching pain aggravated by motion and relieved by rest. Occasionally, hypertrophic spurring in a facet joint may cause unilateral radiculopathy with sciatica.

Treatment: Identify and eliminate provocative activities. Education on back posture, lifting precautions, and abdominal muscle strengthening. APAP or a short course of NSAIDs, including topicals (**Table 82**). Corticosteroid injections may be useful (p 222). Acupuncture and sham acupuncture may provide benefit. In younger persons, additional chiropractic care resulted in moderate short-term improvements in low-back pain intensity and disability. Consider opioids and other pain tx modalities for chronic refractory pain (p 252). Radiofrequency denervation does not benefit chronic low-back pain from facet or Sacroiliac joints or intervertebral disks. Do not prescribe lumbar supports or braces for the long-term tx of low-back pain.[CW]

Lumbar Spinal Stenosis

Symptoms increase on spinal extension (eg, with prolonged standing, walking downhill, lying prone) and decrease with spinal flexion (eg, sitting, bending forward while walking, lying in the flexed position). Only symptom may be fatigue or pain in buttocks, thighs, and legs when walking (pseudoclaudication). May have immobility of lumbar spine, pain with straight leg raises, weakness of muscles innervated by L4 through S1 (**Table 3**). Over 4 y, 15% improve, 15% deteriorate, and 70% remain stable.

Treatment: APAP or a short course of NSAIDs (**Table 82**), PT, and exercises to reduce lumbar lordosis (eg, bicycling) are sometimes beneficial.

Corticosteroid injections have not been demonstrated to have advantage beyond lidocaine-only injections.

Although data are conflicting, surgical decompression (laminectomy and partial facetectomy) may be more effective than conservative tx (eg, PT) in relieving moderate or severe symptoms. If no spondylolisthesis; interspinous spacer insertion (distraction) may be effective and is less invasive. If proven spinal instability is confirmed on flexion-extension radiographs, vertebral destruction, or spinal deformities (eg, scoliosis), fusion may be better than simple decompression. Simple and complex fusion have more complications and higher costs than decompression alone. Recurrence of pain several years after surgery is common and reoperation rates are high.

Depression, comorbidity influencing walking capacity, cardiovascular comorbidity, and scoliosis predict worse surgical outcome. Male sex, younger age, better walking ability and self-rated health, less comorbidity, and more pronounced canal stenosis predict better surgical outcome.

Nonrheumatic Pain (eg, tumors, aneurysms)

Gradual onset, steadily expanding, often unrelated to position and not relieved by lying down. Night pain when lying down is characteristic. Upper motor neuron signs may be present. Involvement is usually in thoracic and upper lumbar spine.

HIP PAIN: DIFFERENTIAL DIAGNOSIS AND TREATMENT
Greater Trochanteric Pain Syndrome (Trochanteric Bursitis)

Pain in lateral aspect of the hip usually due to gluteus medius or minimus tendinopathy that usually worsens when patient sits on a hard chair, lies on the affected side, or rises from a chair or bed; pain may improve with walking. Local tenderness over greater trochanter is often present, and pain is often reproduced on resisted abduction of the leg or internal rotation of the hip. However, trochanteric pain does not result in limited range of motion, pain on range of motion, pain in the groin, or radicular signs.

Treatment: Identify and eliminate provocative activities. Position pillow posterolaterally behind the involved side to avoid lying on bursae while sleeping. Check for leg length discrepancy, prescribe orthotics if appropriate. Trial of up to 2 wk of acetaminophen and, if persistent, 2 wk of NSAIDs. If no improvement, inject a combination of a long-acting corticosteroid with an anesthetic. Refer to surgery if gluteus medius tear on MRI or refractory symptoms for ≥12 mo.

Osteoarthritis

"Boring" quality pain in the hip, often in the groin, and sometimes referred to the back or knee with stiffness after rest. Passive motion is restricted in all directions if disease is fairly advanced. In early disease, pain in the groin on internal rotation of the hip is characteristic.

Treatment: See also Osteoarthritis, p 220. Chondroitin sulfate, glucosamine, and capsaicin are not recommended. Participation in cardiovascular, resistance, or aquatic exercises. Weight loss if overweight. Elective total hip replacement is indicated for patients who have radiographic evidence of joint damage and moderate to severe persistent pain or disability, or both, that is not substantially relieved by an extended course of nonsurgical management.

Hip Fracture

Sudden onset, usually after a fall, with inability to walk or bear weight, frequently radiating to groin or knee. If hip radiograph (Anterior-Posterior with maximal internal rotation and lateral view) is negative and index of suspicion is high, obtain MRI. Fractures are 45% femoral neck, 45% intertrochanteric, and 10% subtrochanteric.

Treatment: Tx is surgical with open reduction and internal fixation (ORIF), hemiarthroplasty, or total hip replacement (THR), depending on the site of fracture and the amount of displacement. Sliding hip screws may have lower complication rates than intramedullary nails for extracapsular fractures. Displaced femoral neck fractures are generally treated with hemiarthroplasty or THR. Subtrochanteric fractures can be treated with intramedullary nails.

Perioperative Care:

- Co-management of hip fracture by geriatrics and orthopedic surgery improves patient outcomes, including risk of delirium. Features of a co-management service usually include:
  - Placement of patient on orthopedic ward with daily visits by orthopedic and geriatrics services
  - Clear delineation of who writes orders for fluid management, pain management, anticoagulation, catheter care, and antibiotics
  - 24-h/d availability of geriatrics
  - Standardized order sets
  - Frequent daily communication between orthopedic and geriatrics services (eg, co-rounding)
- Timing of surgery: Early surgery (within 24 h) is associated with better outcomes but may be due to more comorbidity in those with delayed surgery.

- Treat comorbid conditions (eg, anemia, volume depletion, metabolic abnormalities, infections, HF, CAD).
- Adequate pre- and postoperative analgesia (eg, 3-in-1 femoral nerve block, intrathecal morphine); ultrasound-guided femoral nerve block administered in the emergency department improves pain and functional outcomes compared to conventional analgesics.
- Regional anesthesia if possible
- Antibiotics: Perioperative antibiotics (cefazolin or, if allergic, clindamycin or vancomycin) should be given beginning within 1 h of surgery.
- Pressure-reducing rather than standard mattress; if high risk of pressure sore, use large cell, alternating pressure air mattress.
- Oximetry for at least 48 h with supplemental oxygen prn
- Graduated compression stockings do not add benefit beyond DVT prophylaxis medications.
- Intermittent pneumatic leg compression is recommended for the duration of the hospital stay.
- DVT prophylaxis: Give preoperatively if surgery delay is expected to be >48 h; otherwise begin 12–24 h after surgery. First choices are enoxaparin and dalteparin but other agents can be used (Antithrombotic Therapy and Thromboembolic Disease, p 30, for regimens). Recommended duration is for up to 35 d but at least 10 d and probably 1 mo if patient is inactive or has comorbidities.
- Preoperative traction has no demonstrated benefit.
- Avoid indwelling urinary catheters.
- Nutritional supplements if undernourished
- Transfuse only if symptomatic or Hb <8 g/dL.
- Begin assisted ambulation within 48 h.
- Monitor for the development of delirium, malnutrition, and pressure sores.
- Weightbearing: Usually as tolerated for hemiarthroplasty or THR; toe-touch if ORIF or intertrochanter fracture
- Hip precautions: No adduction past midline; no hip flexion beyond 90%; no internal rotation (toes upright in bed)
- Treat osteoporosis regardless of BMD: Wait 2 wk before starting bisphosphonates; make sure vitamin D is replete (Osteoporosis, p 247).
- Fall prevention: See Fall Prevention, p 123.

For patients who were nonambulatory before the fracture, conservative management is an option.

Nonrheumatic Pain

Referred pain from viscera, radicular pain from the lower spine, avascular necrosis, Paget disease, metastasis. Tx based on identified etiology.

KNEE PAIN: DIFFERENTIAL DIAGNOSIS AND TREATMENT
Osteoarthritis

Pain usually related to activity (eg, climbing stairs, arising from chair, walking long distances). Morning stiffness lasts <30 min. Crepitation is common. Examination should attempt to exclude other causes of knee pain such as hip arthritis with referred knee pain (decreased hip range of motion), chondromalacia patellae (tenderness only over patellofemoral joint), iliotibial band syndrome (tenderness is lateral to the knee at site of insertion in fibular head or where courses over lateral femoral condyle), anserine bursitis (tenderness distal to knee over medial tibia), and determination of malalignment varus (bowlegged) or valgus (knock-kneed).

Treatment: See Osteoarthritis Treatment, p 220. In moderate to severe knee osteoarthritis, surgery is more effective than medical tx but has high rate of complications, especially DVT and stiffness requiring brisement forcé.

HAND AND WRIST PAIN AND RELATED CONDITIONS: DIFFERENTIAL DIAGNOSIS AND TREATMENT

Osteoarthritis

Hand pain (including hand aching or stiffness) plus ≥3 of the following 4 features (ACR):

(1) hard tissue enlargement of 2 of the following: 2nd and 3rd distal interphalangeal (DIP) joints, the 2nd and 3rd proximal interphalangeal (PIP) joints, and the 1st carpometacarpal (CMC) of both hands

(2) hard enlargement of 2 or more DIP joints

(3) fewer than 3 swollen metacarpophalangeal (MCP) joints

(4) deformity of at least 1 of the 10 joints above

X-ray confirmation is not necessary.

Treatment: See Osteoarthritis, p 220. Avoid opioid analgesics and intraarticular tx.

Inflammatory (Rheumatoid and Psoriatic) Arthritis

Typically MCP and PIP joints with morning stiffness often lasting >1 h

Treatment: See Rheumatoid arthritis.

De Quervain Tendinopathy

Pain or tenderness at radial side of wrist

Treatment: Forearm-based thumb splint, NSAIDs, and, if refractory, glucocorticoid injections. If no improvement after injections, consider surgery

Stenosing Flexor Tenosynovitis (trigger finger)

Painless (initially) catching, snapping or locking during flexion due to disparity in the size of flexor tendons and retinacular pulley system overlying the metacarpal-phalangeal joint; may be multiple fingers

Treatment: activity modification, splinting to keep metacarpal-phalangeal joint in slight flexion, short-term NSAIDs for mild cases; glucocorticoid injections if severe or pain; surgery if refractory (less recurrence at 6–12 mo)

Dupuytren Contracture

Loss of full extension of the finger at the metacarpal-phalangeal joint, which is fixed and chronic and is characterized by painless nodular lesions that progress to form a fibrous cord from the palm to the digit

Treatment: modification of hand tools to increase padding or using glove for mild symptoms; glucocorticoid and lidocaine injections if more severe symptoms of recent onset (ineffective if cords); collagenase injections though no long-term studies; surgery or percutaneous needle aponeurotomy for advanced disease if functional impairment but high recurrence rate

Carpal Tunnel Syndrome

Painful tingling or hypoesthesia, or both, in one or both hands in distribution innervated by median nerve. Causes include:

- Repetitive activities
- DM
- Thyroid disease
- Amyloidosis
- RA
- Space-occupying lesions (eg, lymphoma)
- Trauma (eg, Colles fracture)

Physical examination demonstrates decreased sensation in palm, thumb, index finger, middle finger, and thumb side of ring finger, weak handgrip, and tapping over median nerve at wrist causes pain to shoot from wrist to hand (Tinel's sign). An acute flexion of wrist for 60 sec (Phalen's test) should also cause pain.

Laboratory studies should include: fasting glucose, TSH, nerve conduction velocity testing (confirms diagnosis).

Treatment: (combined modalities may be effective if single modalities fail)

Nonpharmacologic

Modify work or leisure activities to avoid repetitive movement, carpal tunnel mobilization (moving bones in wrist through PT or OT), and yoga may provide some symptom relief. Splinting in neutral position, especially at night; surgery (more effective than splinting) is indicated for prolonged (usually >6 mo) of moderate to severe symptoms (pain and numbness, diminished hand function, thenar eminence atrophy) after confirmation of median nerve injury by electrodiagnostic testing. Nerve and tendon gliding maneuvers have not been shown to be effective.

Pharmacologic

Injectable corticosteroids, (eg, methylprednisolone 15 mg) are more effective than oral; oral corticosteroids[BC] (eg, prednisone 20 mg/d for 1 wk followed by 10 mg/d for a 2nd wk). Perineural dextrose (D5%) injections may be helpful.

COMMON FOOT DISORDERS

Calluses and corns: diffuse thickening of the stratum corneum in response to repeated friction or pressure (calluses); corns are similar but have a central, often painful core and are often found at pressure points, especially caused by ill-fitting shoes or gait abnormalities

Equinus: tight Achilles tendon

Hallux valgus (bunion): deviation of the tip of the great toe, or main axis of the toe, toward the outer or lateral side of the foot. No surgery in the absence of symptoms.[CW]

Hammertoes (digiti flexus): muscle tendon imbalance causing contraction of the proximal or distal interphalangeal joint, or both. No surgery in the absence of symptoms.[CW]

Metatarsalgia: usually 2nd and 3rd metatarsal pain (like stepping on a stone) due to collapsed transverse metatarsal heads. Tx is conservative and includes metatarsal pads to relieve distal plantar pressure. If ineffective, order customized orthotics. Surgery is last resort.

Morton neuroma: burning pain usually between 3rd and 4th distal metatarsals. Ultrasound can distinguish between bursal swelling and synovitis. Tx is conservative and includes reducing pressure on metatarsal heads using a support or padded sole insert. If not controlled, inject glucocorticoid. Do not use alcohol injections.[CW] Surgery if symptoms persist >9–12 mo of tx.

Pes cavus: higher than normal arch that can result in excessive pressure, usually placed on the metatarsal heads, and cause pain and ulceration

Tarsal tunnel syndrome: an entrapment neuropathy of the posterior tibial nerve

Treatment:

- Calluses and corns are treated with salicylic acid plaster 40%, available OTC (eg, *Mediplast, Sal-Acid Plaster*) after paring skin with a #15 scalpel blade. Remove dead skin with metal nail file or pumice stone each night before replacing the patch. Do not use in patients with peripheral neuropathy.
- Orthoses can be placed either on the foot or into the shoe to accommodate for a foot deformity or to alter the function of the foot to relieve physical stress on a certain portion of the foot. OTC devices made of lightweight polyethylene foam, soft plastics, or silicone are available for a certain size of foot. Custom-made orthoses are constructed from an impression of a person's foot. In a meta-analysis, orthotics were not effective in improving plantar heel pain and function.
- If conservative methods fail, refer to podiatry or orthopedics for consideration of surgery.

PLANTAR FASCIITIS

Definition

Strain or inflammation in plantar fascia causing foot pain that is worse when getting out of bed in the morning or beginning to walk; 80% resolve spontaneously within 1 y.

Causes/Risk Factors

- Jumping
- Running
- Rheumatic diseases
- Obesity
- Flat feet
- Plantar spurs

Evaluation

Examiner should dorsiflex toes and then palpate plantar fascia to elicit pain points; posterior heel pain is uncommon and suggests other diagnosis.

Treatment

Nonpharmacologic

- Rest and icing
- Exercises (calf plantar fascia stretch, foot/ankle circles, toe curls); strengthening with unilateral heel raises with a towel under the toes may be superior
- Avoid walking barefoot or in slippers
- Foot (low-dye) taping may be of benefit
- Prefabricated silicone heel inserts
- Shoes (running, arch support, crepe sole)
- Short-leg walking cast
- Surgery (rarely needed) and not before trying 6 mo of nonoperative care.[CW]

Pharmacologic

- NSAIDs[BC] (short duration, 2–3 wk)
- Corticosteroid[BC] (eg, methylprednisolone 20–40 mg) and analgesic (eg, 1% lidocaine) injection of fascia; use only if conservative measures fail

OSTEOARTHRITIS

Classification

- Noninflammatory: pain and disability are generally the only complaints; findings include tenderness, bony prominence, and crepitus.
- Inflammatory: may also have morning stiffness lasting >30 min and night pain; findings may include joint effusion on examination or radiograph, warmth, and synovitis on arthroscopy.

MANAGEMENT OF OSTEOARTHRITIS AND GENERAL MUSCULOSKELETAL DISORDERS

- Begin with nonpharmacologic tx

Nonpharmacologic

- Superficial heat: hot packs, heating pads, paraffin, or hot water bottles (moist heat is better): 20 min on, 20 min off
- Deep heat: microwave, shortwave diathermy, or ultrasound
- Superficial cooling using ice packs or fluoromethane spray (eg, Gebauer's Spray and Stretch)
- Biofeedback and transcutaneous electrical nerve stimulation
- Exercises:
  - All programs should include isometric strengthening, stretching, range of motion.
  - Those who can tolerate basics can progress to isotonic strengthening and aerobic exercises.
  - Swimming, bicycling, walking, and tai chi have low joint-loading and may protect the knee. Splints may also help protect the joints.
  - Closed-chain (the limbs are stationary while the body moves) avoid joint torsion.
  - Walking and home-based quadriceps strengthening have comparable effectiveness on pain and disability for knee osteoarthritis.
  - In younger patients, weekly yoga with a recommended 30-min DVD-guided daily practice is as effective as PT for chronic, nonspecific low-back pain.
  - Supervised settings have better adherence than unsupervised home-based exercise.
- PT, OT. PT-prescribed, internet-delivered, home exercise combined with pain coping skills training is effective in knee arthritis.
- Weight loss: especially for low-back, hip, and knee arthritis
- Splinting and orthotics: Avoid splinting for long periods (eg, >6 wk) because periarticular muscle weakness and wasting may occur. For base-of-thumb osteoarthritis, use of a custom-made neoprene splint worn only at night results in decreased pain and disability at 12 mo. Medially wedged insoles if knee lateral compartment osteoarthritis. Don't use lateral wedge insoles if medial compartment knee osteoarthritis.[CW] Bracing (eg, neoprene sleeves over the knee, valgus brace) to correct malalignment is often helpful.
- Assistive devices: Cane should be used in the hand contralateral to the affected knee or hip. Cane length should be to the level of the wrist crease. Use walker if moderate or severe balance impairment, bilateral weakness, or unilateral weakness requiring support of >15–20% of body weight.
- Acupuncture as an adjunct to NSAIDs or analgesics for knee osteoarthritis or chronic low-back pain
- Dry needling performed by physical therapists may provide short-term pain improvement for up to 12 wk.
- Chiropractic care as an adjunct to medical tx for back pain
- Surgical intervention (eg, debridement, meniscal repair, prosthetic joint replacement)

Pharmacologic Overview

- If mild to moderate pain, 3-day trial of scheduled APAP.
- If unsuccessful, moderate to severe, or inflammatory, topical (if 1 or few joints) or oral NSAIDs, with appropriate cautions, at the lowest dose for as short as possible; can add capsaicin if incomplete control of symptoms.
- If inadequately relieved and only one or a few joints, glucocorticoid or hyaluronate (if knee) joint injections.

- If pain is still uncontrolled, consider surgery or opioids (Pain chapter, p 252). Use requires careful risk-benefit analysis. Potent opioids (hydromorphone and oxycodone) are no more effective than tramadol.

Topical Analgesics: (**Table 82**). Liniments containing methyl salicylates (**Table 99**), capsaicin crm, menthol counterirritants, *Aspercreme* lidocaine (4%) crm, *Icy Hot* lidocaine (4%) crm, and other OTC lidocaine pch (4%) *(Balego, LidoPatch, LidoFlex, LenzaPatch)*, lidocaine 5% pch *(Lidoderm)*.

Intra-articular, Bursal, and Trigger-point Injections:

- Corticosteroids (eg, methylprednisolone acetate, triamcinolone acetonide, triamcinolone hexacetonide [longest acting]) may be particularly effective if monoarticular symptoms. May provide moderate short-term improvement of pain and small improvement of function. Typical doses for all these drugs:
  - 40 mg for large joints (eg, knee, ankle, shoulder, hip with fluoroscopy or ultrasound guidance)
  - 30 mg for wrists, ankles, and elbows
  - 10 mg for small joints of hands and feet

Often mixed with lidocaine 1% or its equivalent (some experts recommend giving equal volume with corticosteroids, whereas others give 3–5 times the corticosteroid volume depending on size of joint) for immediate relief. Effect typically lasts 1–2 mo. Usually given no more often than 3×/y.

- Glucocorticoid injections have also been used for back pain due to radiculopathy, spinal stenosis, and nonspecific low-back pain. For spinal stenosis, they have been no more effective than lidocaine injections. Best evidence is for short-term pain relief of radiculopathy due to a herniated disc. Each injection increases the subsequent risk of vertebral fracture. Intradisc and facet injections have not been effective and evidence on sacroiliac joint injections is inconclusive.
- Chemonucleolysis (enzymatic) injections of disc may have limited benefit.
- Etanercept, botulinum toxin, and methylene blue have not been found to be beneficial.
- Blocks and radiofrequency ablation of medial branch of the primary dorsal ramus have limited evidence of effectiveness.
- Prolotherapy (repeated injection of irritants to increase inflammation and strengthen surrounding ligaments) has little evidence of effectiveness.
- Hyaluronate preparations *(Euflexxa, Hyalgan, Orthovisc, Synvisc, Supartz)* 3–5 injections 1 wk apart for knee osteoarthritis. A formulation *(Synvisc-One)* is available that requires only one injection. Benefit is similar to NSAIDs but may last ≥6 mo.

Nutraceuticals: Chondroitin sulfate (400 mg q8h) with or without glucosamine sulfate (500 mg q8h) has a small but clinically significant benefit for knee osteoarthritis, with some evidence that there may a small benefit on slowing disease progression.

APAP (acetaminophen): APAP is ineffective in treating acute low-back pain and has minimal short-term benefit in knee and hip osteoarthritis.

NSAIDs: Topicals are preferred over oral in persons aged >75 with knee or hand arthritis. Diclofenac gel (1%) or pch and ketoprofen (5%, 10%, 20%) have comparable improvement and fewer AEs compared to oral NSAIDs and provide pain relief, but have higher rates of AEs than APAP (**Table 82**). Not recommended for long-term use. If one NSAID is not effective at the maximal dose, switch to a different NSAID. Combining with APAP is slightly more effective but may increase risk of bleeding. Misoprostol▲ 100–200 mg q6h with food [T: 100, 200] or a PPI (**Table 58**) may be valuable prophylaxis against NSAID-induced ulcers in high-risk patients. Celecoxib, a selective COX-2 inhibitor, is less likely to cause gastroduodenal ulcers than nonselective NSAIDs and has no higher cardiovascular adverse effects but may not be as effective in controlling pain as nonselective NSAIDs. All may increase INR in patients receiving warfarin. Avoid in individuals with HTN, HF, or CKD of all causes, including DM.^{CW}

Other:

- Tramadol^{BC} for knee or hip arthritis. Begin with 25 mg [T: 50] q4–6h, not to exceed 300 mg/d if age >75.
- Colchicine (0.6 mg q12h) may be of benefit in inflammatory osteoarthritis with recurrent symptoms.
- Duloxetine^{BC} *(Cymbalta)* [C: 20, 30, 60], beginning at 30 mg/d and increasing to 60 mg/d after 1 wk, may have benefit in chronic low-back pain and osteoarthritis, particularly knee.

Table 82. APAP and NSAIDs

Class, Drug	Usual Dosage for Arthritis	Formulations	Metabolism, Excretion
✓APAP▲	Drug of choice for chronic musculoskeletal conditions; no anti-inflammatory properties and less effective than NSAIDs; hepatotoxic above 4 g/d; at high dosages (≥2 g/d) may increase INR in patients receiving warfarin▲; reduce dosage 50–75% if liver or kidney disease or if harmful or hazardous alcohol intake		
	650 mg q4–6h (q8h if CrCl <10 mg/mL/1.73 m²)	T: 80, 325, 500, 650; C: 160, 325, 500; S: elixir 120/5 mL, 160/5 mL, 167/5 mL, 325/5 mL; S: 160/5 mL, 500/15 mL; Sp: 120, 325, 600	(L, K)
Extended-release	1300 mg q8h	ER: 650	
ASA▲	650 mg q4–6h	T: 81, 325, 500, 650, 975 Sp: 120, 200, 300, 600	(K)
Extended-release▲	1300 mg q8h or 1600–3200 mg q12h	CR: 650, 800	
Enteric-coated▲^{OTC,1}	1000 mg q6h	T: 81, 162, 325, 500, 690, 975	
Nonacetylated Salicylates	Do not inhibit platelet aggregation; fewer GI and renal AEs; no reaction in ASA-sensitive patients; monitor salicylate concentrations		
✓Choline magnesium salicylate▲	3 g/d in 1, 2, or 3 doses	T: 500, 750, 1000 S: 500 mg/5 mL	(K)
✓Choline salicylate *(Arthropan)*	4.8–7.2 g/d divided	T: 325, 545, 600, 650 S: 870 mg/5 mL	(L, K)
✓Magnesium salicylate▲^{OTC,1}	2 tabs q6–8h, max 4800 mg q24h	T: 467, 600, 650	Avoid in kidney failure
✓Salsalate▲	1500 mg to 4 g/d in 2 or 3 doses	T: 500, 750	(K)

(cont.)

Table 82. APAP and NSAIDs (cont.)

Class, Drug	Usual Dosage for Arthritis	Formulations	Metabolism, Excretion
Nonselective NSAIDs	Avoid chronic use without GI protection; avoid in HF.[BC]		
Diclofenac▲	50–150 mg/d in 2 or 3 doses	T: 50, 75; 50, enteric-coated	(L)
(Voltaren-XR)	100 mg/d	T: ER 100	(L)
(Zipsor)	25 mg up to q6h	C: 25	(L)
(Zorvolex)	18–25 mg q8h	C: 18, 35	(L)
(Pennsaid)	apply 40 gtt per knee q6h	sol: 1.5%	(L)
✓Enteric-coated			
(Arthrotec 50)	1 tab q8–12h	50 mg with 200 mcg misoprostol	(L)
(Arthrotec 75)	1 tab q12h	75 mg with 200 mcg misoprostol	(L)
✓Gel▲	2–4 g q6h	1%	(L)
✓Patch *(Flector)*	1 q12h	1.3%	(L)
Diflunisal▲	500–1000 mg/d in 2 doses	T: 500	(K)
✓Etodolac▲	200–400 mg q6–8h	T: 400, 500 ER 400, 500, 600	Fewer GI AEs (L)
(Lodine XL)	400–1000 mg/d	C: 200, 300	
Fenoprofen▲	200–600 mg q6–8h	C: 200, 300; T: 600	Higher risk of GI AEs (L)
Flurbiprofen▲	200–300 mg/d in 2, 3, or 4 doses	T: 50, 100	(L)
✓Ibuprofen▲	1200–3200 mg/d in 3 or 4 doses	T: 100, 200, 300, 400, 600, 800 ChT: 50, 100 S: 100 mg/5 mL	Fewer GI AEs (L)
with famotidine *(Duexis)*	1 tab q8h	T: 800 with 26.6 mg famotidine	
Injectable *(Caldolor)*	400–800 mg IV q6h (max 3200 mg/d)	Inj	
✓Ketoprofen▲	50–75 mg q8h	T: 12.5 C: 50, 75	(L)
Sustained-release *(Oruvail* [Canadian brand])	200 mg/d	C: 200	(L)
gel[OTC]	2–4 g, 2–4×/d (max 15 g)	gel: 2.5%	

(cont.)

Class, Drug	Usual Dosage for Arthritis	Formulations	Metabolism, Excretion
(Active-Ketoprofen, Sound Frotek, Ketophene RapidPaq)	1 g 3×/d	crm: 5% (120 g), 10% (30 mL), 20% (100 g),	
Ketorolac▲	10 mg q4–6h, 15 mg IM or IV q6h	T: 10 Inj	Duration of use should be limited to 5 d (K)
Meclofenamate sodium▲	200–400 mg/d in 3 or 4 doses	C: 50, 100	High incidence of diarrhea (L)
Mefenamic acid▲	250 mg q6h	C: 250	(L)
✓Meloxicam▲	7.5–15 mg/d	T: 7.5, 15 S: 7.5 mg/5 mL	Has some COX-2 selectivity; fewer GI AEs (L)
✓Nabumetone▲	500–1000 mg q12h	T: 500, 750	Fewer GI AEs (L)
✓Naproxen▲	220–500 mg q12h	T: 220, 375, 500, 750 S: 125 mg/5 mL	(L)
Delayed-release *(EC-Naprosyn)*	375–500 mg q12h	T: 375, 500	(L)
Extended-release *(Naprelan)*	750–1000 mg/d	T: 250, 375, 500	(L)
Naproxen sodium▲	275 mg or 550 mg q12h	T: 275, 550	(L)
✓Oxaprozin▲	1200 mg/d	C: 600	(L)
Piroxicam▲	10 mg/d	C: 10, 20	Can cause delirium (L)
Sulindac▲	150–200 mg q12h	T: 150, 200 C: 200	May have higher rate of renal impairment (L)
Tolmetin ▲	600–1800 mg/d in 3 or 4 doses	T: 200, 600 C: 400	(L)
Trolamine salicylate[OTC] *(Aspercreme and others)*	3–4 ×/d	10% sol	
Selective COX-2 Inhibitor	Avoid in HF.[BC]		
✓Celecoxib▲	100–200 mg q12h	C: 50, 100, 200, 400	Increased risk of MI; less GI ulceration; do not inhibit platelets; may increase INR if taking warfarin▲; avoid if moderate or severe hepatic insufficiency; may induce renal impairment; contraindicated if allergic to sulfonamides (L)

✓ = preferred for treating older adults.

[1] Also OTC in a lower tab strength

Evaluation and Diagnosis

Evaluation: RF, anti-CCP, antinuclear antibody (ANA), CBC, ESR, CRP, LFTs, BUN, Cr, eye exam (if starting hydroxychloroquine), hepatitis B screen, hepatitis C screen (if at increased risk), tuberculosis test (if starting biologic), x-rays of hands, wrists, and feet

Table 83. **2010 American College of Rheumatology/European League Against Rheumatism (ACR/EULAR) Criteria for Diagnosis of Rheumatoid Arthritis[1]**

A. Joint involvement (any swollen or tender joint excluding 1st carpometacarpal, metatarsophalangeal, and distal and proximal interphalangeal joints)	
1 large joint (shoulders, elbows, hips, knees, ankles)	0
2 to 10 large joints	1
1 to 3 small joints (with or without involvement of large joints)	2
4 to 10 small joints (with or without involvement of large joints)	3
>10 joints (at least 1 small joint)	5
B. Serology (at least 1 test result is needed for classification)	
Negative RF and negative anticitrullinated protein antibody (ACPA)	0
Low-positive (<3 × upper limit of normal) RF or low-positive ACPA	2
High-positive (>3 × upper limit of normal) RF or high-positive ACPA	3
C. Acute-phase reactants (at least one test result is needed for classification)	
Normal CRP and normal ESR	0
Abnormal CRP or abnormal ESR	1
D. Duration of symptoms (by patient self-report)	
<6 wk	0
≥6 wk	1

Scoring: Add score of categories A–D; a score of ≥6/10 is needed for classification of a patient as having definite RA.

[1] Aimed at classifying newly presenting patients; patients with erosive disease or longstanding disease with a hx of presenting features consistent with these criteria should be classified as having RA.

Adapted from Aletaha D et al. *Arthritis Rheum* 2010;62(9):2569–2581. This material is reproduced with permission of John Wiley & Sons, Inc.

Staging

- Duration: early <6 mo, intermediate 6–24 mo, late >24 mo
- Activity: low, moderate, high by various criteria; see rheumatology.org/Practice-Quality/Clinical-Support/Criteria
- Poor prognostic factors: functional limitation, extra-articular disease, RF positivity ± anti-CCP antibodies, and/or bony erosions by radiography

Management

- See rheumatology.org/Practice-Quality/Clinical-Support/Clinical-Practice-Guidelines
  Note: modifications in guideline for comorbid disease (ie, CHF, hepatitis, malignancy, serious infections); co-management with rheumatology
- All patients with established disease should be offered DMARDs as soon as possible; goal is to induce remission and then lower dosages to maintain remission. Tight control of disease activity is associated with better radiographic and functional outcomes.

- Monitor q1–3 mo if active disease (tight control of tx); if no improvement by 3 mo or target not reached by 6 mo, adjust tx.

Nonpharmacologic

- Patient education
- Exercise
- PT and OT
- Atherosclerosis risk factor modification
- Splints and orthotics
- Surgery for severe functional abnormalities due to synovitis or joint destruction
- Bone protection (see Osteoporosis, p 247)

Pharmacologic

- Analgesics (**Table 82** and Pain, p 252) Opioids typically used only in severe or end-stage disease or in flares. Associated with increased risk for serious infection.
- NSAIDs (**Table 82**) Often used as bridging tx until DMARDs are effective.
- Glucocorticoids (eg, prednisone ≤15 mg/d or equivalent) with osteoporosis prevention measures (Osteoporosis, p 247). Often used as bridging tx until DMARDs are effective. Avoid in delirium.[BC] Low-dose prednisone (10 mg/d) has benefit as an adjunct to methotrexate.
- Methotrexate should be part of 1st tx strategy. Dual and triple nonbiologic DMARD combinations are also used with methotrexate as one component. Use biologic DMARDs only after failure of nonbiologic DMARDs[CW] (**Table 84**). If a 1st biological has failed, treat with a different biological. Consider tofacitinib if other biologicals have failed.
- If in persistent remission after tapering glucocorticoids, consider tapering biologicals.
- Flares can be treated with increased dose of oral or pulse IV glucocorticoids (eg, 3 infusions of up to 1000 mg methylprednisolone per wk).
- Frequent or severe flares should prompt consideration of escalation of dose or modification of regimen.

Table 84. Nonbiologic DMARDs

Medication	Starting/ Usual Dosage	Formulations	Indications	Comments[1]
Hydroxychloroquine▲	Begin 200–400 mg/d; dose at <6.5 mg/kg/d to reduce risk of retinal toxicity	T: 200	Monotx for durations <24 mo, low disease activity, and without poor prognostic features	Baseline and annual eye exam beginning after 5 y of use; contraindicated in G6PD deficiency
Sulfasalazine▲	Begin at 500 mg/d to avoid GI upset; increase dosage by 500 mg every 3–4 d until taking 2–3 g/d split between 2 doses	T: 500	Monotx for all disease durations and all degrees of disease activity, and without poor prognostic features	Check CBC, LFTs q8wk; contraindicated in G6PD deficiency

(cont.)

Table 84. **Nonbiologic DMARDs (cont.)**

Medication	Starting/ Usual Dosage	Formulations	Indications	Comments[1]
Methotrexate▲	10–25 mg/wk, adjust dosage for renal impairment (hold if CrCl <30)	T: 2.5 T: 2.5, 5, 7.5, 10, 15	Monotx for all disease durations and all degrees of disease activity, irrespective of poor prognostic features	Check for hepatitis B and C; check CBC (hold if WBC <3000/mm³), LFTs q8wk; give folic acid 1 mg/d; may cause oral ulcers, hepatotoxicity, pulmonary toxicity, cytopenias; avoid if liver disease or CrCl <30. If oral weekly dosing is ineffective or poorly tolerated, SC can be used.
Leflunomide▲	Begin 100 mg/d × 3 d, then 20 mg/d	T: 10, 20	Monotx for all disease durations and all degrees of disease activity, irrespective of poor prognostic features	Check for hepatitis B and C; check CBC (hold if WBC <3000/mm³), LFTs q8wk; may cause hepatotoxicity, cytopenias; avoid if liver disease

G6PD = glucose-6-phosphate-dehydrogenase; CrCl unit = mL/min/1.73 m²

[1] Check baseline CBC, LFTs, Cr for all.

- Biologic DMARDs: Not used in early RA and only low or moderate disease activity; increased risk of serious infections and reactivation of latent infections. Hold tx for any infection but can start shortly after bacterial infection is successfully treated; may increase risk of skin cancers. Avoid live vaccinations while on biologics.
  - Anti-TNF-α agents: Used if inadequate response to methotrexate, if moderate disease activity and poor prognostic features, or if high activity regardless of poor prognostic features. May be added to or substituted for methotrexate. Combinations of biologic DMARDs are not recommended.
    - Adalimumab *(Humira)*
    - Certolizumab pegol *(Cimzia)*
    - Etanercept *(Enbrel)*
    - Infliximab *(Remicade)*
    - Golimumab *(Simponi)*
  - IL-1 receptor antagonist: anakinra *(Kineret)*
- Medications used when response to DMARD has been inadequate:
  - T-cell activation inhibitor: abatacept *(Orencia)*
  - Anti-CD20 monoclonal antibody: rituximab *(Rituxan)*
  - IL-6 inhibitor: tocilizumab *(Actemra),* sarilumab *(Kevzara)*
  - Janus kinase (JAK) inhibitor: tofacitinib *(Xeljanz),* baricitinib *(Olumiant)*

GOUT

Definition

Urate crystal disease that may be expressed as acute gouty arthritis, usually in a single joint of foot, ankle, knee, or olecranon bursa; intercritical (between flairs), or chronic arthritis and tophaceous gout.

Precipitating Factors

- Alcohol, heavy ingestion
- Allopurinol, stopping or starting
- Binge eating
- Dehydration
- Diuretics (except potassium-sparing)
- Fasting
- Infection
- Serum uric acid concentration, any change up or down
- Surgery

Evaluation of Acute Gouty Arthritis

Joint aspiration to remove crystals and microscopic examination to establish diagnosis; serum urate (can be normal during flare)

If negative and still suspicion, diagnostic rule: male sex (2 points), previous self-reported arthritis flare (2 points), onset within 1 d (0.5 points), joint redness (1 point), 1st metatarsal phalangeal joint involvement (2.5 points), hypertension or CVD (1.5 points), serum urate >5.88 mg/dL (3.5 points). Score ≥8 is high probability, ≥4 and ≤8 is intermediate probability, and <4 is low probability.

Management

Treatment of Acute Gouty Flare: Any of the following are appropriate 1st-line options (ACR):

- Intra-articular injections (p 222) if only 1 or 2 joints involved
- NSAIDs (**Table 82**); avoid ASA, indomethacin[BC]
- Colchicine 1.2 mg (2 tabs) for the 1st dose, followed 1 h later by 0.6 mg (total dose 1.8 mg) unless patient has received this regimen within the last 14 d. Then begin 0.6 mg 1×/d or q12h.
- Prednisone▲ 30–40 mg po daily or in 2 divided doses until flare resolves then taper over 7–10 d. If npo, can give IV or IM.
- If polyarticular or multiple large joint involvement or severe pain, consider combination tx of methylprednisolone 0.5–2 mg/kg po q12h with taper or ACTH 25–40 IU SC; may repeat daily for 3 d
- IL-1 inhibitors (canakinumab [*Ilaris*] and anakinra [*Kineret*]) may be useful if cannot tolerate other options

Pharmacologic anti-inflammatory prophylaxis: Colchicine 0.6 mg/d or 2×/d for 2–4 wk before and for up to 6 mo after beginning any tx in **Table 85**.

Table 85. Medications Useful in Managing Chronic Gout

Medication	Usual Dosage	Formulations	Comments (Metabolism, Excretion)
Xanthine oxidase inhibitors			
✓ Allopurinol ▲	100–900 mg/d in divided doses if >300 mg/d	T: 100, 300	Consider if nephrolithiasis, tophi, Cr ≥2 mg/dL, 24-h urinary uric acid >800 mg. Starting dosage should not exceed 100 mg/d and 50 mg/d in ≥stage 4 CKD. Do not initiate during flare; reduce dosage in renal or hepatic impairment; increase dose by 100 mg every 2–5 wk to normalize serum urate level; monitor CBC; rash is common; if Han Chinese, Thai, or African American, screen for HLA-B*5801 before initiating (K)
Febuxostat (Uloric)	40–80 mg/d	T: 40, 80	Begin 40 mg/d; increase to 80 mg/d if uric acid >6 mg/dL at 2 wk; not recommended if CrCl <30; increased risk of cardiovascular and all-cause mortality (K, L)
Uricosurics			Avoid if urolithiasis and if increase risk of urate nephropathy; less effective in urate overproducers
Probenecid ▲ OTC	500–1500 mg in 2–3 divided doses	T: 500	Contraindicated as 1st-line if hx of urolithiasis. Measure urinary uric acid before initiating and if >800 mg/24 h, contraindicated. Adjust dose to normalize serum urate level or increase urine urate excretion; inhibits platelet function; may not be effective if renal impairment[BC] (CrCl <50) (K, L)
Lesinurad (Zurampic)	200 mg/d	T: 200	Must be taken with allopurinol or febuxostat; should not be started if CrCl <45 (L, K)
Uricase			
Pegloticase (Krystexxa)	8 mg IV q2wk	8 mg/1-mL vial	Effective in reducing flares in patients with high uric acid levels intolerant of or refractory to allopurinol; may cause anaphylaxis, gout flares, and infusion reactions; contraindicated if G6PD deficiency (K)
Rasburicase (Elitek)	0.2 mg/kg IV monthly		Hypersensitivity reactions; do not administer if G6PD deficiency
Other agents			
Colchicine[1] (Colcrys)[2]	0.5–0.6 mg/d	T: 0.5, 0.6 Inj	Lower dose and monitor AEs if CrCl <30.[BC] May also be effective in prevention of recurrent pseudogout; monitor CBC (L)
Losartan (Cozaar)	12.5–100 mg q12–24h	T: 25, 50, 100	Modest uricosuric effect that plateaus at 50 mg/d; may be useful in patients with HTN or HF

✓ = preferred for treating older adults; G6PD = glucose-6-phosphate-dehydrogenase; CrCl unit = mL/min/1.73 m^2

[1] Probenecid (500 mg) and colchicine (0.5 mg) combinations are available as generic.

[2] No longer available as generic.

- If unable to tolerate low-dose colchicine, low-dose NSAIDs with PPI (if indicated)
- If neither of the above are tolerated, or if either are contraindicated or ineffective, low-dose prednisone or prednisolone (<10 mg/d)
- Duration of tx is:
  ◦ 3–6 mo after achieving target urate, if no tophi
  ◦ Until tophi resolve
  ◦ Indefinitely if tophi persist after achieving target urate

Treatment of Chronic Gout

Nonpharmacologic

Lifestyle modification (weight loss if overweight, decrease in saturated fats, substitute low-fat dairy products for red meat or fish, limit alcohol use, avoid organ meats high in purine content [eg, sweetbread, liver, kidney]; avoid high fructose corn syrup–sweetened sodas). D/C nonessential medications that induce hyperuricemia (eg, thiazides and loop diuretics, niacin).

Pharmacologic

Indications for pharmacologic tx: Established diagnosis of gouty arthritis and:
- Tophus or tophi, clinical or on x-ray
- Frequent attacks (≥2/y)
- CKD stage 2 or worse
- Past urolithiasis

Target is <6 mg/dL and often <5 mg/d at no faster rate than 1–2 mg/dL/mo. Most but not all professional societies recommend treating to target and monitoring q12mo if stable, q6mo if ongoing symptoms or tophi (**Table 85**). First-line is allopurinol. If contraindicated or not tolerated, probenecid. Fenofibrate and losartan are also uricosuric. Avoid febuxostat in patients with high cardiovascular risk. Lesinurad is reserved for patients who remain hyperuricemic with allopurinol or febuxostat alone. Pegloticase is reserved for patients with severe gout disease burden and refractory or intolerance to 1st-line agents.

PSEUDOGOUT

Definition

Crystal-induced arthritis (especially affecting knees and wrists) associated with calcium pyrophosphate. A small proportion have pseudo-RA (chronic crystal inflammatory arthritis) with chronic joint inflammation.

Risk Factors

- Advanced osteoarthritis
- DM
- Gout
- Hemochromatosis
- Hypercalcemia
- Hyperparathyroidism
- Hypomagnesemia
- Hypophosphatemia
- Hypothyroidism
- Neuropathic joints
- Older age

Precipitating Factors

- Acute illness
- Dehydration
- Minor trauma
- Surgery

Evaluation of Acute Arthritis

Joint aspiration and microscopic examination to establish diagnosis; radiograph indicating chondrocalcinosis (best seen in wrists, knees, shoulder, symphysis pubis)

Management of Acute Flare

If 1 or 2 joints, aspiration and intra-articular glucocorticoid may be effective. If multiple joints, see Gout, management (p 229). NSAIDs are often used 1st, because colchicine is less effective in pseudogout.

Prevention of Recurrence

If >3 attacks/y, consider colchicine 0.6 mg q12h.

If chronic calcium pyrophosphate crystal inflammatory arthritis (ie, pseudo-RA), NSAIDs +/– colchicines and, if needed, followed by methotrexate (controversial) and/or hydroxychloroquine.

POLYMYALGIA RHEUMATICA, GIANT CELL (TEMPORAL) ARTERITIS

Definitions and Evaluation

Polymyalgia Rheumatica

Proximal limb and girdle stiffness usually lasting ≥30 min without tenderness but with constitutional symptoms (eg, fatigue, malaise, weight loss) for ≥1 mo and sedimentation rate elevated to >50 mm/h (7–22% will have normal sedimentation rate), and CRP; consider ultrasound to demonstrate effusions within shoulder bursae or MRI to demonstrate tenosynovitis or subacromial and subdeltoid bursitis if diagnosis is uncertain.

Provisional ACR/EULAR classification criteria include:
- required criteria: age >50, bilateral shoulder aching, abnormal CRP or ESR
- morning stiffness >45 min (2 points)
- hip pain/limited range of motion (1 point)
- absence of rheumatoid factor and/or anticitrullinated protein antibody (2 points)
- absence of peripheral joint pain (1 point)

Scores ≥4 had 68% sensitivity and 78% specificity. Specificity is higher (88%) for discriminating shoulder conditions from polymyalgia rheumatica and lower (65%) for discriminating RA from polymyalgia rheumatica. A subsequent single-site study demonstrated better test characteristics in an unselected population with early inflammatory articular disease. Clinical usefulness of these criteria remain to be determined.

Other recommended tests include RF, CBC, comprehensive metabolic panel, and dipstick UA.

Giant Cell (Temporal) Arteritis

Medium to large vessel vasculitis that presents with symptoms of polymyalgia rheumatica, headache, unexplained fever or anemia, scalp tenderness, jaw or tongue claudication, visual disturbances, TIA or stroke, and elevated sedimentation rate and CRP. The presence of synovitis suggests an alternative diagnosis. Giant cell arteritis is confirmed by temporal artery biopsy. The value of other diagnostic tests (Color Doppler ultrasound, MRI, positron-emission tomography) is still unproved.

Management

Polymyalgia Rheumatica

- Low-dosage (eg, 12.5–25 mg/d) prednisone[BC] or its equivalent; increase dosage if symptoms are not controlled within 1 wk. If symptoms are not controlled by 20 mg/d, consider alternative diagnosis (eg, giant cell arteritis, paraneoplastic syndrome).
- Individualize dose tapering to oral dose of 10 mg/d within 4–8 wk. If relapse, increase to prerelapse dose and decrease gradually within 4–8 wk. Once-daily dose is 10 mg, taper in 1-mg/4-wk decrements. Minimum duration of tx is 1 y.
- Methylprednisolone[▲BC] 120 mg IM q3–4 wk is an alternative with reduction to 100 mg at wk 12 and reduce by 20 mg every 12 wk until wk 48, then by 20 mg every 16 wk.
- Monitor symptoms and CRP or sedimentation rate.
- Consider the addition of oral methotrexate 7.5–10 mg/wk if high risk of relapse, comorbidities that increase steroid complications, relapse, and for nonresponders. Evidence for TNF inhibitors and IL-6 blockade is still preliminary.
- Consider osteoporosis prevention medication (p 248).

Giant Cell (Temporal) Arteritis

- Tx should not be delayed while waiting for pathologic diagnosis from temporal artery biopsy. Begin prednisone (40–60 mg/d) or its equivalent while biopsy and pathology are pending. Consider GI bleed prophylaxis with PPI.[BC]

- Methotrexate[▲] po 7.5–15 mg/wk and folate 5–7.5 mg/d may reduce the amount of steroid needed and the risk of relapse, but the effect is moderate at best. It may be best for those who have or are at high risk of developing AEs due to prednisone.

- After 2–4 wk, begin taper by 10 mg after 2 wk and another 10 mg prednisone/d at 4 wk, gradual taper (by 10% every 1–2 wk) over 9–12 mo. Once-daily dose is 10 mg, taper in 1-mg/ mo decrements. Monitor Hb, ESR, CRP before dose changes, but treat based on symptoms, not lab tests.

- High-dose pulse parenteral steroids (eg, 1000 mg methylprednisolone IV daily for 3 d) for visual loss is controversial.

- Adding IL-6 receptor inhibitor tocilizumab *(Actemra)* 162 mg SC qwk or every other week or abatacept *(Orencia)* 10 mg/kg days 14, 21, 29, and week 8 increases the rate of glucocorticoid-free remission.

- For relapsing or refractory cases, adding IL-6 receptor inhibitor tocilizumab *(Actemra)* or cyclophosphamide, mean dose 100 mg/d [T: 25, 50] may be helpful. Anti-TNF agents (infliximab, etanercept, and adalimumab) have not been effective.

- Use low-dosage ASA (81–100 mg/d) to reduce risk of visual loss, TIA, or stroke. Combine with PPI or misoprostol.

- Be aware of higher rates of systemic infection during 1st 6 mo of tx and higher rates of CVD.

- Monitor symptoms and CRP or sedimentation rate.

- Maintain tx for 1 y to prevent relapse; 35% relapse within 21 mo.

- Consider osteoporosis prevention medication (p 247).

- Monitor for development of thoracic aortic aneurysm, especially ascending, with CT is on a case-by-case basis.

TREMORS

Table 86. Classification of Tremors

Tremor Type	Hz (cycles/sec)	Associated Conditions	Features	Treatment
Cerebellar	3–5	Cerebellar disease	Present only during movement; ↑ with intention; ↑ amplitude as target is approached	Symptomatic management
Essential	4–12	Familial in 50% of cases	Varying amplitude; common in upper extremities, head, neck; ↑ with antigravity movements, intention, stress, medications	Long-acting propranolol▲ (Table 28); or primidone (Mysoline) 100 mg qhs start, titrate to 250–750 mg/d in 3–4 divided doses [T: 50, 250; S: 250 mg/5 mL]; or gabapentin▲BC (Table 92)
Parkinson	4–7	Parkinson disease, parkinsonism	"Pill rolling;" present at rest; ↑ with emotional stress or when examiner calls attention to it; commonly asymmetric	See Parkinson disease (p 238)
Physiologic	4–12	Normal	Low amplitude; ↑ with stress, anxiety, emotional upset, lack of sleep, fatigue, toxins, medications	Tx of exacerbating factor

BC Avoid if CrCl <60 mL/min/1.73 m²

DIZZINESS

- Medications commonly associated with orthostatic hypotension include:
  - Cardiac: α-blockers, β-blockers, ACEIs, diuretics, nitrates, clonidine, hydralazine, methyldopa, reserpine, dipyridamole
  - CNS: antipsychotics, opioids, medications for Parkinson disease, skeletal muscle relaxants, TCAs
  - Urologic: antimuscarinic agents for UI, PDE-5 inhibitors
- Caffeine, alcohol, nicotine, and head trauma can also cause or contribute to dizziness.

Table 87. Classification of Dizziness

Primary Symptom	Duration	Diagnosis	Management
Dizziness			
Lightheadedness 1–30 min after standing	Seconds to minutes (E)	Orthostatic hypotension	p 70
Wobbly/off balance gait; impairment in >1 of the following: vision, vestibular function, spinal proprioception, cerebellum, lower-extremity peripheral nerves	Occurs with ambulation (C)	Multiple sensory impairments including peripheral neuropathy; Parkinson disease	Correct or maximize sensory deficits; PT for balance and strength training; walking aid

(cont.)

Table 87. Classification of Dizziness (cont.)

Primary Symptom	Duration	Diagnosis	Management
Unsteady gait with short steps; ↑ reflexes and/or tone	Occurs with ambulation (C)	Ischemic cerebral disease	ASA▲; modification of vascular risk factors; PT
Provoked by head or neck movement; reduced neck range of motion	Seconds to minutes (E)	Cervical spondylosis	Behavior modification; reduce cervical spasm and inflammation
Drop attacks			
Provoked by head or neck movement, reduced vertebral artery flow seen on Doppler or angiography	Seconds to minutes (E)	Postural impingement of vertebral artery	Behavior modification
Vertigo			
Brought on by position change, positive Dix-Hallpike test	Seconds to minutes (E)	Benign paroxysmal positional vertigo	Epley or Semont maneuver to reposition crystalline debris[1]
Acute onset, nonpositional	Days	Labyrinthitis/ vestibular neuronitis	Methylprednisolone▲, 100 mg/d po × 3 d with subsequent gradual taper over 3 wk to improve vestibular function recovery; meclizine▲ BC (**Table 61**) for acute symptom relief
Low-frequency sensorineural hearing loss (usually begins unilaterally) and tinnitus, ear pain, sense of fullness in ear	Minutes to hours (E)	Ménière disease	Meclizine▲ BC (**Table 61**) for acute symptom relief; diuretics and/or salt restriction for prophylaxis
Vascular disease risk factors, cranial nerve abnormalities	10 min to several hours (E)	TIAs	ASA▲; modification of vascular risk factors

C = chronic; E = episodic.

[1] youtube.com/watch?v=nX1HU-CCg2Y or youtube.com/watch?v=hiP7ifVxb0Q

MANAGEMENT OF ACUTE STROKE

Examination

- Cardiac (murmurs, arrhythmias, enlargement)
- Neurologic (serial examinations)
- Optic fundi
- Vascular (carotids and other peripheral pulses)

Tests

- Bloodwork: BUN, CBC with platelet count, Cr, electrolytes, glucose, cardiac troponins, INR, PT, PTT, oxygen saturation
- Emergent brain MRI or noncontrast CT
- ECG

- The National Institutes of Health Stroke Scale (NIHSS; stroke.nih.gov/documents/ NIH_Stroke_Scale.pdf) can quantify stroke severity and prognosis. NIHSS score >15 signifies major or severe stroke with high risk of death or significant permanent neurologic disability; NIHSS score <8 has a good prognosis for neurologic recovery.
- Other tests as indicated by clinical presentation:
  - ABG if hypoxia is suspected
  - Thrombin time and/or ecarin clotting time if patient is taking direct thrombin inhibitor or factor Xa inhibitor
  - Intracranial angiography by MRA, CT angiography, or Doppler ultrasound if intraarterial fibrinolysis or mechanical thrombectomy is being contemplated
  - Echocardiography (transesophageal preferred over transthoracic) for detection of cardiogenic emboli
  - Carotid duplex and transcranial Doppler studies for detection of carotid and vertebrobasilar embolic sources, respectively

Provide Supportive Care

- Maintain O_2 saturation >94%.
- Correct metabolic and hydration imbalances.
- Detect and treat coronary ischemia, HF, arrhythmias.
- In patients with ischemic stroke and restricted mobility, implement DVT/PE prophylaxis with UFH[A], LMWH, or fondaparinux[BC] (Avoid if CrCl <30 mL/min/1.73 m²) (**Table 18**).
- Monitor and treat hyperthermia, using antipyretics (eg, APAP) for temperature >100.4°F.
- Monitor for depression.
- Refer to rehabilitation when medically stable.
- Discharge on statin drug (**Table 26** and **Table 27**).

Antithrombotic Therapy for Ischemic Stroke (AHA/American Stroke Association Guidelines)

- Consider IV thrombolysis if patient presents within 180 min of symptom onset.
  - Data on overall risk/benefit ratio of IV thrombolysis in adults aged >75 are limited.
  - Absolute contraindications:
    - BP ≥185/110 mmHg
    - subarachnoid hemorrhage or hx of intracranial hemorrhage
    - intracranial neoplasm, arteriovenous malformation, or aneurysm
    - head trauma or stroke in past 3 mo
    - GI bleed or urinary hemorrhage in past 21 d
    - recent intracranial or intraspinal surgery
    - active bleeding or acute trauma
    - INR >1.7 or PT >15 sec
    - heparin use in past 48 h with supranormal PTT
    - current use of direct thrombin inhibitor or factor Xa inhibitor with elevated tests for anticoagulation (eg, PTT, INR, thrombin time, ecarin clotting time)
    - platelet count <100,000 mm³
    - blood glucose <50 mg/dL
  - Relative contraindications (carefully consider risk/benefit of thrombolysis if 1 or more are present):
    - minor or rapidly improving stroke symptoms
    - seizure at stroke onset with postictal neurologic impairments
    - major surgery or serious trauma in past 14 d

- GI or urinary tract hemorrhage in past 21 d
  - acute MI in past 3 mo
    - Use recombinant tissue plasminogen activator (tPA), 0.9 mg/kg IV, max dose 90 mg.
    - Risk of intracranial hemorrhage 3–7%; age >75 and NIHSS >20 are among risk factors for intracranial hemorrhage.
- IV thrombolysis can be considered 3–4.5 h after symptom onset; additional relative exclusion criteria include age >80 or NIHSS >25.
- Antiplatelet tx: use ASA▲ 162–325 mg/d (initial dose 325 mg), begun within 24–48 h of onset in patients not receiving thrombolytic tx.
- Anticoagulants are not recommended except in DVT/PE prophylactic dosages for medical patients with restricted mobility (**Table 18**).

Management of Acute Hypertension in Ischemic Stroke

- If patient is otherwise eligible for IV thrombolysis (see contraindications, p 236), attempt to lower BP to ≤185/110 mmHg so that patient may undergo reperfusion tx. Options for lowering BP are:
  - Labetalol▲ 10–20 mg IV over 1–2 min, may repeat once; *or*
  - Nicardipine▲ 5 mg/h IV, increasing by 2.5 mg/h q5–15 min to max of 15 mg/h
- If patient is ineligible or not being considered for thrombolytic tx, do not lower BP if SBP ≤220 mmHg or if DBP ≤120 mmHg; higher BP may be lowered gently, with goal of 15% reduction over 1st 24 h. Choice of BP-lowering agent should reflect patient's comorbidities (**Table 28**).

Endovascular Thrombectomy (EVT)

- EVT should be considered in patients with large vessel occlusion presenting within 16 h of symptoms and treated with thrombolytic tx.
- EVT is more likely to be beneficial in larger strokes with more significant deficits (NIHSS >8).
  - Compared to medical tx alone, EVT produces significantly better functional outcomes with no added risks.

Management of Hypertension in Acute Intracranial Hemorrhage

- Do NOT lower BP if SBP is between 150 and 220 mmHg.
- If SBP >220 mmHg, consider lowering BP gently with IV agents and continuous BP monitoring.

STROKE PREVENTION

Risk Factor Modification

- Stop smoking.
- Treat HTN:
  - If previously treated, restart oral antihypertensive medication a few days after TIA or stroke.
  - If hypertensive but not previously treated, initiate oral antihypertensive medication a few days after TIA or stroke.
  - Goal BP <130/80 mmHg; adjust goal upward according to comorbidities, function, and patient preference.
- Treat dyslipidemia (**Table 26** and **Table 27**).
- Start anticoagulation (**Table 18**) or antiplatelet (**Table 17**) tx for AF.
- Low-sodium (≤2.4 g/d), Mediterranean-type diet

- Exercise (≥30 min of moderate-intensity activity daily)
- Weight reduction
- Screen for DM

Antiplatelet Therapy for Patients With Prior TIA or Stroke

- First-line tx is ASA▲ 50–325 mg/d, combination form of ASA and long-acting dipyridamole *(Aggrenox)* 1 tab q12h [T: 25/200], or clopidogrel▲ 75 mg/d [T: 75].
- For patients with minor ischemic stroke or TIA, dual tx with ASA and clopidogrel begun within 24 h of the event and continued for the first 21 d may be of added benefit compared to monotx.
- In the absence of AF, warfarin tx is no more effective and is associated with more bleeding than ASA in preventing strokes.

Table 88. Treatment Options for Carotid Stenosis in Older Adults

Presentation	% Stenosis	Treatment Options	Comments
Prior TIA or stroke	≥70	CA/CE[1] or MM	CE superior to medical tx only if patient is reasonable surgical risk and facility has track record of low complication rate for CE (<6%)
Prior TIA or stroke	50–69	CE or MM	Serial carotid Doppler testing may identify rapidly developing plaques
Prior TIA or stroke	<50	MM	CE of no proven benefit in this situation
Asymptomatic	≥70	CA/CE[CW,1] or MM	CA/CE[1] should be considered over MM only for the most healthy. Don't recommend CE for asymptomatic carotid stenosis unless the complication rate is low (<3%).[CW]
Asymptomatic	<70	MM	CE of no proven benefit in this situation

CA = carotid angioplasty with stent placement in patients with multiple comorbidities and/or at high surgical risk; CE = carotid endarterectomy; MM = medical management.

[1] Younger patients may have a greater risk of stroke with CA and a greater risk of mortality with CE, compared to older patients. Mortality risk for CA and stroke risk for CE are the same in both groups.

PARKINSON DISEASE

Diagnosis Requires:

- Bradykinesia, eg:
  - Slowness of initiation of voluntary movements (eg, glue-footedness when starting to walk)
  - Reduced speed and amplitude of repetitive movements (eg, tapping index finger and thumb together)
  - Difficulty switching from one motor program to another (eg, multiple steps to turn during gait testing)

and one or more of the following:
  - Muscular rigidity (eg, cogwheeling)
  - 4–7 Hz resting tremor
  - Impaired righting reflex (eg, retropulsed during sternal push or shoulder pull test)
- Other clinical features of Parkinson disease:
  - Postural instability and falls
  - Hyposmia
  - Hypophonia
  - Micrographia
  - REM sleep behavior disorder
  - Constipation

- ◦ Masked facies
- ◦ Infrequent blinking
- ◦ Drooling
- ◦ Seborrhea of face and scalp
- ◦ Festinating gait
- Neuropsychiatric conditions are also common usually later in the clinical course: anxiety, depression, dementia, visual hallucinations, dysthymia, psychosis, delirium

Table 89. Distinguishing Early Parkinson Disease From Other Parkinsonian Syndromes

Condition	Tremor	Asymmetric Involvement	Early Falls	Early Dementia	Postural Hypotension
Parkinson disease	+	+	–	–	–
Drug-induced parkinsonism	+/–	–	–	–	–
Vascular parkinsonism	–	+/–	+/–	+/–	–
Dementia with Lewy bodies	+/–	+/–	+/–	+	+/–
Progressive supranuclear palsy	–	–	+	+/–	–
Corticobasal ganglionic degeneration	–	+	+	–	+
Multiple-system atrophy	–	+/–	+/–	–	+

+ = usually or always present; +/– = sometimes present; – = absent.

Source: Adapted from Christine CW, Aminoff MJ. *Am J Med* 2004;117:412–419.

Nonpharmacologic Management

- Patient education is essential, and support groups are often helpful.
- Monitor for orthostatic hypotension (p 70).
- PT/Exercise programs to improve physical functioning, stability, and constipation:
  - ◦ Regular aerobic exercise (eg, treadmill training)
  - ◦ Balance and flexibility exercises (eg, tai chi)
  - ◦ Resistance training
- OT to maximize fine-motor functioning with adaptive equipment (eg, specialized eating utensils) and to perform home safety evaluations
- Speech-language tx to improve dysarthria and hypophonia
- Diet with increased fiber and hydration to minimize constipation; adequate vitamin D and calcium as osteopenia is common

Surgical Treatment—Deep Brain Stimulation (DBS)

- DBS of the globus pallidus or subthalamic nucleus is used for tx of motor complications of Parkinson disease.
- DBS is best suited for patients who have fluctuating motor problems (tremor and other dyskinesias) despite medical tx and who have few comorbidities, especially no dementia.
- Compared with medical tx in selected patients, DBS can significantly increase motor function (several more hours per day of "on" time) and decrease troubling dyskinesias.
- Early (0–3 mo) complications include surgical site infection (~10%), symptomatic intracranial hemorrhage (~2%), death (~1%), cognitive and speech problems (10–15%), and an increased risk of falls.

Pharmacologic Treatment (Tables 90 and 91)

- Begin tx when symptoms interfere with function.
- First-line tx is dopamine or dopamine agonist.
- Start at low dose and titrate upward gradually.
- Monitor orthostatic BP during titration of medications.
- Tailor tx to symptoms.

Table 90. Symptom-Directed Treatment of Parkinson Disease

Category	Symptoms	Treatment Options
Motor	Tremor, bradykinesia, rigidity	Use dopamine, dopamine agonists
	Persistent tremor despite dopamine/dopamine-agonist tx	Add β-blocker or clozapine; consider DBS
	Bradykinesia, motor fluctuations, increased "off time" despite dopamine tx	Increase dopamine dose; add dopamine agonist or COMT inhibitor or MAO B inhibitor (**Table 91**); consider DBS for refractory motor fluctuations
	Postural instability or gait impairment despite dopamine tx	Add amantadine or cholinesterase inhibitor
Nonmotor	Depression	Try SSRI or SNRI; consider careful trial of TCA[BC]; consider trial of pramipexole
	Cognitive impairment/Parkinson disease/Dementia	Consider trial of cholinesterase inhibitor, monitoring carefully for exacerbation of tremor or GI side effects
	Orthostatic hypotension	See Orthostatic (Postural) Hypotension (p 70)
	REM sleep behavior disorder	Try high-dose melatonin 3–15 mg hs (**Table 130** and p 348); if not effective, consider careful trial of clonazepam 0.25–1 mg hs only in healthier patients without dementia or sleep apnea at low risk of falls
Drug-Induced	Dyskinesias	Carefully reduce dopamine dose (if motor symptoms worsen, try adding low dose of dopamine agonist); add amantadine; consider clozapine
	Nausea	Slowly titrate dopamine dose; consider domperidone; avoid metoclopramide, prochlorperazine, and promethazine[BC]
	Impulse-control disorders	Reduce or D/C dopamine agonists; consider trial of amantadine
	Hallucinations/psychosis	Exclude systemic illness; carefully reduce antiparkinsonian drugs; try pimavanserin *(Nuplazid)* 34 mg po qd [T: 17], which can take up to 3 wk to be effective; alternatives are quetiapine or clozapine (avoid all other antipsychotics[BC])

Table 91. Medications for Parkinson Disease

Class, Medication	Initial Dosage	Formulations	Comments (Metabolism, Excretion)
Dopamine			
Carbidopa-levodopa▲	1/2 tab of 25/100 q812h	T: 10/100, 25/100, 25/250	Mainstay of Parkinson disease tx; increase dose by 1/2–1 tab q1–2wk to achieve minimal target dose of 1 tab q8h, then titrate upward gradually prn; watch for GI AEs, orthostatic hypotension, confusion; long-term tx associated with motor fluctuations and dyskinesias (addition of dopamine agonist may attenuate these effects) (L)
(Duopa)	Complex calculation in package insert	sus: 4.63/20 per mL	For use in patients with enteral feeding
Sustained-release carbidopa-levodopa▲	1 tab/d	T: 25/100, 50/200	Useful at daily dopamine requirement ≥300 mg; slower absorption than carbidopa-levodopa; can improve motor fluctuations (L)
(RYTARY)	23.75/95 q8h	C: 23.75/95, 36.25/145, 48.75/195, 61.25/245	
Dopamine Agonists			More CNS AEs than dopamine
Pramipexole▲	0.125 mg/d	T: 0.125, 0.25, 0.5, 1, 1.5	Increase gradually to effective dosage (0.5–1.5 mg q8h) (K)
Extended-release pramipexole▲	0.375 mg/d	T: 0.375, 0.75, 1.5, 2.25, 3, 3.75, 4.5	Increase gradually to effective dosage (1.5–4.5 mg qd) (K)
Ropinirole▲	0.25 mg/d	T▲: 0.25, 0.5, 1, 2, 3, 4, 5 CR: 4, 8	Increase gradually to effective dosage (up to 1–8 mg q8h) (L)
Extended-release ropinirole▲	2 mg/d	T: 2, 4, 6, 8, 12	Increase gradually to effective dosage (up to 6–24 mg qd) (L)
Rotigotine *(Neupro)*	2 mg/24 h for early stage disease; 4 mg/24 h for advanced disease	pch: 1, 2, 3, 4, 6, 8 mg/24 h	Increase weekly to effective dosage (max 6 mg/24 h for early stage disease, 8 mg/24 h for advanced disease) (K)
Catechol *O*-Methyl-transferase (COMT) Inhibitors			Adjunctive tx with L-dopa
Tolcapone *(Tasmar)*	100 mg q8h	T: 100, 200	Monitor LFTs q6mo (L, K)
Entacapone *(Comtan)*	200 mg with each L-dopa dose	T: 200	Watch for nausea, orthostatic hypotension (K)

(cont.)

Table 91. Medications for Parkinson Disease (cont.)

Class, Medication	Initial Dosage	Formulations	Comments (Metabolism, Excretion)
Anticholinergics			
Benztropine▲ ᴮᶜ	0.5 mg/d	T: 0.5, 1, 2	Can cause confusion and delirium; helpful for drooling. Avoid.ᴮᶜ (L, K)
Trihexyphenidyl▲ ᴮᶜ	1 mg/d	T: 2, 5 S: 2 mg/5 mL	Same as above. Avoid.ᴮᶜ (L, K)
Dopamine Reuptake Inhibitor			
Amantadine▲	100 mg q12–24h	T: 100 C: 100 S: 50 mg/5 mL	Useful in early and late Parkinson disease; watch closely for CNS AEs; do not D/C abruptly (K)
Extended-release Amantadine *(Gocovri)*	137 mg qhs	C: 68.5, 137	Can be used for tx of dyskinesia in patients on dopamine tx; many behavioral AEs (K)
(Osmolex ER)	129 mg/d	T: 129, 193, 258	
Monoamine Oxidase B (MAO B) Inhibitors			
Rasagiline *(Azilect)*	0.5 mg/d	T: 0.5, 1	Interactions with numerous drugs and tyramine-rich foods; expensive (L, K)
Safinamide *(Xadago)*	50 mg/d	T: 50, 100	Use as adjunctive tx with dopamine to treat "off" episodes; many AEs and drug interactions (K)
Selegiline▲	5 mg qam; 1.25 mg/d for ODT	T: 5 ODT: 1.25	Use as adjunctive tx with dopamine; do not exceed a total dosage of 10 mg/d; metabolized to amphetamine derivatives (L, K)
Combination Medication			
Carbidopa-levodopa + entacapone *(Stalevo)*	1 tab/d	T: 12.5/50/200, 25/100/200, 37.5/150/200	Should be used only after individual dosages of carbidopa, L-dopa, and entacapone have been established (L, K)

✓ = preferred for treating older adults

MULTIPLE-SYSTEM ATROPHY (MSA)

Diagnosis (see also **Table 89**)

- Diagnosis is made on hx and physical findings.
- May have early nonmotor phase characterized by urinary and/or sexual dysfunction, orthostatic hypotension, REM sleep behavior disorder.
- Clinical hallmarks are (in varying combinations):
  - Progressive autonomic failure – erectile dysfunction, genital hyposensitivity in women, urinary dysfunction, orthostatic hypotension.
  - Parkinsonism – bradykinesia, rigidity, falls; resting pill-rolling tremor is not usually seen but may have postural action tremor.
  - Cerebellar dysfunction – wide-based gait ataxia, uncoordinated limb movements.

- Other common features include:
  - Inspiratory stridor
  - Pronounced neck flexion (antecollis)
  - Depression and/or anxiety
  - Absence of dementia and hallucinations
  - Frontal lobe executive dysfunction and attention deficits

Clinical Course
- Rapid progression of motor symptoms once they appear (about half of patients will require a walking aid within 3 y after onset of motor manifestations)
- Progressive course over approximately 6–10 y, culminating in death
- Late stage characterized by frequent falls, profound bradykinesia, unintelligible speech, recurrent aspiration pneumonia

Management
- Tx is for symptom management of above conditions; there are no known disease-altering tx.
- Up to 40% of patients will respond transiently to L-dopa tx, which should be continued if there are no side effects.
- Neurorehabilitation programs can be helpful for maximizing mobility, preventing falls, increasing communication ability, and preventing choking episodes.

SEIZURES

Classification
- Generalized: All areas of brain affected with alteration in consciousness
- Partial: Focal brain area affected, not necessarily with alteration in consciousness; can progress to generalized type

Initial Evaluation, Assessment
- History: neurologic disorders, trauma, drug and alcohol use
- Physical examination: general, with careful neurologic
- Routine tests: BUN, calcium, CBC, Cr, ECG, EEG, electrolytes, glucose, head CT, LFTs, magnesium
- Tests as indicated: head MRI, lumbar puncture, oxygen saturation, urine toxic or drug screen

Common Causes
- Advanced dementia
- CNS infection
- Drug or alcohol withdrawal
- Idiopathic causes
- Metabolic disorders
- Prior stroke (most common)
- Toxins
- Trauma
- Tumor

Management
- Treat underlying causes.
- Institute anticonvulsant tx (**Table 92**). Virtually all anticonvulsant medications can cause sedation and ataxia.
- Avoid the following drugs, which can lower seizure threshold: bupropion, chlorpromazine, clozapine, maprotiline, olanzapine, thioridazine, thiothixene, and tramadol.[BC]

Table 92. Anticonvulsant Therapy in Older Adults

Medication	Dosage (mg)	Target Blood Concentration (mcg/mL)	Formulations	Comments (Metabolism, Excretion)
◆ Carbamazepine▲	200–600 q12h	4–12	T: 200▲ ChT: 100 S: 100/5 mL▲ T: 100, 200, 400▲ C: ER 100, 200, 300	Many drug interactions; mood stabilizer; may cause SIADH[BC], thrombocytopenia, leukopenia (L, K)
◆ Gabapentin▲	300–600 q8h or q12h	NA	C: 100, 300, 400 T: 600, 800 S: 250/5 mL	Used as adjunct to other agents; reduce dosage if CrCl <60[BC] (K)
Lacosamide *(VIMPAT)*	50–200 q12h	NA	T: 50, 100, 150, 200 S: 10/mL	Used as adjunct to other agents for partial-onset seizures; not studied in older adults (L, K)
Lamotrigine▲	100–300 q12h	2–4	T: 25, 100, 150, 200 ChT: 2, 5, 25	Prolongs PR interval; risk of severe rash; when used with valproic acid, begin at 25 mg q48h, titrate to 25–100 mg q12h (L, K)
Levetiracetam▲	500–1500 q12h	NA	T: 250, 500, 750 S: 100/mL CR: 500, 750	Reduce dosage in renal impairment[BC]: CrCl 30–50: 250–750 q12h CrCl 10–29: 250–500 q12h CrCl <10: 500–1000 q24h (K)
Oxcarbazepine *(Trileptal)*	300–1200 q12h	NA	T▲: 150, 300, 600 ChT: 2, 5, 25 S: 300/5 mL	Can cause hyponatremia[BC], leukopenia (L)
Phenobarbital▲	30–60 q8–12h	20–40	T: 15, 16, 30, 32, 60, 100 S: 20/5 mL	Many drug interactions; not recommended for use in older adults (L)
Phenytoin▲	200–300/d	5–20	C: 30, 100 ChT: 50 S: 125/5 mL	Many drug interactions; exhibits nonlinear pharmacokinetics (L)
◆ Pregabalin *(Lyrica)*	50–200 q8–12h		C: 25, 50, 75, 100, 150, 200, 225, 300	Indicated as adjunct tx for partial-onset seizures only; adjust dosage on basis of CrCl[BC] (K)
Tiagabine *(Gabitril)*	2–12 q8–12h	NA	T: 2, 4, 12, 16, 20	AE profile in older adults less well described (L)
Topiramate▲	25–100 q12–24h	NA	T: 25, 100, 200 C, sprinkle: 15, 25	May affect cognitive functioning at high dosages (L, K)
Extended-release topiramate▲	25–200/d	NA	C: 25, 50, 100, 150, 200	
Valproic acid▲	250–750 q8–12h	50–100	T: 125, 250, 500 C: 125, 250 S: 250/5 mL	Can cause weight gain, tremor, hair loss; several drug interactions; mood stabilizer; monitor LFTs and platelets (L)
(Depakote ER)			T: 500	
Zonisamide▲	100–400/d	NA	C: 25, 100	Anorexia; contraindicated in patients with sulfonamide allergy (K)

NA = not available   ◆ = also has primary indication for neuropathic pain. CrCl unit = mL/min/1.73 m^2

Table 93. Aphasias in Which Repetition Is Impaired

Type	Fluency	Auditory Comprehension	Associated Neurologic Deficits	Comments
Broca	–	+	Right hemiparesis	Patient aware of deficit; high rate of associated depression; message board helpful for communication
Wernicke	+	–	Often none	Patient frequently unaware of deficit; speech content usually unintelligible; tx often focuses on visually based communication
Conduction	+	+	Occasional right facial weakness	Patient usually aware of deficit; speech content usually intelligible
Global	–	–	Right hemiplegia with right field cut	Most commonly due to left middle cerebral artery thrombosis, which has a poor prognosis for meaningful speech recovery

+ = present; – = absent.

PERIPHERAL NEUROPATHY

History and Physical Exam

- Time course – acute (<4 wk), subacute (1-3 mo), chronic (>3 mo)
- Family hx – Charcot-Marie-Tooth disease is most common hereditary neuropathy
- Drug and toxin exposure hx – alcohol, amiodarone, antibiotics (eg, metronidazole, dapsone), chemotherapeutic agents, phenytoin, statins, solvents, heavy metals, insecticides
- Distribution (focal, multifocal, symmetric/asymmetric) and type (sensory, motor, and/or autonomic) of deficit

Diagnosis

- Most neuropathies can be diagnosed clinically (**Table 94**)
- Reasonable blood screening tests would include CBC, glucose, Cr, BUN, TSH, LFTs, vitamin B_{12} level, ESR, SPEP
- Nerve conduction studies can help distinguish the more common axonal pathologies (DM, medication effects, alcohol, kidney failure, malignancy) from demyelinating ones (including Guillain-Barré syndrome and chronic inflammatory demyelinating polyneuropathy [CIDP])
- About 30% of cases are idiopathic.

Table 94. Diagnostic Features of Selected Neuropathies

Distribution	Type of Deficit	Common Causes
Lower extremities symmetric polyneuropathy	Sensory predominant (burning, tingling, numbness)	DM (~30% of all neuropathies), idiopathic, B_{12} deficiency, MGUS, CKD, alcohol, chemotherapy
Upper and lower extremities symmetric polyneuropathy	Sensory +/- motor +/- autonomic	Idiopathic, Guillain-Barré, CIDP, Lyme disease, HIV
Mononeuropathy or radiculopathy	Sensory +/- motor	Carpal tunnel, ulnar neuropathy, Bell palsy, radiculopathy
Asymmetric polyneuropathy	Sensory +/- motor +/- autonomic	Vasculitis, DM, ALS

CIDP = chronic inflammatory demyelinating polyneuropathy; MGUS = monoclonal gammopathy of undetermined significance.

Prevention of Complications

- Protect distal extremities from trauma—appropriate shoe size, daily foot inspections, good skin care, avoidance of barefoot walking.
- Prevent falls (p 123–130)
- Maintain appropriate glycemic control in diabetic neuropathy.

Medications for Painful Neuropathy

- Expected to achieve a 30–50% reduction in pain in roughly 1/3 of patients
- Help only pain, not other neurologic symptoms
- Should be started at low dosage and increased as needed and tolerated
- In older adults, anticonvulsants are reasonable as 1st-line oral agents:
  - Gabapentin▲ can begin 100–200 mg qhs but may need up to 100–600 mg q8h; lower dosage according to CrCl if CrCl <60 mL/min/1.73 m^2 ^{BC} [C: 100, 300, 400; T: 600, 800; S: 250/5 mL]
  - Pregabalin *(Lyrica)* 75–300 mg po q12h; lower dosage according to CrCl if CrCl <60 mL/min/1.73 m^2 ^{BC} [C: 25, 50, 75, 100, 150, 200, 225, 300]: primary indication is for management of postherpetic neuralgia, diabetic peripheral neuropathy, or fibromyalgia
  - Carbamazepine▲ 200–400 mg q8h [T: 200; ChT: 100; S: 100 mg/5 mL]; (carbamazepine ER) 200 mg q12h [T: 100, 200, 400; C: CR 200, 300]
- Other oral agents that may be effective include:
  - TCAs^{BC}; eg, nortriptyline▲ 10–100 mg qhs [T: 10, 25, 50, 75] or desipramine▲ 10–75 mg qam [T: 10, 25, 50, 75]; benefits often outweighed by side effects in older adults
  - Duloxetine^{BC} *(Cymbalta)* 20–60 mg/d [C: 20, 30, 60]; avoid if CrCl <30 mL/min/1.73 m^2
  - SSRIs^{BC} have not been shown to be as effective as TCAs (**Table 42**)
  - Lamotrigine *(Lamictal,* **Table 92**) 400–600 mg/d
  - Opioids^{BC}: watch for AEs of itching, mood changes, weakness, confusion
  - Tramadol▲^{BC} 100–300 mg/d; reduce dose for IR^{BC} or avoid for ER^{BC} if CrCl <30 mL/min/1.73 m^2
- Topical agents that may be effective include:
  - Capsaicin▲ applied q6–8h, starting at low dose and titrating upward as needed [crm: 0.025%, 0.035%, 0.075%, 0.1%; gel: 0.025%; liquid 0.15%; lot: 0.025%; pch: 0.025%, 0.0375%, 0.05%]
  - Capsaicin cutaneous pch *(Qutenza)* applied by health professional, using a local anesthetic, to the most painful skin areas (max of 4 pch). Apply for 30 min to feet, 60 min for other locations. Risk of significant rise in BP after placement; monitor patient for at least 1 h [pch: 8%].
  - Transcutaneous electrical nerve stimulation
  - Lidocaine 5% pch *(Lidoderm)* 1–3 patches covering the affected area up to 24 h/d [700-mg pch]; lidocaine 4% patches are available OTC
  - Other topical lidocaine preparations 2–4×/d [crm: 3%, 4%; gel: 3%, 4%, lot: 3%; oint 5%: spr: 0.5%]

COMMONLY USED DEFINITIONS

- Established osteoporosis: occurrence of a minimal trauma fracture of any bone (WHO).
- Osteoporosis: a skeletal disorder characterized by compromised bone strength (bone density and bone quality) predisposing to an increased risk of fracture
- Osteoporosis: BMD 2.5 SD or more below that of younger normal individuals (T score) (WHO). Scores between 1 and 2.5 SD below young normals are termed osteopenia. For each SD decrement in BMD, hip fracture risk increases about 2-fold; for each SD increment in BMD, hip fracture risk is about halved.

RISK FACTORS FOR OSTEOPOROTIC FRACTURE

- Increasing age[1]
- Female sex[1]
- BMI (both low and high)[1]
- Previous low-trauma fracture as adult[1]
- Parent fractured hip[1]
- Current smoking[1]
- Oral glucocorticoids (ever used ≥3 mo at a dose of prednisolone of 5 mg daily or equivalent)[1]

- RA[1]
- Secondary osteoporosis (type I DM, osteogenesis imperfecta in adults, untreated long-standing hyperthyroidism, hypogonadism or premature menopause (<45 y), chronic malnutrition, or malabsorption and chronic liver disease; if BMD entered into FRAX, no need to enter these variables[1]

- Alcohol (>3 drinks/d)[1]
- Lower BMD[1]
- Frailty
- Dementia
- Depression
- Impaired vision
- Low physical activity
- Recurrent falls
- Nocturia
- CKD (GFR <45 mL/min/1.73 m²) BSA

[1]indicates risk factors included in the WHO Fracture Risk Assessment Tool (FRAX)

TOXINS AND MEDICATIONS THAT CAN CAUSE OR AGGRAVATE OSTEOPOROSIS

- Alcohol
- ADT
- Anticonvulsants
- Antipsychotics
- Corticosteroids
- Heparin

- Lithium
- Nicotine (ie, smoking)
- Phenytoin
- PPIs (if ≥1 y; Controversial. Observational studies with mixed results.)

- SSRIs (Controversial. Observational studies with mixed results.)
- Thyroxine (if over-replaced or in suppressive dosage)

EVALUATION

- BMD at least once in all women after age 65; insufficient evidence to support screening in men (USPSTF) but National Osteoporosis Foundation (NOF) recommends BMD in all men after age 70, and in men with prior clinical fracture after age 65 (**Table 103**). Uncertain how often to repeat. Some suggest in 3 y for patients with osteopenia and in 5 y for those with normal bone density. Do not routinely repeat more than once every 2 y.^cw
  ○ The value of monitoring BMD in patients already receiving tx is unproved, and professional societies differ in recommendations. Even patients who continue to lose BMD during tx have benefits in fracture reduction.
  ○ A measure of bone microarchitecture, Trabecular Bone Score, can generated with software add-ons to some BMD systems and can be entered into FRAX (see below). It should not be used independently to make clinical decisions or monitor.
  ○ Although NOF recommends screening with vertebral imaging (dual-energy x-ray absorptiometry or x-ray) for women ≥70 and men ≥80 with any T score ≤-1.0 and women

65–69 and men 70–79 with any T score ≤1.5, this is controversial and is not covered by Medicare.
- Routine screening for serum 25(OH)D deficiency is not recommended.**ᶜʷ**
- Some experts recommend excluding secondary causes (serum PTH, TSH, calcium, phosphorus, albumin, alkaline phosphatase, bioavailable testosterone in men, kidney function tests, LFTs, CBC, UA, electrolytes, protein electrophoresis). Less consensus on 24-h urinary calcium excretion, cortisol, and antibodies associated with gluten enteropathy.

MANAGEMENT
Universal Recommendations

Elemental calcium, 1200 mg/d (diet plus supplement) for women aged >50 and men aged >70, 1000 mg/d for men aged <70. The amount of elemental calcium in supplements is listed on the product label under "Supplement Facts." Better absorbed when doses are ≤600 mg, so give 2×/d. For most patients, calcium carbonate (40% elemental calcium) is sufficient and least expensive.

For patients on H2RA or PPIs (**Table 58**) or who have achlorhydria, calcium citrate (20% elemental calcium) should be used.

- For patients who have difficulty swallowing calcium citrate tabs, smaller tabs of 125 mg *(Freeda Mini Cal-citrate)* and granules, 1 tsp = 760 mg *(Freeda Calcium Citrate Fine Granular)*, are available.
- Dietary sources of calcium include:
  ◦ Milk (per 8 oz): whole 276 mg; reduced fat 293 mg; low fat 305 mg; nonfat 316 mg
  ◦ Yogurt (per 6 oz): whole 209 mg; low fat 311 mg
  ◦ Cheese: American (per slice) 293 mg; cheddar (per 1 oz) 201 mg; Swiss (per 1 oz) 252 mg
  ◦ Cottage cheese (per cup): 174–187 mg
  ◦ Ice cream (per cup): 144–168 mg
- Calcium supplementation probably does not increase risk of CVD. Data on the risk of dementia and stroke-related dementia are inconclusive. Risk of kidney stones is increased.
- Vitamin D 800–1000 IU (Institute of Medicine); Each 8-oz glass of milk or fortified orange juice has approximately 100 IU. D_3 (cholecalciferol) is the preferred form of supplementation.
- OTC calcium plus vitamin D preparations vary considerably in amounts of each, so ask patients to read labels (look for elemental calcium) to ensure they are getting adequate amounts.
- Avoid tobacco.
- Falls prevention, including exercise for muscle strengthening and balance training (**Table 56**)
- No more than moderate alcohol use (≤1 drink/d in women, ≤2 drink/d in men)

Pharmacologic Prevention and Treatment

Indications for Pharmacologic Treatment
- Prior fragility fracture is defined as those occurring from a fall from a standing height or less, or due to minor trauma (eg, not a car or sports accident). Fragility fractures occur particularly at the spine, hip, wrist, humerus, rib, and pelvis. Certain skeletal locations, including the face, skull, cervical spine, fingers, and toes are not considered fragility sites.
- No prior fracture but osteoporosis by BMD (below –2.5)
- Osteopenia (BMD –1 to –2.5) with an estimated 10-y probability of hip fracture >3% or 10-y risk of all major osteoporotic fracture (cervical spine, forearm, hip, or shoulder) >20%

based on risk factors using FRAX (shef.ac.uk/FRAX/) (NOF guidelines). Practitioners in some countries use FRAX 1st and perform BMD only if tx decision is equivocal.

○ Some question NOF thresholds because application would result in pharmacotherapy for 72% of white women aged >65 and 93% of women aged >75 compared with bone density criteria alone, which would result in pharmacotherapy for 50% of women in both age groups. Also should consider patient's expected survival and whether patient will live long enough to accrue benefit of tx.

Treatment Principles

- Vitamin D levels should be normal before initiating pharmacotherapy because bisphosphonates and denosumab can precipitate symptomatic hypocalcemia if vitamin D levels are low.
- When initiating tx with bisphosphonates or denosumab, discuss the risk factors for developing osteonecrosis of the jaw (ONJ) (eg, IV administration, cancer and cancer tx, glucocorticoid tx, smoking, DM, and preexisting dental disease) and review the symptoms of ONJ. A routine dental visit before starting tx is not necessary; if the patient has any active and unevaluated dental problems, a preinitiation dental visit is advisable. If an invasive dental procedure (eg, dental implant or extraction) is planned, many experts delay bisphosphonate tx for a few months until healing of the jaw is complete.

Bisphosphonates

- 1st-line tx but are contraindicated in renal failure. If CrCl <35 mL/min/1.73 m^2, denosumab is an alternative.
- IV bisphosphonates if GI contraindications (eg, esophageal disorders, feeding tubes) or are unable to sit up after oral dosing.
- Some experts recommend using bisphosphonates that have demonstrated efficacy in reducing hip fractures and shorter-acting agents as preferred initial tx (**Table 95**).
- PPIs reduce the effectiveness of oral bisphosphonates, and some experts recommend holding the PPI the day before bisphosphonate administration and not administering the PPI until >60 min after the bisphosphonate has been taken.
- Bisphosphonates are more effective in preventing hip fracture when adherence is >80% (compared with adherence <50%). Adherence is better with weekly, compared to daily, regimens.
- Although bisphosphonates increase the risk of atypical femoral fractures, for every 1000 patients treated for 3 y, 11 hip fractures would be prevented, and 1.25 atypical fractures would occur.
- The optimal duration of bisphosphonate tx is uncertain. The risk of subtrochanteric or femoral shaft fractures increases with tx beyond 3 y. An FDA analysis concluded neither clear benefit nor harm for overall osteoporotic fracture risk by continuing bisphosphonates beyond 5 y. Some recommend discontinuing temporarily after 5 y of oral tx or 3 y of IV tx. After bisphosphonates have been discontinued, there are no data on whether or when to resume tx.

Denosumab

- An alternative for those who are intolerant of bisphosphonates or have CKD. However, little data support denosumab efficacy in Stage 4 and 5 CKD, and CKD increases risk of hypocalcemia with denosumab tx.
- Risk of atypical fracture is expected to be similar to that of bisphosphonates.
- Discontinuation of denosumab results in bone loss to pretreatment levels within 2 y and vertebral fractures within a short period (8–16 mo). Hence, starting a bisphosphonate is appropriate if denosumab is discontinued.

Parathyroid Hormone and Hormone-related Protein Analog Therapy
- For high-risk patients with multiple fractures who continue to fracture after 1 y of bisphosphonate tx or who are intolerant of bisphosphonates, consider teriparatide (PTH) or abaloparatide (parathyroid hormone-related protein analog). Some evidence supports teriparatide to accelerate bone healing, but this evidence is preliminary and use for this purpose is not standard practice. Some experts use teriparatide for prolonged fracture-related pain or nonhealing.
- Maximum duration of use is 2 y and usually a bisphosphonate or denosumab is started after stopping PTH-based tx.
- Teriparatide is more effective than risedronate at preventing vertebral and clinical (nonvertebral and symptomatic vertebral) but not nonvertebral fractures.

Osteoporosis in Men
- For men, nonpharmacologic tx, indications for pharmacologic tx, and choices of drugs, other than estrogen, are the same as for women. Bisphosphonate tx has been evaluated less in men. Zoledronic acid reduces the risk of morphometric vertebral fractures.
  - If symptomatic hypogonadism or a medical reason for hypogonadism, testosterone replacement. (p 327)

Table 95. Pharmacologic Prevention and Treatment of Osteoporosis[1]

Medication	Dosage	Formulations	Administration/Comments
Bisphosphonates	*Class effect:* Esophagitis; bone, joint, or muscle pain; osteonecrosis of jaw (estimated 1–28 cases/100,000 patient-years with oral tx)[2]; occipital inflammation; possibly AF); association with atypical femoral fractures rare. Consider discontinuing or suspending after 5 y.		
Alendronate▲	Prevention: 5 mg/d or 35 mg/wk Tx: 10 mg/d or 70 mg/wk	T: 5, 10, 35, 40, 70; S:70/100 mL/d. Drink with 2 oz water.	Must be taken fasting with water; patient must remain upright and npo for ≥30 min after taking; do not use if CrCl <35; relatively contraindicated in GERD
Effervescent (Binosto) with cholecalciferol	70 mg/wk 1 tab/wk	T: 70 T: 70/2800 U 70/5600 U	Same as above
Ibandronate▲	Tx and prevention: po: 150 mg/mo or 2.5 mg/d IV: 3 mg q3mo	T: 2.5, 150 IV: 1 mg/mL (available in 3-mL prefilled syringes)	Must be taken fasting with 6–8 oz water; patient must remain upright and npo for ≥60 min after taking; do not use if CrCl <30. IV can cause acute phase reaction (flu-like symptoms) in 1/3 after 1st infusion; rare in subsequent infusions.
Risedronate▲	Tx and prevention: 35 mg/wk, 5 mg/d, or 150 mg/mo	T: 5, 30, 35, 150	Must be taken fasting or ≥2 h after evening meal; patient must remain upright and npo for 30 min after taking; do not use if CrCl <30
Delayed-release (Atelvia)	35 mg/wk	T: 35 DR	
Zoledronic acid▲	5 mg IV given over >15 min every y for 3–6 y for tx or q2y for prevention	5 mg/100 mL	Causes acute phase reaction (flu-like symptoms) in 1/3 after 1st infusion; rare in subsequent infusions. May cause acute renal failure in patients using diuretics do not use if CrCl <35

(cont.)

Table 95. Pharmacologic Prevention and Treatment of Osteoporosis[1] (cont.)

Medication	Dosage	Formulations	Administration/Comments
Others			
Raloxifene *(Evista)*	60 mg/d	T: 60	Reduces spinal and all nonspinal fractures. Used more often for prevention because of reduced risk of breast cancer; may cause hot flushes, myalgias, cramps, and limb pain
Calcitonin▲	Tx and prevention: 100 IU/d SC (human) or 200 IU intranasally (salmon) in alternate nostrils q48h	Inj: human *(Miacalcin)* 0.5 mg/vial Intranasal▲: salmon 200 U/mL *(Miacalcin, Fortical)*	Not shown to reduce hip or all nonspinal fractures. Rhinitis in 10–12%; increased risk of cancer. FDA advisory panel concluded that calcitonin's benefits do not outweigh its risks.
Estrogen▲	p 362		For use in select patients; for risks and benefits, see p 362
Teriparatide *(Forteo)*	Tx: 20 mcg/d for up to 24 mo	Inj: 3 mL, 28-dose disposable pen device	Avoid in patients with Paget disease, prior skeletal radiation tx, hx of skeletal malignancies, hypercalcemic disorders, or metabolic bone disease other than osteoporosis; can cause hypercalcemia (L, K); tx for 1 y followed by 1 y of bisphosphonates or raloxifene can maintain 1-y gains in BMD
Abaloparatide *(Tymlos)*	80 mg SC qd	Inj: 3120 mcg/1.56 mL (pen injector)	Avoid in patients with Paget disease, prior skeletal radiation tx, hx of skeletal malignancies, hypercalcemic disorders, or metabolic bone disease other than osteoporosis; can cause hypercalcemia (L, K); tx for no more than 2 y; may cause orthostatic hypotension, hypercalcemia (K)
Denosumab *(Prolia)*	60 mg SC q6mo	Inj: 60 mg/mL in prefilled syringe	Skin infections, dermatitis, osteonecrosis of jaw, hypocalcemia especially if CrCl <30, hypoparathyroidism, malabsorption, or uncorrected calcium. Risk of atypical fracture is expected to be similar to bisphosphonates. Rapid bone loss when drug is discontinued.
Combination			
Conjugated estrogens/bazedoxifene *(Duavee)*	1 tab/d	T: 45/20 (conjugated estrogens/bazedoxifene)	In clinical trials, no increase in vaginal bleeding, breast, endometrial, or ovarian cancer, VTE, or MI. Long-term risk for VTE or ischemic stroke uncertain.

CrCl unit = mL/min/1.73 m^2

[1] Unless specified, medication can be used for prevention or tx.

[2] Risk factors include IV tx (little data on osteoporosis doses); cancer; dental extractions, implants, and poor-fitting dentures; glucocorticoids; smoking; and preexisting dental disease. Some experts recommend that bisphosphonates be stopped for several months before and after elective complex oral procedures, or, if procedures are emergent, that bisphosphonates be held for several months after.

PAIN

DEFINITION

An unpleasant sensory and emotional experience associated with actual or potential tissue damage (International Association for Study of Pain taxonomy)

Acute Pain

Distinct onset, usually evident pathology, short duration; self-limiting; common causes: trauma, postsurgical pain

Persistent or Chronic Pain

Pain that does not remit in the expected amount of time; due to ongoing nociceptive, neuropathic, or mixed pathophysiologic processes, often associated with functional and psychologic impairment; may occur in absence of any past injury or evident body damage; can fluctuate in character and intensity over time (**Table 96**). Chronic pain occurs on at least half of the days for 6 mo or more (National Pain Strategy 2016, iprcc.nih.gov/National-Pain-Strategy/Objectives-Updates), referred to as persistent pain hereafter.

Table 96. Types of Pain, Examples, and Treatment

Type of Pain and Examples	Typical Description	Nonpharmacologic Treatments and Effective Drug Classes
Peripheral		
Nociceptive: somatic (eg, tissue injury of bones, soft tissue, joints, muscles)		
Arthritis, low-back pain, myofascial pain	Well localized, constant; aching, stabbing, gnawing, throbbing	Exercise, PT and CBT, other nondrug tx, APAP, topical anesthetics/NSAIDs, intraarticular corticosteroid, salsalate, NSAIDs, duloxetine, tramadol, hydrocodone/APAP, oxycodone, fentanyl, methadone
Acute postoperative, fracture, bone metastases	Well localized, constant; aching, stabbing, gnawing, throbbing	APAP, topical anesthetics/NSAIDs, nondrug tx (eg, massage, music), NSAIDs, opioids
Nociceptive: visceral (eg, tissue injury of visceral organs including heart, lungs, testes, and biliary system)		
Renal colic	Diffuse, poorly localized, referred to other sites, intermittent, paroxysmal; dull, colicky, squeezing, deep, cramping; often accompanied by nausea, vomiting, diaphoresis	Tx of underlying cause, APAP, IV NSAID, opioids with nondrug tx

(cont.)

Table 96. Types of Pain, Examples, and Treatment (cont.)

Type of Pain and Examples	Typical Description	Nonpharmacologic Treatments and Effective Drug Classes
Neuropathic: peripheral nervous system (eg, injury to nervous system—nerves and spinal cord)		
Cervical or lumbar radiculopathy, postherpetic neuralgia, trigeminal neuralgia, diabetic neuropathy, phantom limb pain, herniated intervertebral disc, drug toxicities	Prolonged, usually constant, but can have paroxysms; sharp, burning, pricking, tingling, pins and needles, shooting electric-shock–like; associated with other sensory disturbances, eg, paresthesias and dysesthesias; allodynia, hyperalgesia, impaired motor function, atrophy, or abnormal deep tendon reflexes	Nondrug tx, topical anesthetics, TCAs, SNRIs, opioids
Central, Undetermined, or Mixed (eg, pain from neurological dysfunction or combined and uncertain causes)		
Myofascial pain syndrome, somatoform pain disorders, fibromyalgia; poststroke; temporomandibular joint dysfunction, tension HA	No identifiable pathologic processes or symptoms out of proportion to identifiable organic pathology; widespread musculoskeletal pain, stiffness, and weakness; fatigue, sleep disturbance; taut bands of muscles and trigger points; sensitivity to sensory stimuli	Exercise, PT and CBT, other nondrug tx, antidepressants, antianxiety agents, and psychological tx

Note: Cancer pain may present with any of the types described above.

EVALUATION

Key Points, Approach

- Perform comprehensive evaluation for underlying cause of pain, pain characteristics, and impact on physical and psychosocial function and quality of life. Identify multiple factors (eg, anxiety, depression, beliefs, insomnia, fear avoidance, biomechanical issues) that when combined with pain can cause impairment or dysfunction.
- Geriatricpain.org for provider and caregiver tools and resources for pain assessment
- Use multidisciplinary assessment and tx (eg, pharmacists, physical therapists, psychologists) when possible, particularly for persistent pain.
- Patient's report is the most reliable evidence of pain intensity and impact on function.
- Assess for pain on each presentation (older adults may be reluctant to report pain).
- Use synonyms for pain (eg, burning, aching, soreness, discomfort).
- Use a standard pain scale (eg, Numeric Rating Scale, Verbal Descriptor Scale, or Faces Pain Scale); adapt for sensory impairments (eg, large print, written vs spoken).
- Reassess regularly for improvement, deterioration, and complications/AEs, and document.

Assessment in Cognitively Impaired Patients

- Use simple pain tools (eg, scale with none, mild, moderate, or severe pain) or questions with yes/no answers to solicit self-report of pain in persons with moderate cognitive impairment.
- Assess pain in persons with severe cognitive impairment or inability to communicate pain using the Pain Assessment algorithm (**Figure 10**), including medical hx and physical examination to identify potential pain etiologies.
- In cognitively impaired persons with behavioral disturbances/agitation suspected of an underlying pain etiology for which other causes have been ruled out and behaviors not responding to nondrug intervention, try an analgesic trial for diagnostic purposes to evaluate pain as etiology. The following is a guide to be adjusted based on individual comorbidities and/or contraindications:
  - Try APAP 1st (if no hepatic dysfunction). Order scheduled rather than prn. APAP is often effective in improving behaviors and/or function.
    - If no response to APAP after 24–48 h and localized inflammatory pain suspected, try topical NSAIDs and/or lidocaine.
    - If no response after 24 h, try oral morphine sulfate sol (5–10 mg q4–6h) or oxycodone 5–10 mg oral q6–8h. Consider buprenorphine transdermal pch (5 mcg/h to max 10 mcg/h) if unable to take oral analgesic.
  - If no response to APAP after 24–48 h and neuropathic pain is suspected, try gabapentin 100 mg 3×/d (Reduce dose if CrCl <60 mL/min/1.73 m^2 ^{BC}). If pain diagnosis supported by response to pregabalin, consider a tx plan that includes gabapentin.
- Carefully monitor response to analgesics with each change as agent and dose are titrated to achieve pain relief yet avoid undesirable AEs.
- If behavior improves with pain tx, establish pain tx plan considering risks/benefits/costs of tx options.

History and Physical Examination

- Evaluate underlying diseases that are known to be painful in older persons (**Table 96**).
- Consider potential drug toxicities (eg, amiodarone, bortezomib, leflunomide, ixabepilone, chemotherapeutic agent neuropathy, antibiotic-induced neuropathies). Note if neuropathy is acute after starting medication, or if there is an increase in existing neuropathy after adding a new medication.
- Focus on a complete examination of pain source and on musculoskeletal, peripheral vascular, and neurologic systems as well as any body part that might be the source of referred pain.
- Physical exam essential to identify physical pain contributions (eg, leg length discrepancy, hip OA, myofascial pain, sacroiliac joint syndrome).
- Distinguish new illness from chronic condition.
- Analgesic hx: effectiveness and AEs, current and previous prescription drugs, OTC drugs, "natural" remedies.

Figure 10. Pain Assessment in Older Adults with Severe Cognitive Impairment

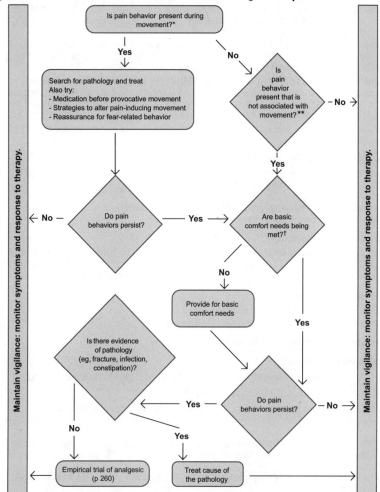

* Examples: grimacing, guarding, combativeness, groaning with movement; resisting care

** Examples: agitation, fidgeting, sleep disturbance, diminished appetite, irritability, reclusiveness, disruptive behavior, rigidity, rapid blinking

† Examples: toileting, thirst, hunger, visual or hearing impairment

Sources: American Geriatrics Society. *J Amer Geriatr Soc* 2002; 50(6 Suppl):S205–S240; and Weiner D, Herr K, Rudy T, eds. *Persistent Pain in Older Adults: An Interdisciplinary Guide for Treatment,* 2002, Copyright Springer Publishing Company, Inc., New York NY 10036.

- Assess effectiveness of prior nondrug tx.
- Laboratory and diagnostic tests to establish etiologic diagnosis. More than half of patients who report being pain-free have radiographic evidence of degenerative joint disease, thus not useful as evidence of pain etiology.
  - Avoid imaging studies (MRI, CT, or x-rays) for acute low-back pain without specific indications.[CW] *Note:* Comparative plain film x-ray may be highly important in identifying new vertebral compression fractures in symptomatic patient.
  - Don't recommend advanced imaging (eg, MRI) of the spine within the 1st 6 wk in patients with nonspecific acute low-back pain in the absence of red flags (eg, trauma hx, unintentional weight loss, immunosuppression, cancer hx, IV drug use, steroid use, osteoporosis, age >50, focal neurologic deficit, and progression of symptoms).[CW]
  - Do not use electromyography and nerve conduction studies to determine cause of axial lumbar, thoracic, or cervical spine pain.[CW]

Characteristics of Pain Complaint

Provocative (aggravating) and **P**alliative (relieving) factors
Quality (eg, burning, stabbing, dull, throbbing)
Region (eg, pain map)
Severity (eg, scale of 0 for no pain to 10 for worst pain possible)
Timing (eg, when pain occurs, frequency and duration)

Psychosocial Assessment

- Depression, anxiety, mental status (p 5 for screen). Impact on family or significant other. Enabling behaviors by others (eg, over-solicitousness, codependency, reinforcing debility).
- Evaluate pain coping, fear avoidance, and pain self-efficacy that impact tx success.

Functional Assessment

- ADLs, impact on activities, and quality of life
- Evaluate sleep pattern and perception of quality sleep.

Assessing Pain and Impact on Function

Brief Pain Inventory (BPI)

Use for comprehensive assessment of pain and its impact (geriatricscareonline.org).

PEG Scale (VA-developed 3-item version of BPI)

Average 3 individual question scores. 30% improvement from baseline is clinically meaningful.
  Q1:
  What number from 0–10 best describes your pain in the past week?
  0 = "no pain", 10 = "worst you can imagine"
  Q2:
  What number from 0–10 describes how, during the past week, pain has interfered with your enjoyment of life?
  0 = "not at all", 10 = "complete interference"
  Q3:
  What number from 0–10 describes how, during the past week, pain has interfered with your general activity?
  0 = "not at all", 10 = "complete interference"

MANAGEMENT

Goal: To find optimal balance in pain relief, functional improvement, and AEs. Nondrug (complementary and alternative tx) can be beneficial and considered early in tx plan, particularly in managing persistent pain problems. Combination of drug and nondrug approaches may lower dosing of analgesics and reduce drug-related AEs.

- Establish realistic measurable tx goals and expectations with patient (eg, 30% pain reduction or significantly improved function), social and family supports, before initiating tx.
- Develop a therapeutic alliance and reinforce positive outcomes at each visit.
- Involve caregivers and seek out resources (eg, community-based programs) to help reinforce adherence to tx plans.

Acute Pain and Short-term Management

- Identify cause of pain and treat if possible.
- Use fixed schedule of APAP, NSAIDs (consider nonselective vs celecoxib depending on risk factors and comorbidities, **Figure 10**), or opioids (**Table 99**). Combination of APAP and NSAIDs may offer superior analgesic than either alone.
  - Do not exceed 3000 mg maximum daily dose of APAP.
  - IV acetaminophen (*Ofirmev*; 15 mg/kg q6h or 12.5 mg/kg q4h adult dose) option if no other route available; expensive.
  - *Exparel* is a liposome injection of bupivacaine, an amide-type local anesthetic, indicated for administration into the surgical site to produce postsurgical analgesia (ie, one-time intraoperative injection). Caution with hepatic and renal disease. Monitoring of cardiovascular and respiratory (adequacy of ventilation) vital signs and the patient's state of consciousness should be performed after injection of bupivacaine and other amide-containing products.
  - When opioids required, use should taper with healing of injury.
    - Prescribe lowest dose of IR opioids and no greater quantity than needed for expected duration of pain severe enough to require opioids. No more than a 5-d supply for initial acute injury with follow-up evaluation for further need.
    - Do not prescribe ER or LA opioids for acute pain.
    - Do not exceed daily opioid po MS equiv of 90 mg without justification.
- Teach patient the use of nonpharmacologic techniques (eg heat/cold, relaxation, TENS).
  - Do not recommend bed rest for more than 48 h when treating low-back pain.[CW]
- Refer to PT for selected nonpharmacologic strategies (eg, joint mobilization, stabilizing exercises, assistive devices).
- Patient-controlled analgesia (PCA): Requires patient comprehension of PCA instructions.
  - Indications
    - Acute pain (eg, postoperative pain, trauma)
    - Persistent pain in patients who are npo
  - Dosing strategies (**Table 97**)
    - Titrate up PCA dose 25–50% if pain still not well controlled after 12 h.
    - Unless patient is awakened by pain during sleep, continuous opioid infusion is not recommended because of increased risk of opioid accumulation and toxicity.
    - If basal rate used, hourly monitoring of sedation and respiratory status is warranted. If low respiratory rate (≤8) and moderate sedation (difficulty arousing patient from sleep) after expected peak of opioid, withhold further opioid until respiratory rate rises or pain returns. If needed, a small dose of dilute naloxone can be given and repeated.
    - D/C PCA when patient is able to take oral analgesics or unable to self-medicate due to altered mental status or physical limitations.

Table 97. Typical Initial Dosing of PCA for Older Adults with Severe Pain

Medication (usual concentration)	Usual Dose Range[1]	Usual Lockout (min)
Morphine▲ (1 mg/mL)	0.5–2.5 mg	5–10
Hydromorphone▲ (0.2 mg/mL)	0.05–0.3 mg	5–10

[1]For opioid-naïve patients, initiate tx at lower end of dosage range.

Persistent Pain

- Identify and treat local causes of pain with local tx (eg, manipulation, massage, heat, PT, TENS), topical anesthetics (eg, lidocaine oint/pch or diclofenac gel/pch/gtt), minor interventions (eg, steroid joint injection), or surgery.
- Educate patient and promote self-management and coping. Include caregiver when possible.
  - Use positive messaging and establish realistic expectations and goals for pain relief. Complete absence of pain may not be possible, but reduction in severity to maximize function and quality of life is priority.
  - Identify attitudes and beliefs that interfere with tx success (eg, concerns about pain, beliefs that impact willingness to try a pain tx, concerns about tx considered).
  - Identify and schedule pleasurable activities as part of core coping skill development. Identify barriers and develop plan.
  - Geriatricpain.org for provider and caregiver tools and resources for pain management
  - Promote healthy behaviors including physical activity, weight control, and sleep.
  - Establish exercise or movement-based program and consider barriers to adherence (eg, lack of time, fear of exacerbating pain, lack of perceived need, lack of motivation). Ask about exercise habits at each visit.
  - Strength training, aerobic conditioning, and flexibility exercises optimal
    - Intensities up to 80% of 1 repetition maximum (RM) for resistance training and 60% maximum HR or maximum oxygen update are safe for patients with OAs.
  - Progressive exercise key component
    - Isometric exercises progressed gradually from 30–75% muscle maximum voluntary contraction
    - Isometric resistance training increased by 5–10% weekly
    - Aerobic intensity increased by 2.5% weekly
  - Individual measures of intensity frequency and duration should be specified and gradually increased.
  - Refer to Pain Self-Management program and resources (healthinaging.org/aging-and-health-a-to-z/topic:pain-management).
  - Programs to emphasize exercise, pain education, and pain-coping strategies.
  - Refer to Arthritis Foundation or community resources such as senior centers (arthritis.org/living-with-arthritis/pain-management/)
- In those overweight with mild to moderate pain, start with weight loss (eg, MOVE!® Weight Management program, cardiovascular and/or resistance land-based exercises, aquatic program).
- Emphasize self-administered tx (eg, heat, cold, massage, liniments, and topical agents, distraction, relaxation, music) and self-management approaches (eg, CBT). Prescribe exercise for analgesic effects (p 293).
- Prescribe assistive devices for joint unloading.
- Combine pharmacologic and nonpharmacologic strategies.
  - Add tx taught and/or conducted by professionals (eg, coping skills, biofeedback, imagery, hypnosis) as needed.

Nondrug Treatment

Table 98. Nondrug Interventions for Persistent Pain in Older Adults

Intervention	Outcomes	Problems Studied
Physical		
Exercise (walking, tai chi, yoga)	+	LE OA; CLBP, chronic pain, fibromyalgia
Acupuncture	+	Back, knee, shoulder, neck
TENS	+/−	Knee, back
Qigong	+/−	Back, neck
Massage	+	Back, neck
Heat	+	CLBP
Spinal manipulation	+/-	CLBP
Psychosocial		
Cognitive-Behavioral Therapy	+	Chronic pain
Acceptance and Commitment Therapy	+	CLBP, chronic pain
Guided Imagery with Progressive Muscle Relaxation	+	Chronic OA pain
Music	+	Chronic pain
Mindfulness-based Meditation	+/−	CLBP
Self-Management Education	+	Chronic pain, CLBP
Internet-delivered exercise and pain-coping skills training and education	+	Knee pain

+ = positive outcomes; +/− = mixed outcomes; CLBP = chronic low-back pain; LE OA = lower extremity osteoarthritis; TENS = transcutaneous electrical nerve stimulation.

Notes: Short-term efficacy, good tolerance, low risk, low cost; Best format, intensity, duration, content not established; Studies in older adults limited; No clear consensus on best.

- Treat comorbid psychiatric conditions associated with persistent pain, including anxiety, depression, and posttraumatic stress disorder.
  ○ Options include psychotherapy, biofeedback, mindfulness training, counseling (relationship, social, financial, substance abuse)
- Consider therapeutic injections to treat acute and persistent pain syndromes (see Musculoskeletal chapter for specific indications).
  ○ Injections are rarely sole tx.
  ○ Diagnostic value can be determined by response to an injected local anesthetic.
  ○ Spinal cord stimulation may be useful for failed back syndrome (ie, postlaminectomy), complex regional pain syndrome, and neuropathic pain.
  ○ Intrathecal infusions may be indicated for both cancer and noncancer pain.
- When appropriate, refer for:
  ○ Consult PT and OT for mechanical devices to minimize pain and facilitate activity (eg, splints), transcutaneous electrical nerve stimulation, range-of-motion and ADL programs.
  ○ Pain clinic with interdisciplinary team approach for complex pain syndromes with poor response to 1st-line tx.

- ○ Psychiatric pain management consult for somatization or severe mood or personality disorder.
- ○ Anesthesia pain management consult for possible interventional tx (eg, neuroaxial analgesia, injection tx, neuromodulation) when more conservative approaches are ineffective.
- ○ Pain or chemical dependency specialist referral for management of at-risk patients and ongoing chemical dependency, "chemical coping," aberrant drug-related behaviors, and drug withdrawal.

Pharmacologic Treatment

Approach

- Base initial choice of analgesic on the severity and type of pain and impact on function; consider cost, availability, patient preference, comorbidity, impairments, safety, and adverse outcomes (**Figure 10** and **Table 99**)
- For ongoing analgesic tx, careful risk/benefit analysis should be completed when determining appropriate drug and use.

Table 99. Principles of Analgesic Management for Persistent Pain in Older Adults

Drug Class and Dosing	Practical Considerations
Step 1: Treatment of Mild Pain (Score of 1–3 and limited functional impairment)	
Acetaminophen (APAP) (**Table 82**)	Continue evaluating risk/benefit for prescribing APAP due to recent evidence of uncertain analgesic benefit and increased safety concerns. Renal impairment, hepatic dysfunction, and alcohol abuse are known risk factors for ADR. APAP in treating persistent mild to moderate musculoskeletal pain with maximal dose of 4 g in healthy patients and 3 g in frail older adults. Advise against alcohol use; schedule around-the-clock. Ask about all OTC with acetaminophen.
	NOT anti-inflammatory; leading cause of acute liver failure (including accidental overdose); monitor for severe liver injury and acute renal failure.
Nonacetylated salicylates (eg, salsalate, trisalicylate) (**Table 82**)	Consider if inflammatory pain. Does not interfere with platelet function. Educate regarding salicylism and monitor Cr. Avoid in patients with advanced renal disease or hepatic impairment.
Counterirritants	Many available OTC with limited evidence to support use. Use in localized musculoskeletal pain. May be effective for arthritic pain, but effect limited when pain affects multiple joints. Apply to affected area and monitor for skin injury, especially if used with heat or occlusive dressing. Ideal for minor pains due to minimal side effects.
✓ Camphor-menthol-phenol▲OTC	lot: camphor 5%, menthol 5%, phenol 5% prn; max q6h
✓ Camphor and phenol▲OTC	S: camphor 5%, phenol 4.7% prn; max q8h
✓ Methyl salicylate and menthol▲	Monitor for salicylate toxicity if used over several areas.
(eg, *BenGay* oint^OTC, *Icy Hot* crm^OTC)	methyl salicylate 18.3%, menthol 16% q6–8h
(eg, *BenGay* extra strength crm ^OTC)	methyl salicylate 30%, menthol 10% q6–8h

(cont.)

Table 99. Principles of Analgesic Management for Persistent Pain in Older Adults (cont.)

Drug Class and Dosing	Practical Considerations
✓Trolamine salicylate▲ (*Aspercreme* rub[OTC])	trolamine salicylate 10% q6h or more frequently
OTC counterirritants	
Icy Hot pch 5% menthol[OTC]	May moderately reduce musculoskeletal or neuropathic pain
Icy Hot Advanced[OTC] pch 7.5% menthol	Burning is common, but decreases with time. Do not leave patch on for >1 h (max 2 pch/24 h)
BenGay Pain Relieving[OTC] pch 5% menthol	Patches may have advantage in nongreasy
Salonpas Pain Relief[OTC] pch 3% menthol/10% methyl salicylate *Salonpas Pain Relieving Patch*[OTC] 3.1% camphor/6% menthol/10% methyl salicylate *Salonpas Original*[OTC] 1.2% camphor/5.7% menthol/6.3% methyl salicylate	Caution applying near eyes, genitals
Topical Analgesics	Temporary tx of minor pain associated with muscles and joints due to backache, strains, sprains, cramps, arthritis; pain associated with diabetic neuropathy OTC compounded topical analgesics available, although no evidence to support use Never apply over broken or compromised skin. Wash hands after applying or use glove. Do not use heating pad.
✓Capsaicin▲ (eg, *Capsin, Capzasin, No Pain-HP, R-Gel, Zostrix, Qutenza*) crm, lot, gel, roll-on: 0.025%, 0.075%; cutaneous pch 8% q6–8h	Evidence for localized peripheral neuropathic pain, particularly postherpetic neuralgia and HIV neuropathy. Only use in dermal neuropathic pain. Renders skin and joints insensitive by depleting and preventing reaccumulation of substance P in peripheral sensory neurons; may cause burning sensation (which is intolerable to some) up to 2 wk; instruct patient to wash hands after application to prevent eye contact; do not apply to open or broken skin. Pch should be applied by health professional, using a local anesthetic, to the most painful skin areas (max of 4 pch). Apply for 30 min to feet, 60 min to other locations. Repeat no more often than every 3 mo. Risk of significant rise in BP after placement; monitor patient for at least 1 h. Crm effective in osteoarthritis.
Salonpas Hot[OTC] pch 0.025% capsaicin	
✓Lidocaine *(Lidoderm)* transdermal pch 5% 12 h on, 12 h off; up to 24 h on	*Lidoderm* safe, effective for localized peripheral neuropathic pain, approved for postherpetic neuralgia. Limited evidence for other painful conditions (low-back pain, osteoarthritis). Monitor for rash or skin irritation; potential for systemic absorption; dosing limit of 3 pch applied up to 24 h/d *Application pch:* May be cut to smaller sizes. Avoid occlusive dressings and heat, but clothing may be worn. Avoid contact with water, wash hands after application, and fold pch adhesive sides together on removal.

(cont.)

Table 99. Principles of Analgesic Management for Persistent Pain in Older Adults (cont.)

OTC lidocaine patches <5% available   OTC products: no comparative studies. Apply up to 12 h.

Drug Class and Dosing	**Practical Considerations**
Balego^OTC 4% lidocaine/1% menthol	
LenzaPatch^OTC 4% lidocaine/ 1% menthol	
Lidocare^OTC 4% lidocaine	
LidoPatch^OTC 3.99% lidocaine/1.25% menthol	
LidoFlex^OTC 4% lidocaine	
OTC lidocaine cream	
Aspercreme Pain Relieving Creme with Lidocaine^OTC 4% lidocaine	
Icy Hot Lidocaine^OTC crm 4% lidocaine/1% menthol	

Topical NSAIDs **(Table 82)**	As effective as oral NSAIDs with fewer systemic and GI AE for chronic localized musculoskeletal pain, particularly hand and knee OA. Lack of clear efficacy data in acute or chronic low-back pain, neuropathic pain.
	Don't combine topical plus oral NSAIDs.
	Evaluate serum Cr as some systemic absorption.
	Diclofenac 1% gel, 1.5% topical sol, 1.3% pch
	Note: Some topical tx are expensive and insurer may not cover.
	Application: Gel rubbed into skin with dosing card to determine correct amount. Elbow, wrist, or hand: use 2-g dose 4×/d; Knee, ankle, or feet: use 4-g dose 4×/d. Maximum amount per day not to exceed 32 g.
	Do not apply heat nor occlusive dressing postapplication.
	Application: Pch applied 2×/d to most painful area with intact skin. Reinforce peeling edges with tape. Mesh sleeve or netting can be used. Remove pch during bathing (reduces adhesiveness).
	Wash hands after applying, touching, or removing pch.
	Application: Sol applied via pump or dropper; typically 40 gtt to each painful knee (10 gtt per time and rub in to avoid spillage). Do not apply clothing until totally dry.

(cont.)

Table 99. Principles of Analgesic Management for Persistent Pain in Older Adults (cont.)

Drug Class and Dosing	Practical Considerations
NSAIDs/Cox-2 anti-inflammatory drug (**Table 82**)	Avoid nonselective NSAIDs for chronic use (>6 wk) and in patients with hx of gastric or duodenal ulcers, unless other alternatives are not effective and patient can take gastroprotective agent.[BC] Avoid preexisting HTN, CKD, HF, and/or peptic ulcer disease, or those taking concomitant warfarin or corticosteroids.[BC] Use NSAIDs with caution in highly selected patients (eg, acute-on-chronic pain flare or new acute pain problem [eg, gout] in existing persistent pain disorder [eg, CLBP]) for short-term use (<2 wk) with nonacetylated salicylate, or ibuprofen or celecoxib. Use misoprostol or PPI with nonselective NSAIDs to reduce GI bleeding risk. Avoid scheduled use of PPI for >8 wk unless for high-risk patients (eg, chronic NSAID use).[BC] Consider celecoxib for patients who would benefit from anti-inflammatory medication with no cardiovascular risk based on risk/benefit assessment (**Figure 11** and **Table 82**). Long-term use not recommended. Avoid in HF.[BC] Avoid in renal impairment (CrCl <30).[BC] Caution in patients with CVD or at risk for CVD.

Drug Class and Dosing	Practical Considerations

Step 2: Treatment of Moderate Pain (Score 4–7 and interference with active function (eg, exercise, mobility-related), pain not alleviated with medicine from Step 1, and/or if pain worsens

Marijuana (Substance Use Disorders, p 349)	*Chronic pain:* Limited evidence but effective in controlling cancer and noncancer persistent pain. Debate is ongoing over its use. Medical marijuana is legal most US states and provides an alternative to opioids for moderate to severe pain. No cannabinoid is currently FDA-approved as analgesic, although there is evidence of efficacy. Little information on optimal dosing. Monitor for signs of excessive use/abuse; neurologic/psychiatric AEs (eg, dysphoria, euphoria, somnolence, vertigo).
Dronabinol *(Marinol)* C: 2.5, 5, 10; 10 mg 3×/d to 4×/d Nabilone *(Cesamet)* C: 1 mg; 1 mg 2×/d	Titrate dose slowly and monitor for adverse effects Titrate gradually at weekly increments of 0.5 mg until target relief attained of max dosing of 1 mg 2×/d
Short-Acting Opioids	See section on Opioid Use (p 266). Morphine sulfate equivalent dose (MS equiv)[1] provided to use in converting from one opioid to another due to differences in opioid potency.

Drug/Formulations	MS Equiv[1] (Route)	Starting Dosage for Opioid-Naïve	Comments
Hydrocodone + APAP▲ T: 5/325, 10/325; S: 2.5/167/5 mL (contains 7% alcohol) (eg, *Vicodin*) T: 5/300, 7.5/300, 10/300	30 mg (po)	2.5–5 mg q4–6h	*Caution:* Total APAP dosage should not exceed 3 g/d

(cont.)

Drug/Formulations	MS Equiv[1] (Route)	Starting Dosage for Opioid-Naïve	Comments
Hydrocodone + ibuprofen▲ T: 7.5/200	30 mg	7.5/200	Monitor renal function and use gastric protection ER tablets without abuse-deterrent formulation
Oxycodone▲ T: 5, 15, 30; C: 5; S: 5 mg/mL, 20 mg/mL	20 mg (po)	2.5–5 mg q4–6h	Limited information on dosing in renal failure; use caution despite weak active metabolites and avoid if CrCl <30 ER abuse-deterrent products available
Oxycodone + APAP▲ T▲: 2.5/325, 5/325, 7.5/325, 10/325 S: 5/325/5 mL	20 mg (po)	2.5–5 mg oxycodone q6h including 325 mg APAP	
(Magnacet) T: 2.5/400, 5/400, 7.5/400, 10/400	20 mg (po)	2.5–5 mg oxycodone q6h including 400 mg APAP	
Oxycodone + ASA▲ T: 2.25/325, 4.5/325	20 mg (po)	2.25–4.5 mg oxycodone q6h	Monitor renal function and use gastric protection
Oxycodone + ibuprofen▲ T: 5/400	20 mg (po)	1 tab po q6h; do not exceed 4 tabs in 24 h	Monitor renal function and use gastric protection. Tx not to exceed 7 d.
Tramadol▲BC T: 50	150–300 mg (po)	25 mg q4–6h; increase 25–50 mg in divided doses over 3–7 d to max dose of 100 mg 4×/d; not >300 mg for those aged >75	Not 1st-line tx; consider before starting pure opioids. Avoid in seizure disorders.[BC] Risk of seizures (↑ risk with higher doses and combination with SSRI/TCA) and orthostatic hypotension; withdrawal symptoms can occur. Risk of serotonin syndrome when combined with SSRIs. Risk of suicide for patients who are addiction prone, taking tranquilizers or antidepressant drugs, and at risk of overdosage. Additive effects with alcohol and other opioids. Risk of hyponatremia and falls. When CrCl <30, reduce dose for IR; Avoid ER.[BC]
Tramadol[BC] + APAP▲ T: 37.5/325	150-300 mg (po)	2 tabs q4–6h; max 8 tabs/d	Caution: total APAP dosage should not exceed 3 g/d.

(cont.)

Table 99. Principles of Analgesic Management for Persistent Pain in Older Adults (cont.)

Drug Class and Dosing	Practical Considerations
Adjuvants (Table 100)	Consider adjuvant analgesics, including antidepressants and anticonvulsants, for patients with neuropathic pain or mixed pain syndromes, or refractory persistent pain. Tailor to pain characteristics/etiology and risk factors. Effects may be enhanced when used in combination with other analgesics and/or nondrug strategies. Select agents with lowest AE profiles. Begin low and titrate slowly; allow adequate therapeutic trial (eg, 2–3 wk for onset of efficacy).

Step 3: Treatment of Moderate to Severe Pain (Score 6–10), pain not alleviated with nondrug interventions and medicine from Step 2, and severe enough to impact function and quality of life

Opioids	Avoid if hx falls or concurrent benzodiazepine use.[BC] See section on Opioid Use (p 266).

Drug/Formulations	MS Equiv[1] (Route)	Starting Dosage for Opioid-Naïve	Comments
Morphine *(MSIR, Astramorph PF, Duramorph, Infumorph, Roxanol, OMS Concentrate, MS/L, RMS, MS/S)* C: 15, 30 soluble T: 15, 30 S: 10 mg/5 mL, 20 mg/5 mL, 100 mg/5 mL, 4 mg/mL, 20 mg/mL Sp: 5, 10, 20, 30 Inj	30 mg (po), 10 mg (IV, IM, SC)	5 mg po q4h; 1–2 mg IV q3–4h; 2.5–5 mg IM, SC q4h; 5–10 mg Sp q3–4h	Not recommended in renal failure; metabolites accumulate
Hydromorphone▲ T: 2, 4, 8; S: 5 mg/5 mL Sp: 3 Inj	7.5 mg (po), 1.5 mg (IV, IM, SC), 6 mg (rectal)	1–2 mg po q3–6h; 0.1–0.3 mg IV q2–3h; 0.4–0.5 mg IM, SC q4–6h; 3 mg Sp q4–8h	Considered safer in renal insufficiency
Oxymorphone *(Opana, Opana injectable)* T: 5, 10 Sp: 5 Inj	10 mg (po), 1 mg (IV, IM, SC)	5 mg po q4–6h; 0.5 mg IM, IV, SC q4–6h; Sp 5 mg q4–6h	Use carefully in renal failure and liver impairment ER option with abuse-deterrent properties

(cont.)

Drug Class and Dosing	Practical Considerations
Extended-Release and Long-Acting Opioids ER Hydrocodone bitartrate *(Zohydro ER)* ER Hydromorphone *(Exalgo)* ER Morphine▲ ER Oxycodone▲ Oxycodone/acetaminophen ER *(Xartemis XR)* Tramadol ER[BC] *(Ultram ER, ConZip)* Tapentadol ER *(Nucynta ER)* Transdermal buprenorphine *(Butrans Transdermal System CIII)* Transdermal fentanyl▲	When opioids are indicated, ER products reduce dosing frequency and may be useful in adherence and in those with cognitive impairment. Given that the long-term use of opioids is not recommended unless clearly warranted, ER and LA opioids are less often used. FDA label indication for ER opioids for management of pain severe enough to require daily, around-the-clock, long-term opioid tx and for which alternative tx options are inadequate. ER formulation should ONLY be used in opioid-tolerant patients (ie, those taking at least 60 mg/d of oral morphine, 25 mcg/h of transdermal fentanyl, 30 mg/d of oral oxycodone, 8 mg/d of oral hydromorphone, 25 mg/d of oral oxymorphone, or an equianalgesic dosage of another opioid for ≥1 wk). For opioid-tolerant patients, calculate based on conversion factors. See product information for starting dose for ER products. *Note:* Conversion from any oral immediate-release opioid should be based on conversion ratios; start by administering 50% of calculated total daily dose of ER opioid, and titrate until adequate pain relief is achieved with tolerable adverse effects.
Methadone	Methadone is an option if other long-acting agents are not affordable, but should be used with extreme caution and only with expertise and monitoring ability because of highly variable half-life, risk of dose accumulation, and high interpatient variability. Associated with prolonged QTc interval. Acceptable in renal insufficiency. Consult palliative care or pain service. For details on methadone prescribing and monitoring, see geriatricscareonline.org
Abuse-deterrent Products ER Morphine/naltrexone *(Embeda)* ER Morphine▲ *(eg, Arymo ER, MorphaBond ER)* Oxycodone/naloxone *(Targiniq ER)* Oxycodone/naltrexone HCl *(Troxyca ER)*	These products contain an opioid antagonist intended to decrease misuse and abuse. If the product is taken as intended and taken whole, analgesia is not affected. If the product is altered (eg, chewed, crushed, dissolved), the opioid antagonist is released and can reverse the analgesic effect. See product information.
Rapid-acting opioids Fentanyl *(Actiq, Abstral, Fentora, Lazanda, Subsys, Onsolis)*	Do not use in opioid-naïve patients. Use is for breakthrough pain in those on opioid tx. May be used in oncology and palliative care. Consult package information and consult with palliative care or pain specialist.

NA = not applicable; CrCl unit = mL/min/1.73 m²

[1] MS equiv = dose of opioid equivalent to 10 mg of parenteral morphine or 30 mg of oral morphine with chronic dosing.

Opioid Use in Persistent Pain

Considerations in Opioid Use

- Nonpharmacological and nonopioid tx are preferred for persistent pain. Consider opioids only if expected benefits for both pain and function are anticipated to outweigh risks to patient. Careful risk-benefit analysis is essential.
  - Establish potential benefits of opioid use in improved function and quality of life.

- Assess for medical risks (eg, respiratory, sleep apnea), potential for misuse or abuse of opioid medication, and potential adverse effects of opioids.
  - Before starting opioids for chronic pain, establish tx goals for pain and function and consider how opioid tx will be discontinued if benefits do not outweigh risks. See below for creating an opioid plan and abuse-prevention approaches.
  - Before starting opioid tx, discuss with patients known risks and realistic benefits of opioid tx as well as patient and clinician responsibilities for managing tx.
  - Establish standard expectations for use to reduce risks and protect others from unintentional or intentional diversion in practice setting. Communicate to patients verbally and in simple written materials.
  - Screen for risks of opioid misuse with thorough hx, medical record review, prescription drug monitoring program (PDMP) review, and standard opioid risk tool (eg, ORT, SOAPP-R).
- Select patients who may benefit from low-dose opioid tx in combination with other tx (eg, specific somatic, peripheral, or neuropathic pain).
  - Avoid opioids in chronic central or visceral pain syndromes such as fibromyalgia, headaches, or abdominal pain.
- Evaluate benefits and harms within 1–4 wk of initiating opioid tx for persistent pain or of dose escalation. Evaluate continued tx every 90 d or more frequently.
  - Continue opioid tx only if there is clinically meaningful improvement in pain and function that outweighs risks to patient safety.
  - If benefits do not outweigh harms, optimize other tx and work to taper opioids to lower dosages or to taper and D/C opioids.

Initiating

- Select least invasive route (usually oral) and fast-onset, short-acting analgesics for episodic or breakthrough pain.
- Begin with lowest dose possible, usually 25–50% adult dose, increasing slowly. Reassess individual benefits and risks when considering doses 50 MS equiv/d or higher, and justify decision to titrate dosage to >90 MS equiv/d. Dosing higher than 90 MS equiv/d should trigger reevaluation of tx plan.
- Start with IR opioids, instead of ER or LA.
- Start stimulant laxative to prevent tx-related constipation. Docusate not recommended with limited efficacy.
- Combination products not recommended for chronic use.
- Total dose limited by maximum dose for APAP; all combination products now contain ≤325 mg of APAP per unit dose, consistent with FDA guidance.
- Titrate dose on basis of persistent need for and use of medications for breakthrough pain. If using ≥3 doses/d of breakthrough pain medication, consider increased dosage of ER medication.

Changing

- Use long-acting or SR analgesics for continuous pain after stabilizing dose with short-acting opioid. Administer around-the-clock for continuous pain.
- Use morphine equivalents (MS equiv) as a common denominator for all dose conversions to avoid errors, and titrate to effectiveness. See hopweb.org/index.cfm?cfid=101993669.
- When changing opioids, decrease equivalent analgesic dose by 25–50% because of incomplete cross-tolerance.

Tapering

- Opioid analgesics should not be discontinued abruptly. Gradual tapering is necessary to avoid withdrawal symptoms (eg, agitation, anxiety, muscle aches, runny nose/tearing, nausea, insomnia, abdominal cramps, diaphoresis, tachycardia, HTN).
- Opioid doses exceeding 100 mg of MS equivalents increase risk of overdose and should prompt consideration of tapering and referral to pain specialist.
- Approach to weaning off long-term opioid use can range from a slow 5–10% dose reduction every 1–4 wk (or even every 2–3 mo for those receiving high doses) to a more rapid 25–50% reduction every 2–3 d. Decreasing the daily dosage by 10–20% each day for 10 d can wean most patients without adverse responses. Adapt based on comorbidities and withdrawal symptoms when process is begun. It is not unreasonable to take months to wean off those on chronic opioid tx.
- Tapering may require conversion to short-acting opioids. For patients at cardiovascular risk, a slower taper with close monitoring for sympathetic hyperactivity is recommended, and low-dose clonidine may be useful in preventing some of the physiologic (and symptomatic) stress related to opioid withdrawal.
- Educate patient that resurgence of pain may occur that is withdrawal-mediated, time-limited, and not usually life-threatening. Psychological support may be needed.

Management of Opioid Adverse Events

- Anticipate, prevent, and vigorously treat AEs; older adults more sensitive to AEs.
- Begin prophylactic, osmotic, or stimulant laxative when initiating opioid tx **(Table 60)**. Titrate laxative dose up with opioid dose.
- Warn about risk of APAP toxicity when using combination products and importance of including all OTC products with APAP in daily APAP total (not to exceed 4 g/d in healthy and 3 g/d in frail older adults).
- Monitor for dry mouth, constipation, sedation, nausea, delirium, urinary retention, and respiratory depression. Growing evidence of concerns related to cognitive impairment, sleep, endocrine dysfunction (hypogonadism), immunosuppression, and hyperalgesia.
- Tolerance can develop to most adverse effects of opioids, except constipation. Reduce dosage and/or consider adding medication to counter medication-related AEs, if troublesome, until tolerance develops.
- Warn patient about risk of sedation with opioids that gradually resolves within 1 wk.
- Opioid-induced constipation (OIC) can result. If prophylactic and 1st-line interventions (dietary changes, OTC tx, exercise) not effective, evaluate for OIC using Bowel Function Index focused on 3 items rated on 0–100 scale: In the past 7 d, ease of defecation, feeling of incomplete bowel evacuation and personal judgement of constipation. Score of 30 or higher merits consideration of prescription OIC medication.
- Opioid antagonists approved to treat OIC. Careful titration and observation are necessary because some patients may experience partial analgesia reversal (also p 137).
- Instances of severe OIC may respond to oral naloxone 0.8–2 mg q12h, titrated to a max of 12 mg/d given in water or juice, along with routine bowel regimen.
  - Methylnaltrexone bromide *(Relistor)* approved for the tx of OIC in adults with chronic, noncancer pain and those with advanced illness receiving palliative care SC 8 mg (38–62 kg) to 12 mg (62–114 kg) and 0.15 mg/kg for other weights with one dose q48h or 450 mg po 1×/d.
  - Oral naloxegol *(Movantik)* 25 mg po 1×/d is indicated for the tx of OIC in adult patients with chronic noncancer pain. D/C all maintenance laxative tx before initiating naloxegol. Laxatives can be used as needed if no response to naloxegol after 3 d.

Prevention of Opioid Harm, Misuse, Abuse, and Withdrawal

Opioids should be initiated as a trial, to be continued if progress is documented toward functional goals, and if there is no evidence of complications, including misuse or diversion. An ongoing tx plan for all patients receiving opioid tx that includes the following is good practice:

- Evaluate for risk of harm. Known risk factors include:
  - Illegal drug use; prescription drug use for nonmedical reasons
  - Hx of substance use disorder or overdose
  - Mental health conditions (eg, depression, anxiety)
  - Sleep-disordered breathing
  - Concurrent benzodiazepine use
- Assess for risk of opioid misuse or abuse (eg, ORT or SOAPP-R); Substance Abuse, p 349, drugabuse.gov/sites/default/files/files/OpioidRiskTool.pdf.
  - Score of 8 or higher on the ORT is considered high risk. Prescribe opioids only after all other tx modalities exhausted, under close supervision—ideally in consultation with a pain or addiction specialist.
  - In at-risk patients requiring opioid management, abuse-deterrent agents may be useful (eg, *Embeda, Targiniq ER*).
- Consider offering prescription for naloxone hydrochloride *(Narcan)* when factors that increase the risk of opioid overdose, such as hx of overdose, hx of substance abuse disorder, higher opioid dosages (≥50 MS equiv/d) or concurrent benzodiazepine use. Naloxone hydrochloride, an opioid antagonist, is available in some states OTC for emergency reversal of opioid adverse effects including respiratory depression. Naloxone can precipitate acute opioid withdrawal and potential pain crisis.
- Use state PDMP to determine if patient is receiving opioid dosages or dangerous combinations that increase the risk of overdose. Review when starting tx for persistent pain and periodically (eg, every prescription to every 3 mo).
- Consider urine drug testing before initiating opioid tx and at least yearly to confirm the presence of prescribed substances and for undisclosed prescription drug or illicit substance use (be aware that false-negative and -positive results are possible, so cautious interpretation is needed).
- Consider a written opioid agreement (drugabuse.gov/sites/default/files/files/SamplePatientAgreementForms.pdf).
- Physical dependence is expected with long-term opioid use (can occur with several weeks of around-the-clock use); it is not the same as substance abuse or addiction.
- In at-risk patients, adjust prescribing boundaries (eg, weekly pickup at local pharmacy).
- Risk evaluation and mitigation strategy (REMS) requires companies to provide educational materials for patients on safe use of long-acting or extended-release opioids and for all immediate-release opioids. Prescriber training provided but not required.
- Monitor pain and signs of misuse during ongoing opioid use (eg, Current Opioid Misuse Measure [COMM]; painedu.org).
- Evaluate for caregiver diversion and neglect or abuse related to opioids. Advise regarding locking of opioids; note requests for early refills.
- Offer or arrange tx for opioid use disorder if needed.
- Consult CDC for resources and tools to support safe opioid prescribing and education of patients (cdc.gov/drugoverdose/prescribing/guideline.html).

Adjuvant Medication Use

- Medications not typically used for pain may be helpful for its management, depending on the etiology (eg, antidepressants, antiseizure medications).
- Use alone or in combination with nonpharmacologic tx and other analgesics (**Table 100**).

Table 100. Adjuvant Medications for Pain Relief in Older Adults[1]

Class, Medication	Indications/Comments
Anticonvulsants (also **Table 92** and p 244)	Indicated for neuropathic pain, fibromyalgia
	If one does not work, try another.
	Numerous drug interactions (fewer for gabapentin and pregabalin); adverse effects include sedation, dizziness, peripheral edema
	Increased risk of falls due to dizziness and somnolence. Avoid if hx of falls or fractures.[BC]
Carbamazepine▲ *(Tegretol XR; Carbatrol)*	Many drug interactions; mood stabilizer; used for trigeminal or glossopharyngeal neuralgia; may cause SIADH[BC], thrombocytopenia, leukopenia
Oxcarbazepine *(Trileptal, Oxtellar XR)*	
Gabapentin▲[BC] (p 246)	Recommended as 1st line or as co-analgesic in postherpetic neuralgia and/or dermatosis papulosa nigra.
	Slow titration based on analgesic response increasing every 3–7 d (may take several mo). If CrCl >15–29, dose at 200–700 mg/d; if CrCl >30–59, dose at 200–700 q12h; if CrCl ≤15, dose at 100–300 mg/d; reduce dose if CrCl <60.[BC]
Pregabalin *(Lyrica)*[BC] (p 246)	Primary indication is for management of postherpetic neuralgia, diabetic peripheral neuropathy, and fibromyalgia; fewer AEs and titration to analgesic effect more rapid. Start 100 mg/d in divided doses increasing to 300 mg/d over several wk. Effect in 3–4 wk. Reduce dose if CrCl <60.[BC]
Lamotrigine▲	Prolongs PR interval; risk of severe rash
Antidepressants (Table 42)	Indicated for neuropathic pain, fibromyalgia, chronic musculoskeletal pain, including osteoarthritis and chronic low-back pain, depression. TCAs often helpful for migraine or tension headaches and arthritic conditions. Avoid tertiary amines due to increased AEs.[BC]
	Of TCAs, low-dose desipramine▲ or nortriptyline▲ best side-effect profile, however avoid due to anticholinergic, sedating, and orthostatic hypotension.[BC]
	Older adults more sensitive to anticholinergic effects, use cautiously with comorbid disease.
	SNRIs lower anticholinergic properties. Avoid if hx of falls or fractures.[BC]
	Data on SSRIs for pain management lacking, but may increase bleeding risk if combined with ASA or NSAIDs; taper dose before discontinuing. Avoid if hx of falls or fractures.[BC]
Duloxetine▲	Preferred SNRI for older adults, typically well tolerated with reduced side effects
	Most common AEs: nausea, dizziness, dry mouth, constipation, diarrhea, urinary hesitancy; significant drug-drug interactions. Monitor for serotonin syndrome.
	Slow taper when discontinuing, may require 10 mg for days (open capsule and put half in applesauce).
	Avoid if CrCl <30.[BC] Avoid if hx of falls or fractures.[BC]
Venlafaxine▲ *(Effexor XR)*	Low anticholinergic activity; minimal sedation and hypotension; may increase BP and QTc; may be useful when somatic pain present; EPS, withdrawal symptoms, hyponatremia
	Analgesic effect is dose dependent and often requires higher dosing than for antidepressant effect. Avoid if hx of falls or fractures.[BC]

(cont.)

Table 100. Adjuvant Medications for Pain Relief in Older Adults[1] (cont.)

Class, Medication	Indications/Comments
Milnacipran *(Savella)*	Dual reuptake inhibitor; used to treat pain of fibromyalgia; contraindicated with MAOI or within 2 wk of MAOI discontinuation
Corticosteroids (Table 50)	Low-dose medical management may be helpful in inflammatory pain conditions. Intraarticular injection 1st- line tx for hip OA; taper dose if discontinuing
Skeletal Muscle Relaxants[BC]	Limited evidence of effectiveness, predominantly sedating with limited analgesic effect. High risk for older adults due to anticholinergic ADRs, excessive sedation, and weakness.
	Recommended for short-term use to relieve acute pain associated with true spasticity (baclofen and tizanidine may be useful).
	Avoid or use with caution in older adults due to limited efficacy and adverse effects.[BC]
	Monitor for muscle weakness, urinary function, cognitive effects, sedation, orthostasis; potential for many drug-drug interactions. Avoid abrupt discontinuation because of CNS irritability.
Baclofen▲	T: 10, 20; Inj 5 mg up to q8h
Carisoprodol *(Soma)*[BC]	T: 350; 250–350 mg 3×/d and bedtime
Methocarbamol *(Robaxin)*[BC]	T: 500, 750; 1.5 g 4×/d for 2–3 d
Tizanidine▲	T: 2, 4; 2 mg up to q8h
Neuromuscular Blocking Agent	Injected into muscles to treat myofascial pain syndrome resulting from skeletal muscle spasm and migraines when source is neck or facial muscles
Onabotulinum toxin A *(Botox)*	Dosing individualized based on muscle affected, severity of muscle activity, and prior experience; not to exceed 360 U q12–16 wk

✓ = preferred for treating older adults

[BC]Avoid

[1] Useful for moderate and/or severe pain depending on pain etiology.

CrCl unit = mL/min/1.73 m^2

DEFINITION

Palliative care is a patient- and family-centered approach that optimizes quality of life by anticipating, preventing and treating suffering associated with serious life-threatening or terminal illness. Palliative care occurs throughout the continuum of illness addressing physical, psychosocial, and spiritual needs to facilitate patient autonomy, access to information, and choice. Hospice care is palliative care provided by an interprofessional tx delivery team for patients who are no longer seeking disease-modifying treatment and who have a prognosis of <6 mo if the disease follows its normal trajectory.

APPROACH

- Initiate palliative care at the time of diagnosis of serious or life-threatening disease.
- Advocate comprehensive palliative care for all suffering patients with serious illness, especially those dying.
- Educate, plan, and document advance directives; final wishes; healthcare and financial proxy; family awareness of decisions.
- Support, educate, and treat both patient and family.
  - Communicate, listen, and support decision making
  - Focus on attainable goals
  - Teach stress management skills, coping
  - Encourage conflict resolution
  - Help complete unfinished business
  - Urge focus on non–illness-related affairs and one day at a time
- Address physical, psychologic, social, and spiritual needs.
  - Promote physical and psychological comfort
  - Encourage spiritual practices
  - Anticipate grief, losses, and completion of unfinished business
  - Refer to PT
- Provide therapeutic environment (palliation can be given in any location).
- Use comprehensive, interprofessional team (physicians, nurses, social workers, chaplain, pharmacist, physical and occupational therapists, dietitian, family and caregivers, volunteers) as appropriate and available.
- Coordinate care among providers. Help integrate potentially curative, disease-modifying, and palliative tx.
- Focus on the continuum of needs, from symptom management, comfort, meeting goals, completion of "life business," healing relationships, and bereavement.
- Offer bereavement support.

PAYMENT

- Except for hospice, all palliative care services are reimbursed though public or private payers using the same mechanism used for physician payment, or have a variety of funding from grants and healthcare system subsidy.
  - Hospices are funded primarily through the Medicare Hospice Benefit (that is also observed by most private insurers).

DECISIONS ABOUT PALLIATIVE CARE

Palliative care is a low risk intervention and has been shown to improve many patient-facing outcomes. It should be recommended without reservation.

Follow principles involved in informed decision making (**Figure 2**) to determine decisional capacity of the patient (p 11).

When to Communicate Bad News

Patients need to be alerted to the expected trajectory of their serious or life-threatening disease, and advanced care planning should be initiated at the time of first diagnosis. Updates on the progression of the patient's disease along the trajectory of the illness should be communicated with the patient and their family at least annually or more frequently depending on the needs of the patient. Focus on living as well as you can for as long as you can.

Communicating Bad News (SPIKES)

S=Setting: Prepare for discussion by ensuring all information/facts/data are available. Deliver in person in private area without interruptions or physical barriers. Determine individuals who patient may want involved.

P=Establish patients' perception of their illness (knowledge and understanding) by asking open-ended questions. Use vocabulary patient uses when breaking bad news.

I=Secure invitation to impart medical information. Determine what/how much patient wants to know.

K=Deliver knowledge and information in sensitive, straightforward manner; avoid technical language and euphemisms. Check for understanding after small chunks of information and clarify concepts and terms.

E=Use empathetic and exploratory responses; use active listening, encourage expression of emotions, acknowledge patient's feelings.

S=Strategize and summarize and organize an immediate tx plan addressing patient's concerns and agenda. Provide opportunity to raise important issues. Reassess understanding of condition and tx plan and determine need for further education and follow-up with patient and family.

Advance Directives

- Any written or verbal statement that provides guidance of what tx the patient might desire. Living wills document tx patient might refuse in a life-threatening situation and typically require the patient's witnessed signature.
- Designed to respect patient's autonomy and determine his or her wishes about future life-sustaining medical tx if unable to indicate wishes. (See Informed Decision-making and Patient Preferences for Life-sustaining Care, p 11.)
- Written by the patient and documented, although not accepted by emergency medical services as legally valid forms; vary from state to state.
- Spoken conversations with relatives, friends, and clinicians should be thoroughly documented in the medical record for later reference; carry the same ethical and legal weight as those recorded if properly verified.
- The role of the team in assisting with advance directives and advance care planning is to ensure that the patient's wishes are met, wherever they may lie on the spectrum of aggressiveness.

Durable Power of Attorney (POA) for Healthcare or Healthcare Proxy

- A written document that enables a capable person to appoint someone else to make future medical tx choices for him or her in the event of decisional incapacity (**Figure 2**).

Instructional Advance Directives (DNR Orders, Living Wills, MOLST, POLST, POST)

- Do-Not-Resuscitate (DNR) orders written by the physician based on the wishes previously expressed by the individual in his or her advanced directive or living will.
- Physician Orders for Life-Sustaining Treatment (POLST), Physician Orders for Scope of Treatment (POST) or Medical Orders for Life-Sustaining Treatment (MOLST) include written instructions about the initiation, continuation, withholding, or withdrawal of particular forms of life-sustaining medical tx.
- POLST documents differ from state to state, but are designed to be recognizable (eg, bright pink; posted on refrigerator), used by first responders, and transferred across settings.
- Clinicians who comply with such directives are provided legal immunity for such actions.
- POLST form can be very useful in formalizing patient preferences (polst.org). May be revoked or altered at any time by the patient.
- Key elements of POLST Plan of Care address: cardiopulmonary resuscitation; level of medical intervention desired in the event of an emergency (comfort only, limited tx, or full tx); and use of artificial nutrition and hydration. Some states include use of antibiotics, hospitalization, and mechanical ventilation.
- To determine whether POLST should be completed, ask "Would I be surprised if this person died in the next year?" If no, the POLST is appropriate.

Key Interventions, Treatment Decisions to Include in Advance Directives

- Resuscitation procedures
- Mechanical respiration
- Chemotherapy, radiation tx
- Dialysis
- Simple diagnostic tests
- Pain control
- Blood products, transfusions
- Intentional deep sedation
- ICD and pacemakers

Withholding or Withdrawing Therapy

- Any person can refuse tx at any time. Withholding tx (not starting) has same legal and ethical standing as withdrawing tx (stopping it after it has been started), although withdrawal is clinically and emotionally more challenging.
- Beginning a tx does not preclude stopping it later; a time-limited trial may be appropriate.
- Palliative care should not be limited, even if life-sustaining tx are withdrawn or withheld.
- Decisions on artificial feeding should be based on the same criteria applied to the use of ventilators and other medical tx.
- Initiate discussion about pacemaker deactivation only if there is a potential patient benefit; consider the potential negative effects of deactivation before disabling the pacemaker. *Note*: Pacemaker is not a resuscitative device and usually does not keep palliative-care patients alive.
- Reanalyze risk-to-benefit ratio of ICD tx in patients with terminal illness. Life-prolonging tx may no longer be desired.

Death Certificate Completion (see Assessment and Approach chapter, p 4)

- Certification of death at the end of life may be completed by the hospice medical director or primary provider and provides personal information about the decedent and about circumstances and cause of death.
- Information is important for settlement of estate and provides family members closure, peace of mind, and documentation of the cause of death.

HOSPICE

Hospice is comprehensive and coordinated bio-psycho-social-spiritual approach to interdisciplinary care at the end of life that also incorporates grief and bereavement services.

Referral and Eligibility

- Patients, families, or other healthcare providers can make a referral to hospice; eligibility for service is confirmed by a physician's certification of terminal illness (CTI) from primary physician or hospice medical director (**Table 101**).
  - CTI must state the objective reasons the physician has established the prognosis, which often includes the diagnosis, its rate of change, the patient's functional status, and various biometric markers of decline.
  - **Table 101** provides guidelines for disease specific prognosis, but multiple comorbidities and unique circumstances necessitate the physician's carefully documented statement of best rationale for admission. Patient may not be referred simply because "they need more help." Some states may have expanded eligibility criteria or concurrent care demonstration projects, though most follow the recommendations in **Table 101.**
  - Patients are evaluated for eligibility on admission and every 60–90 days thereafter.
- Referral is appropriate when curative tx is no longer indicated (ie, ineffective, AEs too burdensome) and life is limited to months.

Approach

- Hospice is designed for people who have a prognosis of <6 mo, but there is no limit on how long a person may spend is hospice as long as their illness continues to cause decline.
- Patients may rescind hospice if their illness improves, and then return to hospice without penalty at a later point.
- Hospice must be accepted by the patient or family, or both, and can be rescinded at any time.
- Hospice provides palliative medications, medical supplies and durable medical equipment, team member visits as needed and desired by patient and family (physician, nurses, home health aide, social worker, chaplain), and volunteer services. Refer to Medicare Conditions of Participation that define requirements (eg, interdisciplinary team composition [expertise/credentials], levels of care, visits, team meetings, plan of care, documentation).
- Optimal hospice care requires adequate time in the program; referral when death is imminent does not take full advantage of hospice care.
- Hospice care is usually delivered in patient's home, but it can be delivered in a nursing home or residential care facility (long-term care, assisted living) or in an inpatient setting (hospice-specific or contracted facility) if acuity or social circumstances warrant.
- Coverage of hospice services variable (eg, inpatient availability, amount of home care, sites for care), so determine and discuss with patient/family.

Disease	Typical Determinants for Hospice Eligibility[1]
Cancer	Clinical findings of malignancy with widespread, aggressive, or progressive disease evidenced by increasing symptoms, worsening laboratory values, and/or evidence of metastatic disease Impaired performance status with a Palliative Performance Scale (PPS value of ≤70% Refuses further curative tx or continues to decline in spite of definitive tx
Dementia	• FAST Scale Stage 7 (p 78) **and** Have had 1 of the following in the past 12 mo: • aspiration pneumonia • pyelonephritis or other upper UTI • decubitus ulcer (multiple, stage 3–4) • fever (recurrent after antibiotics) • inability to maintain sufficient fluid and calorie intake with 10% weight loss during previous 6 mo, or serum albumin < 2.5 g/dL • septicemia
Failure to thrive[2]	BMI <22 kg/m^2 and either declining enteral/parenteral nutritional support or not responding to such support, despite adequate caloric intake **and** Karnofsky score ≤40 or PPS value ≤40% **and** Must have chronic disease diagnosis (eg, HF, COPD)
End-stage heart disease	Optimally treated for HD or either not candidates for surgical procedures or who decline those procedures (optimally treated: not on vasodilators have a medical reason for refusing [eg, hypotension or renal disease]) **and** Significant symptoms of recurrent HF at rest and classified as NYHA Class IV (ie, unable to carry on any physical activity without symptoms, symptoms present at rest, symptoms increase if any physical activity is undertaken) Documentation of following will support eligibility but not required: • tx-resistant symptomatic supraventricular or ventricular arrhythmia • hx of cardiac arrest or resuscitation or unexplained syncope • brain embolism of cardiac origin • concomitant HIV disease • documented ejection fraction of ≤20%
End-stage pulmonary disease	Disabling dyspnea at rest, poorly or unresponsive to bronchodilators, resulting in decreased functional capacity, eg, bed to chair existence, fatigue, and cough (documentation of FEV_1, after bronchodilator, <30% of predicted is objective evidence for disabling dyspnea, but is not necessary to obtain) **and** Progression of end-stage pulmonary disease, as evidenced by *prior* increased visits to emergency department or *prior* hospitalization for pulmonary infections and/or respiratory failure or increasing physician home visits before initial certification (documentation of serial decrease of FEV_1 >40 mL/y is objective evidence for disease progression, but is not necessary to obtain) **and** Hypoxemia at rest on room air, as evidenced by pO_2 ≤55 mmHg or O_2 sat ≤88% or hypercapnia, as evidenced by $PaCO_2$ ≥50 mmHg. Values may be obtained from MR within 3 mo. Documentation of the following will support eligibility, but not required: • right HF secondary to pulmonary disease (cor pulmonale) • unintentional progressive weight loss of >10% of body weight over preceding 6 mo • resting tachycardia >100 bpm

(cont.)

Table 101. Typical Trajectory and Hospice Eligibility for Selected Diseases (cont.)	
Disease	**Typical Determinants for Hospice Eligibility[1]**
Chronic renal failure	Not seeking dialysis or renal transplant or discontinuing dialysis **and** CrCl <10 mL/min/1.73 m2 (<15 mL/min for DM) **or** Serum Cr >8 mg/dL (>6 mg/dL for DM) (<15 mL/min with comorbid CHF; <20 mL/min for diabetics) Documentation of the following signs and symptoms of renal failure lend support for eligibility: • uremia • intractable hyperkalemia (>7) not responsive to tx • hepatorenal syndrome • oliguria (<400 mL/d) • uremic pericarditis • intractable fluid overload not responsive to tx

[1] May vary depending on fiscal intermediary; additional supportive indications available for most diagnoses. Source: Adapted from montgomeryhospice.org/health-professionals/end-stage-indicators (extracted from CMS documentation LCD for Hospice-Determining Terminal Status [L13653]).

[2] Adult failure to thrive can be used to determine hospice eligibility, but should not be listed as principal diagnosis.

MANAGEMENT OF COMMON END-OF-LIFE SYMPTOMS

Pain

- Primary goal: to alleviate suffering at end of life. See Pain chapter (p 252) for assessment and interventions.
- The most distressing symptom for patients and caregivers
- Placement of Foley catheters, limited repositioning to prevent increased pain are acceptable for comfort measures at the end of life.
- If intent is to relieve suffering, the risk that sufficient medication appropriately titrated will produce an unintended effect (hastening death) is morally acceptable (double effect).
- Alternate routes may be needed (eg, transdermal, transmucosal, rectal, vaginal, topical, epidural, IT).
- Recommend expert pain management consult if pain not adequately relieved with standard analgesic guidelines and interventions.
- Additional tx may include:
  ∘ radionuclides and bisphosphonates (for metastatic bone pain)
  ∘ radiation tx or chemotherapy directed at source of pain
- Pain crisis: Palliative sedation for intractable pain and suffering is an important option to discuss with patients. Ketamine▲ 0.1 mg/kg IV bolus. Repeat prn q5min. Follow with infusion of 0.015 mg/kg/min IV (if IV access not available, SC at 0.3–0.5 mg/kg). Decrease opioid dosage by 50%. Benzodiazepines may be used to induce sleep state in the event of excruciating pain unrelieved by other options. Observe for problems with increased secretions and treat (p 280).

Altered Mental Status, Delirium (Delirium, p 72)

- Regular screening with validated tool (CAM, DSM-5, ICD-10)
- Collateral hx from caregiver with Single Question in Delirium (SQiD): Do you feel that (person's name) has been more confused lately?
- Optimize nondrug approaches including orientation, therapeutic activities, optimized sleep, mobilize, avoid sensory input and deprivation; monitor hydration and nutrition, bladder and bowel function

- Investigate and manage reversible factors (if consistent with agreed-upon goals of care), including deprescribing opioid rotation, treating infection, fluid replacement, addressing environmental and other factors
- Consider pharmacologic strategies if needed for distress and safety
- The use of benzodiazepines is controversial. Cautious use as a trial in patients with agitation who are not responding to haloperidol.
- Although commonly used to manage delirium in palliative care, recent evidence suggests that antipsychotics are associated with both increased delirium symptoms and reduced patient survival.
- Lorazepam (3 mg) IV in addition to haloperidol (2 mg) IV upon onset of an agitation episode may decrease agitated delirium in patients with advanced cancer.
- Provide communication, education, and emotional support to patients, family, and healthcare team.

Anorexia, Cachexia, Dehydration

See also Malnutrition (p 203) and volume depletion (p 198). Universal symptom of patients with serious and life-threatening illness.

Note: Percutaneous feeding tubes are not recommended in patients with dementia; instead offer oral assisted feeding.[CW]

Reassure patient and caregivers that appetite abates with age and dehydration is not uncomfortable.

Nonpharmacologic

- Educate patient and family on effects of disease progression that result in lack of appetite and weight loss.
- Promote interest, enjoyment in meals (eg, alcoholic beverage if desired, involve patient in meal planning, small frequent feedings, cold or semi-frozen nutritional drinks).
- Good oral care is important.
- Alleviate dry mouth with ice chips, popsicles, moist compresses, or artificial saliva.

Pharmacologic

- Corticosteroids: dexamethasone[▲] 1–2 mg po q8h; methylprednisolone[▲] 1–2 mg po q12h; prednisone[▲] 5 mg po q8h. Systematic review found beneficial in palliative care patients with cancer, but no evidence for use in end-stage nonmalignant disease. Insufficient evidence to recommend any particular corticosteroid or dosing regimen.

Note: Avoid prescription appetite stimulants or high-calorie supplements for tx of anorexia or cachexia in older adults; instead, optimize social supports, provide feeding assistance, and clarify patient goals and expectations.[CW]

Anxiety, Depression

- Provide opportunity to discuss feelings, fears, existential concerns.
- Referral to appropriate team members (spiritual, nursing)
- Medicate (Anxiety, p 41, and Depression, p 86)
- Methylphenidate or ketamine can be used for depression in palliative care.

Bowel Obstruction

Indications for Radiographic Evaluation

- To differentiate between constipation and mechanical obstruction
- To confirm the obstruction, determine site and nature if surgery is being considered

Nonpharmacologic Management

- Nasogastric intubation: only if surgery is being considered, for high-level obstructions, and poor response to pharmacotherapy
- Percutaneous venting gastrostomy: for high-level obstructions and profuse vomiting not responsive to antiemetics
- Palliative surgery
- Hydration: IV or hypodermoclysis

Pharmacologic Management (aimed at specific symptoms)

- Nausea and vomiting: haloperidol▲ po, IM 0.5–5 mg (≤10 mg) q4–8h prn; ondansetron▲ IV (over 2–5 min) 4 mg q12h, po 8 mg q12h [inj; T: 4, 8, 24; S: 4 mg/5 mL] (**Table 61**).
- Spasm, pain, and vomiting: scopolamine▲ IM, IV, SC 0.3–0.65 mg q4–6h prn; po 0.4–0.8 mg q4–8h prn; transdermal 2.5 cm^2 pch applied behind the ear q3d [inj; T: 0.4; pch 1.5 mg] *or* hyoscyamine▲ sl [T: 0.125; S: 0.125 mg/mL] 0.125–0.25 q6–8h.
- Diarrhea and excessive secretions: loperamide▲ (**Table 62**); octreotide▲ SC 0.15–0.3 mg q12h [inj], very expensive.
- Pain: **Table 100**.
- Inflammation due to malignant obstruction: dexamethasone▲ po 4 mg q6h × 5–7 d.

Constipation (p 137)

- Most common cause: adverse effects of opioids, medications with anticholinergic adverse effects. Use stimulant or osmotic laxative (**Table 60**). Consider enema if no bowel movement for 4 d. Evaluate for bowel obstruction or fecal impaction.
- OIC not responsive to laxative tx: methylnaltrexone bromide *(Relistor)* SC 8 mg (38–62 kg) to 12 mg (62–114 kg) and 0.15 mg/kg for other weights with 1 dose q48h; also newly approved oral naloxegol *(Movantik)* (**Table 60**).

Cough (p 306)

Dysphagia (also p 131)

Nonpharmacologic

- Feed small, frequent amounts of pureed or soft foods.
- Avoid spicy, salty, acidic, sticky, and extremely hot or cold foods.
- Keep head of bed elevated for 30 min after eating. If possible, feed patient sitting upright.
- Instruct patient to wear dentures and to chew thoroughly.
- Use suction machine when necessary.
- Have speech therapist do a bedside swallowing assessment to develop techniques for mouth positioning, swallowing techniques, assistive equipment, and correct consistency of food and beverages.
- For painful mucositis: Do not use magic mouthwash.^{CW} Use frequent and consistent oral hygiene; salt or soda mouth rinses.

Pharmacologic

- For oral candidiasis: clotrimazole 10-mg troches▲, 5 doses/d, *or* fluconazole▲ 150 mg po followed by 100 mg/d po × 5 d.
- For severe halitosis: antimicrobial mouthwash; fastidious oral and dental care; treat putative respiratory tract infection with broad-spectrum antibiotics.

Dyspnea (p 308)

Nonpharmacologic

- Teach positions to facilitate breathing, elevate head of bed or sitting position leaning on table, pursed lips breathing with COPD.
- Teach relaxation techniques.
- Eliminate smoke and allergens.
- Ensure brisk air circulation (facial breeze) with a room fan; oxygen is indicated only for symptomatic hypoxemia (ie, SaO_2 <90% by pulse oximetry) or if comfort perceived by patient.
- Do not administer supplemental oxygen to relieve dyspnea in patients with cancer who do not have hypoxia.[CW]
- Use olive oil or swabs, and humidified oxygen, for dry mouth.

Pharmacologic

- Opioids: oral morphine▲ concentration (20 mg/mL: 1/4 to 1/2 mL sl, po; repeat in 15–30 min prn) *or* morphine tabs 5–10 mg po q2h; if oral route not tolerated, nebulized morphine 2.5 mg in 2–4 mL NS *or* fentanyl 25–50 mcg in 2–4 mL NS; *or* IV morphine 1 mg or equivalent opioid q5–10min.
- Bronchodilators (**Table 120**).
- Diuretics, if evidence of volume overload (**Table 29**).
- Anxiolytics (eg, lorazepam▲ po, sl, SC 0.5–2 mg q2–4h or prn); titrate slowly to effect.
- Guaifenesin *(Robitussin)* or nebulized saline to loosen thick secretions.

Excessive Secretions

Nonpharmacologic: Positioning and suctioning, prn

Pharmacologic: Glycopyrrolate▲ 0.1–0.4 mg IV, SC q4h prn *or* scopolamine▲ 0.3–0.6 mg SC prn *or* transdermal scopolamine pch q72h *or* atropine▲ 0.3–0.5 mg SC, sl, nebulized q4h prn

Existential Suffering

- Often present in terminal illness and associated with reduced quality of life, depression, anxiety, suicidal ideation, and desire for hastened death.
- Descriptions include lack of meaning and purpose, loss of connectedness to others, thoughts about dying process, difficulty finding sense of self, loss of hope, autonomy, or temporality.
- It is helpful to know patient's spiritual beliefs using questions based on the FICA spiritual history tool gathering information on faith and belief, importance, community, and address in care (https://smhs.gwu.edu/gwish/clinical/fica/spiritual-history-tool).
- Symptom interventions (eg, antidepressants, CBT) work in palliative care setting, as well.
- Clarify new-onset symptoms, such as insomnia, for evidence of anxiety and existential suffering that require a broader approach.
- Assist patients to see that many things haven't changed since diagnosis and help reframe (eg, relationship with children changing from giving care to receiving care).
- Support family member distress from losing loved one and caregiving roles.
- Adjust tx boundaries to communicate connectedness or caring (eg, hold hand of dying patient, gentle hand on shoulder).
- Recommend formalized interventions such as meaning-centered psychotherapy, dignity tx, and other manualized therapies for existential distress.
- Help patients find a silver lining (eg, still alive, time to explore relationships and beauty).

Nausea, Vomiting (p 140)

Determine cause to select appropriate antiemetic based on pathway-mediating symptoms and neurotransmitter involved (**Table 61**). For refractory nausea and vomiting (ie, not amenable to other tx), a trial of dexamethasone (2 mg q8h) can be tried; risks are dyspepsia, altered mental status. Taper when discontinued.

Do not use topical lorazepam *(Ativan)*, diphenhydramine *(Benadryl)*, haloperidol *(Haldol)* ("ABH") gel for nausea.[CW]

Olanzapine▲ for chemotherapy-induced nausea (See Malnutrition).

Skin Failure

An event in which the skin and underlying tissue die due to hypoperfusion that occurs concurrent with severe dysfunction or failure of other organs

See Skin Ulcers (p 331) for Chronic Wound Assessment.

Management

- Interdisciplinary approach focused on resident-centered and caregiver-centered outcomes
- Engage in frank discussions regarding prognosis, tx of symptoms, and goals of care
- Manage pain determining if acute pain associated with debridement, associated with care routines, or chronic
- Repositioning to off-load pressure
- Dietary consultation regarding amount of calories and fluid to promote healing, if healing is considered possible
- Avoid wet-to-dry dressings, which can increase bacterial burden and infection
- Recommended dressings: nonadhesive, absorptive, and odor-controlling that prevent desiccation of wound bed, protect periwound from maceration, and can be left in place for longer periods (eg, hydrogels, foams, polymeric membrane foams, silicones, alginates)
- Control odor by removing necrotic debris and using antimicrobials, activated charcoals, and external odor absorbers

Weakness, Fatigue

Nonpharmacologic

- Modify environment to decrease energy expenditure (eg, placement of phone, bedside commode, drinks).
- Adjust room temperature to patient's comfort.
- Teach reordering tasks to conserve energy (eg, eating first, resting, then bathing).
- Modify daily procedures (eg, sitting while showering rather than standing).

Pharmacologic

- Treat remediable causes such as pain, medication toxicity, insomnia, anemia, and depression.
- Consider psychostimulants (eg, dextroamphetamine▲ [Avoid[BC]] 2.5 mg po qam or q12h, methylphenidate▲ 2.5 mg po qam or q12h to start titrate upward to 3×/d or 4×/d prn, or modafinil *[Provigil]* 200 mg qam); monitor for signs of psychosis, agitation, or sleep disturbance. Prescribe doses before noon especially for ER to avoid insomnia. Avoid in insomnia.[BC]

PHYSICIAN-ASSISTED DYING AND ACTIVE EUTHANASIA

Physician-assisted Dying

Although not recognized or promoted as acceptable palliative care practice, providers need to be aware of the status of physician-assisted dying (also called aid in dying, death with dignity, right to die, compassionate dying, assisted suicide) to respond to a request from patients. Physician-assisted dying is the patient's intentional, willful ending of his or her own life with the assistance of another; it may involve providing knowledge, means, or both, to end one's life, including counseling about lethal doses of drugs, prescribing such lethal doses, or supplying the drugs; a criminal offense in most states.

- In states where legal (CA, CO, OR, WA, VT, MT, DC), eligibility must be established and may include: (1) aged 18 y or older, (2) resident of the state, (3) capable of making and communicating healthcare decisions for oneself, and (4) diagnoses with terminal illness that will lead to death within 6 mo.
- The patient must verbally request the medication at least twice and contribute to at least 1 written request.
- Physician must notify the patient of alternatives (eg, palliative care, hospice, pain management).
- Finally, physician is to request—but not require—that the patient notify his or her next of kin about the request of a prescription for a lethal dose of medication.

Active Euthanasia

Direct intervention, such as lethal injection, intended to hasten a patient's death (also called mercy killing); a criminal act of homicide in all United States.

PREOPERATIVE CARE

Surgical Decision Making

- With the prospect of potential surgery, the patient's tx goals should be determined before surgical consultation.
- Goal setting is predicated on decision-making capacity, patient preferences, and life expectancy (see *Goal-Oriented Care, Life Expectancy, and Medical Decision Making and Informed Decision Making and Patient Preferences for Life-Sustaining Care,* p 9).
- Cognitive impairment, functional dependence, malnutrition, and frailty are risk factors for adverse outcomes of surgery (eg, mortality, functional decline, institutionalization).
- If surgery is determined to be a potential option that is in accordance with tx goals, additional cardiac, pulmonary, cognitive, functional, nutritional, and metabolic assessments should be conducted to further estimate surgical risk (see next 3 sections).

Cardiac Risk Assessment in Noncardiac Surgery (2014 ACC/AHA Guidelines)

- Risk of perioperative cardiac complications (eg, MI, death) is related to patient characteristics and type of surgery.
  - Major patient-related risk factors include active HF, LV dysfunction, CAD, and valvular disease.
  - Other patient-related factors include age, renal dysfunction, DM, and poor functional status.
  - Surgeries conferring increased risk include open aortic or other vascular, cardiac, intrathoracic, intraabdominal, major orthopedic, and major GU procedures.
  - Low-risk surgeries (<1% perioperative risk of MI or death) include cataract, endoscopic, breast, dermatologic, and superficial procedures.
- Several tools are available for formal assessment of cardiac risk, including:
  - Revised Cardiac Risk Index (RCRI): score 1 point each for: Cr ≥2 mg/dL, HF, DM, hx of stroke or TIA, CAD, and undergoing intrathoracic, intraabdominal, or suprainguinal vascular surgery. Total score ≥2 confers increased risk.
  - Two risk calculators from the American College of Surgeons are available at riskcalculator.facs.org and surgicalriskcalculator.com/miorcardiacarrest.
- **Figure 11** shows a suggested algorithm for assessment of cardiac risk.
- Obtain a preoperative ECG for patients with known CAD, arrhythmia, PAD, prior stroke or TIA, or other structural heart disease. ECG is not indicated in patients undergoing low-risk surgery.

Choosing Wisely Recommendations for Preoperative Cardiac Assessment

- Don't perform stress cardiac imaging or advanced noninvasive imaging as a preoperative assessment in patients scheduled to undergo low-risk noncardiac surgery.[CW]
- Patients who have no cardiac hx and good functional status do not require preoperative stress testing before noncardiac thoracic surgery.[CW]
- Don't perform preoperative medical tests for eye surgery unless there are specific medical indications.[CW] See Eye chapter (p 114).

Figure 11. Assessing Cardiac Risk in Noncardiac Surgery (adapted from 2014 ACC/AHA Guidelines)

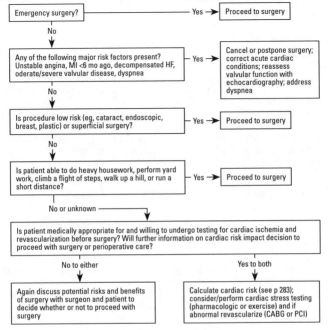

- Avoid echocardiograms for preoperative/perioperative assessment of patients with no hx or symptoms of heart disease.**CW**
- Don't order coronary artery calcium scoring for preoperative evaluation for any surgery, irrespective of patient risk.**CW**
- Don't initiate routine evaluation of carotid artery disease before cardiac surgery in the absence of symptoms or other high-risk criteria.**CW**

Pulmonary Risk Assessment

Major risk factors for postoperative pulmonary complications:
- COPD
- ASA Class II – V (I – healthy; II – mild systemic disease; III – moderate/severe systemic disease; IV – life-threatening systemic disease; V – moribund)
- ADL dependence
- HF

- Prolonged (>3 h) surgery; abdominal, thoracic, neurologic, head and neck, or vascular surgery; AAA repair; emergency surgery
- General anesthesia
- Serum albumin <3.5 mg/dL

Minor risk factors:
- Confusion/delirium
- Weight loss >10% in previous 6 mo
- BUN >21 mg/dL or Cr >1.5 mg/dL
- Alcohol use
- Current cigarette use
- Sleep apnea
- Pulmonary hypertension

Reducing risk of postoperative pulmonary complications:
- Smoking cessation 6–8 wk before surgery
- Before cardiac surgery, there is no need for pulmonary function testing in the absence of respiratory symptoms.[CW]
- Preoperative training in incentive spirometry, active-cycle breathing techniques, and forced-expiration techniques
- Postoperative incentive spirometry, chest PT, coughing, postural drainage, percussion and vibration, suctioning and ambulation, intermittent positive-pressure breathing, and/or CPAP
- Nasogastric tube use for patients with postoperative nausea or vomiting, inability to tolerate oral intake, or symptomatic abdominal distention

Other Preoperative Assessments

Screen for Conditions Associated with Postoperative Complications:
- Cognitive impairment: Mini-Cog (p 5)
- Depression: PHQ-2
- Delirium risk factors: p 72
- Alcohol and substance abuse: CAGE questionnaire (p 350)
- Functional impairment: ADLs, IADLs
- Malnutrition: BMI <18.5 kg/m^2, >10% unintentional weight loss in past 6 mo, serum albumin <3.0 g/dL
- Frailty syndrome: at least 3 of the following: ≥10 lb unintentional weight loss in past year (shrinkage), decreased grip strength (weakness), self-reported poor energy and endurance (exhaustion), low weekly energy expenditure (low physical activity), slow walking (slowness)

Routine Laboratory Tests
- Recommended: Hb, Cr, BUN, albumin, or basic metabolic panel if it includes these tests and is cheaper
- Not routinely recommended as should be obtained selectively according to the patient's conditions: electrolytes, CBC, platelets, ABG, PT, PTT
- Don't obtain preoperative chest radiography in the absence of clinical suspicion for intrathoracic pathology.[CW]

Cataract Surgery: Routine laboratory testing or cardiopulmonary risk assessment is unneccessary for cataract surgery performed under local anesthesia. If patient is on anticoagulation tx, it should not be interrupted. Use of α$_1$-blockers for BPH (p 294) within 14 d of cataract surgery is associated with increased risk of complications (intraoperative floppy iris syndrome), but it is unknown if cessation of α_1-blockers before surgery lowers risk.

Antiplatelet Therapy: If surgery poses high bleeding risk (eg, CABG, intracranial surgery, prostate surgery), D/C antiplatelet tx 5–9 d before procedure.

Patients With Bare Metal Stents (BMS) or Drug-Eluting Stents (DES) on Dual Antiplatelet Therapy:

• If possible, postpone surgery until 30 d after BMS were placed and 12 mo after DES were placed.

• If surgery cannot be delayed until 30 d after BMS or 12 mo after DES placement:
  ◦ For most surgeries, which are at low risk of bleeding, continue dual antiplatelet tx.
  ◦ Continue dual antiplatelet tx during the 1st 6 wk after placement of stent unless risk of bleeding is judged to be higher than benefit of stent thrombosis prevention.
  ◦ For surgeries at intermediate risk of bleeding in patients with DES placement >12 mo previous, D/C clopidogrel or prasugrel 5–7 d before procedure and maintain ASA tx. Because the platelet inhibition of ticagrelor is reversible, it should be stopped 1 d before procedure.
  ◦ For surgeries at high risk of catastrophic bleeding (intracranial, spinal canal, or posterior chamber eye surgery), D/C clopidogrel or prasugrel 5 d before procedure, D/C ticagrelor 1 d before procedure, and consider D/C of ASA 5 d before procedure. Stopping ASA is an individual decision based on patient's risk factors for stent thrombosis and on assessed bleeding risk.
  ◦ If both antiplatelet agents need to be stopped, consider bridging tx (requires admitting patient 2–4 d before surgery) with tirofiban or eptifibatide (**Tables 12** and **18**) in patients felt to be at very high risk of stent thrombosis (consult with cardiology).
  ◦ If antiplatelet tx is discontinued, resume it the day of the surgical procedure.

Anticoagulation:

• For procedures at minimal risk of bleeding (eg, cataract surgery, dermatologic procedures), maintain anticoagulation before surgery.

• Cessation of oral anticoagulation tx before surgery that is assessed to be of significant bleeding risk (eg, abdominal, thoracic, or orthopedic surgery, spinal puncture, liver or kidney biopsy, TURP, or placement of spinal or epidural catheter/port):
  ◦ Stop warfarin 5 d before surgery.
  ◦ Bridging tx with LMWH is based on VTE risk (**Table 102**).
  ◦ DVT tx doses of LMWH (**Table 18**) should be used for bridging tx. Begin LMWH 3 d before surgery; give last preoperative LMWH dose at one-half of total daily dose 24 h before surgery.
  ◦ Stop dabigatran 1–3 d before surgery (2–4 d if CrCl <50 mL/min/1.73 m^2) and stop apixaban or rivaroxaban 1–2 d before surgery.

• Resumption of anticoagulation tx after surgery:
  ◦ If bridging, resume LMWH 24 h after surgery, longer (48–72 h) with major surgical procedures or difficulty with hemostasis.
  ◦ Resume warfarin, apixaban, edoxaban, rivaroxaban, or dabigatran 12–24 h after surgery if adequate hemostasis.

• Minor dental procedures: stop warfarin 2–3 d before procedure and recommend administration of prohemostatic agent (eg, tranexamic acid) by dentist.

Table 102. Indications for Perioperative Anticoagulation Bridging Therapy (ACCP Guidelines)

Thromboembolic Risk	Patient Conditions Determining Risk	Recommendations for LMWH Bridging Therapy
Low	• No VTE in past 12 mo • AF without prior TIA/stroke and 0–2 SRF • Bileaflet mechanical aortic valve without AF, prior TIA/stroke, or SRF	Not recommended
Intermediate	• VTE in past 3–12 mo • Recurrent VTE • Active malignancy • AF without prior TIA/stroke and with 3–4 SRF • Bileaflet mechanical aortic valve with AF, prior TIA/stroke, or any SRF	Optional according to individual thrombotic and bleeding risk
High	• VTE within past 3 mo • TIA/stroke within 3 mo • Rheumatic heart disease • AF with prior TIA/stroke and 3–4 SRF • Mechanical mitral valve or ball/cage mechanical aortic valve	Recommended

ACCP = American College of Chest Physicians; SRF = stroke risk factors: age ≥75, HTN, DM, HF.

Diuretics and Hypoglycemic Agents: Withhold on day of surgery.

NSAIDs: despite its common practice, there is no direct evidence to support cessation of NSAIDs before surgery. Coordinate decision to maintain or discontinue NSAID with surgeon.

SSRIs: SSRIs increase risk of bleeding with surgery, but discontinuing them before surgery is not recommended unless routine medication review indicates no tx need.

Advance Directives: Establish or update.

Reducing Cardiovascular Complications of Surgery (MI, Ischemia, Death, Infection)

- **β-blockers**: if chronically stable on β-blocker, continue perioperatively at usual dose. In patients with intermediate- or high-risk myocardial ischemia found on stress testing or with RCRI score >3 (p 283), consider initiating long-acting β-blocker days to weeks before surgery (target HR=60) and continuing throughout postoperative period.
- **Statins**: continue as usual dosage for patients already on a statin. Strongly consider prescribing a statin for all patients undergoing vascular surgery or for patients with multiple cardiac risk factors undergoing non–low-risk surgery.
- **Antiplatelets**: before CABG and other high-risk procedures for bleeding (p 286), D/C ASA, clopidogrel, or prasugrel 5 d before surgery and D/C ticagrelor 1 d before surgery. Resume antiplatelets as soon as possible after surgery, within 24 h after CABG.
- **Anticoagulants**: for VTE prophylaxis, see **Tables 13** and **14**. For patients already on an anticoagulant, see **Table 102** for management guidelines.
- **Antibiotics**: for endocarditis prophylaxis, see p 291.

PRINCIPLES OF GERIATRIC CO-MANAGEMENT OF COMPLEX PATIENTS

- Both geriatrician and other specialist write orders with clearly demarcated areas of responsibility; care is co-managed.
- Both geriatrician and other specialist see patient daily.
- Patient goals are elucidated and shared with co-managing teams.
- Standard protocols are used as much as possible.

- In surgical cases, geriatrician performs/facilitates comprehensive preoperative assessment.
- Geriatrician often manages medical regimen to minimize adverse drug effects.

POSTOPERATIVE DELIRIUM (also DELIRIUM, p 72)

Epidemiology and Risk Factors

- Occurs after 15–50% of surgeries depending on type of procedure.
- Most episodes occur in 1st 2 postoperative days.
- Occurrences after postoperative day 2 are usually due to surgical complications or alcohol/sedative withdrawal.
- Major risk factors:
  - age ≥80
  - dementia
  - recent or unresolved delirium
  - major cardiac, open vascular, major abdominal surgery
  - emergency surgery
  - major surgical complication (eg, cardiogenic shock, prolonged intubation)
  - postoperative ICU stay ≥2 d
- Minor risk factors:
  - age 70–79
  - mild cognitive impairment
  - hx of stroke
  - poor functional status
  - significant comorbidity
  - alcohol or sedative use
  - depressive symptoms
  - abdominal, orthopedic, ENT, gynecologic, urologic surgery
  - general anesthesia
  - regional anesthesia with IV sedation
  - minor surgical complication (eg, infection, minor bleeding)
  - poorly controlled pain
  - exposure to opiates or sedatives
  - postoperative ICU stay <2 d

Diagnosis and Management

- Systematic **preoperative** assessment and risk-lowering interventions have been shown to reduce the rate of postoperative delirium. This can be accomplished through proactive geriatrics team consultation/co-management, nurse-run programs to detect and prevent delirium, and the Hospital Elder Life Program (HELP) intervention (hospitalelderlifeprogram.org).
- See pp 72–74 for delirium diagnosis (Confusion Assessment Method or CAM) and management.
- If workup finds bacteriuria, do not automatically ascribe a UTI as the cause of the delirium as asymptomatic bacteriuria is very common in older adults (p 176).

PREVENTIVE TESTS AND PROCEDURES

Table 103. Recommended Primary and Secondary Disease Prevention for People Aged 65 and Older

Preventive Strategy	Frequency
USPSTF Grade A/B[1] or CDC[1] Recommendations for Primary Prevention	
BMD (women)	at least once after age 65
BP screening	yearly
DM screening	every 3 y in people aged 40–70 who are overweight or obese
Exercise	adults aged ≥65 at increased risk of falls
Hepatitis A vaccination	at least once in adults at high risk (Section 12 of cdc.gov/vaccines/schedules/hcp/imz/adult-conditions.html)
Hepatitis B vaccination	at least once in adults at high risk (Section 13 of cdc.gov/vaccines/schedules/hcp/imz/adult-conditions.html)
Herpes zoster vaccination	after age 50 for recombinant zoster vaccine *(Shingrix)* or after age 60 for live zoster vaccine *(Zostavax)* in immunocompetent people[2]
Influenza vaccination	yearly
Lipid disorder screening	every 5 y, more often in CAD, DM, PAD, prior stroke
Pneumonia vaccination	once at age 65 with PCV13 pneumococcal conjugate vaccine *(Prevnar),* followed 6–12 mo later by dose of PPSV23 pneumococcal polysaccharide vaccine *(Pneumovax)*[3]
Smoking cessation	at every office visit
Tetanus vaccination	every 10 y
Weight management multicomponent intensive behavioral tx	Offer to or refer for adults with BMI ≥30
USPSTF Grade A/B[1] Recommendations for Secondary Prevention	
AAA ultrasonography	once between age 65–75 in men who have ever smoked
Alcohol abuse screening	unspecified but should be done periodically
Depression screening	yearly
FOBT; Fecal immunochemical test (FIT); FIT-DNA test; CT colonography; sigmoidoscopy; colonoscopy[4]	Yearly for FOBT and FIT; every 1–3 y for FIT-DNA; every 5 y for CT colonography and sigmoidoscopy; every 10 y for colonoscopy from age 50 to age 75
Hepatitis B screening	at least once in adults at high risk (uspreventiveservicestaskforce.org/Page/Document/UpdateSummaryFinal/hepatitis-b-virus-infection-screening-2014)
Hepatitis C screening	at least once in adults at high risk (uspreventiveservicestaskforce.org/Page/Document/UpdateSummaryFinal/hepatitis-c-screening)
HIV screening	at least once in persons aged ≥65 with risk factors for HIV

(cont.)

Preventive Strategy	Frequency
Low-dose CT scanning for lung cancer	yearly in persons aged 55–80 with ≥30 pack-y of smoking and currently smoke or have quit in the past 15 y
Mammography[5]	every 2 y in women aged 50–74

USPSTF C/I[1] or Other[6] Recommendations for Primary Prevention

ASA to prevent MI and/or stroke[7]	daily in persons aged 60–69 for whom benefit of stroke risk reduction outweighs risk of GI bleeding
Calcium (1200 mg) and vitamin D (≥800 IU) to prevent osteoporosis/fractures	daily
Falls prevention: risk assessment and management	at least once after age 65
FOBT; FIT; FIT-DNA test; CT colonography; sigmoidoscopy; colonoscopy[4]	Yearly for FOBT and FIT; every 1–3 y for FIT-DNA; every 5 y for CT colonography and sigmoidoscopy; every 10 y for colonoscopy in adults aged 76–85
Measurement of serum CRP	at least once in people with one CAD risk factor
Obesity/undernutrition screening	yearly
Omega-3 fatty acids to prevent MI, stroke	at least 2×/wk (see MI care, p 47)

USPSTF Grade C/I[1] or Other[6] Recommendations for Secondary Prevention

Skin examination	yearly
Cognitive impairment screening	yearly
Glaucoma screening	yearly
Hearing impairment screening	yearly
TSH, especially in women	yearly
Visual impairment screening	yearly

[1] US Preventive Services Task Force (www.uspreventiveservicestaskforce.org/Home/GetFileByID/989) grade recommendations: A = recommended, substantial benefit; B = recommended, moderate benefit; C = selectively offer based on professional judgment and patient preferences; I = evidence is inconclusive regarding benefits and harms of service. Centers for Disease Control and Prevention (cdc.gov/vaccines/schedules/hcp/adult.html)

[2] *Shingrix*, administered in 2 doses 2–6 mo apart, is recommended as a 1st choice over *Zostavax*, which is administered as a single dose. *Shingrix* may be given in persons who have already received *Zostavax* (wait at least 8 wk after *Zostavax* to give 1st *Shingrix* dose). Compared to *Zostavax*, *Shingrix* more frequently causes side effects (pain and swelling at injection site, muscle aches, fatigue, and/or mild fever for 2–3 d). Patients with history of herpes zoster infection may be vaccinated.

[3] Adults aged >65 who have already received PPSV23 should receive a dose of PCV13 at least 1 y after PPSV23 vaccination.

[4] Do not repeat colorectal cancer screening (by any method) for 10 y after a high-quality colonoscopy is negative in average-risk individuals.[CW]

[5] Mammograms to age 70 are almost universally recommended; many organizations recommend that mammography should be continued in women over 70 who have a reasonable life expectancy.

[6] Not endorsed by USPSTF/CDC for all older adults, but recommended in selected patients or by other professional organizations.

[7] Use with caution in adults aged ≥70.[BC]

For individualized age- and sex-specific USPSTF prevention recommendations, see ahrq.gov/professionals/clinicians-providers/guidelines-recommendations/guide.

USPSTF GRADE D RECOMMENDATIONS (AGAINST PERFORMING PREVENTIVE ACTIVITY)

Against screening for:
- Asymptomatic bacteriuria with UA
- Bladder cancer with hematuria detection, bladder tumor antigen measurement, NMP22 urinary enzyme immunoassay, or urine cytology
- CAD with ECG, exercise treadmill test, or electron-beam CT in people with few or no CAD risk factors
- Carotid artery stenosis with duplex ultrasonography
- Cervical cancer in women aged ≥65 who have had adequate prior screening or who have had a hysterectomy for benign disease
- Colon cancer with FOBT/sigmoidoscopy/colonoscopy in people aged ≥85. Screening may be modestly beneficial in people aged 76–85 with long life expectancy and no or few comorbidities.
- COPD
- Ovarian cancer with transvaginal ultrasonography or CA-125 measurement
- PAD with measurement of ABI
- Pancreatic cancer with ultrasonography or serologic markers
- Prostate cancer with PSA and/or digital rectal examination in men aged 70 and over
- Don't use PET/CT for cancer screening in healthy individuals.**CW**

Also against:
- Beta-carotene or vitamin E supplementation to prevent CVD or cancer
- Use of estrogen/progestin tx to prevent chronic conditions
- Vitamin D supplementation to prevent falls in community-dwelling older adults

CANCER SCREENING AND MEDICAL DECISION MAKING
- Many decisions about whether or not to perform preventive activities are based on the estimated life expectancy of the patient. Refer to **Table 7** for life expectancy data by age and sex.
- Most cancer screening tests do not realize a survival benefit for the patient until after 10 y from the time of the test. Cancer screening should be discouraged or very carefully considered in patients with ≤10 y of estimated life expectancy.
- Don't recommend screening for breast or colorectal cancer, or prostate cancer (with the PSA test), without considering life expectancy and the risks of testing, overdiagnosis, and overtreatment.**CW**

ENDOCARDITIS PROPHYLAXIS (AHA GUIDELINES)
Antibiotic Regimens Recommended (Table 77)

Table 104. Endocarditis Prophylaxis Regimens	
Situation	**Regimen (Single Dose 30–60 Min Before Procedure)[1]**
Oral	Amoxicillin▲ 2 g po
Unable to take oral medication	Ampicillin▲ 2 g, cefazolin▲ 1 g, or ceftriaxone▲ 1 g IM or IV
Allergic to penicillins or ampicillin	Cephalexin▲ 2 g, clindamycin▲ 600 mg, azithromycin▲ 500 mg, or clarithromycin▲ 500 mg po
Allergic to penicillins or ampicillin and unable to take oral medication	Cefazolin▲ 1 g, ceftriaxone▲ 1 g, or clindamycin▲ 600 mg IM or IV

[1] For patients undergoing invasive respiratory tract procedures to treat an infection known to be caused by *Staph aureus*, or for patients undergoing surgery for infected skin, skin structures, or musculoskeletal tissue, regimen should include an antistaphylococcal penicillin or cephalosporin.

Cardiac Conditions Requiring Prophylaxis (all others do not)

- Prosthetic cardiac valve
- Previous infective endocarditis
- Cardiac transplant recipients who develop cardiac valvulopathy
- Unrepaired cyanotic congenital heart disease
- Repaired congenital heart disease with residual defects at the site or adjacent to the site of a prosthetic patch or device
- Congenital heart disease completely repaired with prosthetic material or device (prophylaxis needed for only the 1st 6 mo after repair procedure)

Procedures Warranting Prophylaxis (only in patients with cardiac conditions listed above)

- Dental procedures requiring manipulation of gingival tissue, manipulation of the periapical region of teeth, or perforation of the oral mucosa (includes extractions, implants, reimplants, root canals, teeth cleaning during which bleeding is expected)
- Invasive procedures of the respiratory tract involving incision or biopsy of respiratory tract mucosa
- Surgical procedures involving infected skin, skin structures, or musculoskeletal tissue

Procedures Not Warranting Prophylaxis

- All dental procedures not listed above
- All noninvasive respiratory procedures
- All GI and GU procedures

ANTIBIOTIC PROPHYLAXIS FOR PATIENTS WITH TOTAL JOINT REPLACEMENTS (TJR)

Procedures/Conditions Prompting Consideration of Antibiotic Prophylaxis

- The American Academy of Orthopedic Surgeons in conjunction with the American Dental Association recommend that clinicians consider discontinuing the practice of routine antibiotic prophylaxis in patients with prior TJR who are undergoing dental procedures (www.orthoguidelines.org/topic?id=1002).
  - Bacteremias are produced not just by dental procedures, but also by common daily activities such as tooth brushing.
  - While antibiotic prophylaxis reduces bacteremia after dental procedures, there is no evidence that withholding antibiotics or dental procedures themselves are associated with prosthetic knee or hip infections.
- Antibiotic prophylaxis should be considered for patients with prior TJR, regardless of when joint was replaced, who are undergoing ophthalmic, orthopedic, vascular, GI, head and neck, gynecologic, or GU procedures.
- Additional risk factors for considering prophylaxis in patients with prior TJR: immunocompromised state; disease-, radiation-, or drug-induced immunosuppression; inflammatory arthropathies; malnourishment; hemophilia; HIV infection; type 1 DM; malignancy; megaprostheses; comorbidities (eg, DM, obesity, smoking)
- Conditions not requiring prophylaxis: patients with pins, plates, or screws

Suggested Prophylactic Regimens

- Dental procedures (see those listed above for endocarditis): amoxicillin▲, cephalexin▲, or cephradine▲ 2 g po 1 h before procedure
- Prophylactic antibiotic recommendations for other types of procedures vary by procedure (Antimicrobial Prophylaxis for Surgery. *The Medical Letter, Treatment Guidelines* 2006;4[52]:83–88).

EXERCISE PRESCRIPTION

Before Giving an Exercise Prescription

Screen patient for:

- Musculoskeletal problems: decreased flexibility, muscular rigidity, weakness, pain, ill-fitting shoes
- Cardiac disease: consider stress test if older adult is beginning a vigorous exercise program and is sedentary with symptoms of active CVD (eg, angina, HF, PAD), DM, end-stage renal disease, or chronic lung disease.

Individualize the Prescription

Initiating low-intensity (rated 1–4 on a 10-point scale by the patient) to moderate-intensity (rated 5–6 on a 10-point scale) exercise is generally safe in older adults with multiple chronic conditions. Guidelines below should be adjusted according to patient's ability to tolerate each activity. Specify short- and long-term goals; include the following components (CDC and American College of Sports Medicine/AHA recommendations):

Endurance: Moderate-intensity activity, ≥30 min ≥5×/wk

- Moderate-intensity activities such as brisk walking are those that increase HR and would be rated 5–6 on a 10-point intensity scale by the patient.
- It is never too late to start exercising. Brisk walking in previously sedentary older adults significantly lowers risk of disability.
- Using pedometers to record the number of steps in a walking program has been demonstrated to increase physical activity, lower BMI, and lower BP.

Strength: Weight (resistance) training at least 2×/wk, 10 exercises on major muscle groups, 10–15 repetitions per exercise

Flexibility: Static stretching, at least 2×/wk for ≥10 min of flexibility exercises, 10–30 sec per stretch, 3–4 repetitions of major muscle/tendon groups

Balance: Balance exercises are recommended for people with mobility problems or who fall frequently.

Patient information: See go4life.nia.nih.gov. See also Assessment and Management of Falls, **Figure 5**.

PROSTATE DISORDERS

BENIGN PROSTATIC HYPERPLASIA (BPH)

Lower urinary tract symptoms (LUTS; increased frequency of urination, nocturia, hesitancy, urgency, and weak urinary stream) may or may not be associated with enlarged prostate gland, bladder outlet obstruction (eg, urinary retention, recurrent infection, renal insufficiency), or histological BPH.

Evaluation

Evaluation of the severity of symptoms (International Prostate Symptom Score for BPH): Detailed medical hx focusing on physical exam of the urinary tract, including abdominal exam, digital rectal exam, and a focused neurologic exam; UA and culture if pyuria or hematuria. Postvoid residual (PVR) if neurologic disease or prior procedure that can affect bladder or sphincter function, UI, or reports of incomplete emptying. PVR should be performed before initiating antimuscarinic tx (below). Measurement of prostate-specific antigen (PSA) is controversial, but should not be measured if life expectancy is <10 y. Don't order Cr or upper tract imaging if only LUTS.[CW]

INTERNATIONAL PROSTATE SYMPTOM SCORE (IPSS) SYMPTOM INDEX FOR BPH

Questions to be answered (circle one number on each line)	Not at all	Less than 1 time in 5	Less than half the time	About half the time	More than half the time	Almost always	
1. Over the past month or so, how often have you had a sensation of not emptying your bladder completely after you finished urinating?	0	1	2	3	4	5	
2. Over the past month or so, how often have you had to urinate again less than 2 hours after you finished urinating?	0	1	2	3	4	5	
3. Over the past month or so, how often have you found you stopped and started again several times when you urinated?	0	1	2	3	4	5	
4. Over the past month or so, how often have you found it difficult to postpone urination?	0	1	2	3	4	5	
5. Over the past month or so, how often have you had a weak urinary stream?	0	1	2	3	4	5	
6. Over the past month or so, how often have you had to push or strain to begin urination?	0	1	2	3	4	5	
7. Over the last month, how many times did you most typically get up to urinate from the time you went to bed at night until the time you got up in the morning?	none	1 time	2 times	3 times	4 times	>5 times	
8. If you knew you were going to live the rest of your life with your urinary problems, how would you feel?[1]	Very satisfied	Satisfied	Mostly Satisfied	Neither satisfied	Mostly dissatisfied	Dissatisfied	Terrible

[1] The last question is about quality of life and is not entered into the scoring.

AUA Symptom Score = sum of responses to questions 1–7 =___.

0–7 points	Mild symptoms
8–19 points	Moderate symptoms
20–35 points	Severe symptoms

Management

Mild Symptoms: (eg, AUA IPSS <8;) watchful waiting

Moderate to Severe Symptoms: (eg, AUA score ≥8) watchful waiting, medical or surgical tx

Nonpharmacologic Treatment: Avoid fluids before bedtime, reduce mild diuretics (eg, caffeine, alcohol), double voiding to empty bladder completely, voiding in sitting position (if LUTS). For some patients with obstruction causing urinary retention who are not surgical candidates, clean intermittent catheterization can be used.

Pharmacologic Treatment: If mild to moderate symptoms, can start with α_1-blockers alone. Combining drugs from different classes may have better long-term effectiveness than single-agent tx. Because of immediate onset of benefit, many recommend beginning with α-adrenergic blockers. If overactive bladder symptoms without evidence of bladder outlet obstruction or high PVR, consider beginning with antimuscarinics or combination α-blocker and antimuscarinic.

If large prostate (eg, >30 g) or severe symptoms, consider beginning with combined tx (α-adrenergic blockers and 5-α reductase inhibitors). No dietary supplements have been demonstrated to be effective.

- **α_1-Blockers** reduce dynamic component by relaxing prostatic and bladder detrusor smooth muscle. Nonselective and selective agents are equally effective. Do not start in men with planned cataract surgery until after surgery is completed. First-generation drugs appear to have lower rates of intraoperative floppy iris syndrome. Use of PDE5 inhibitors (sildenafil, tadalafil, vardenafil) with α_1-blockers can potentiate hypotensive effect.
  - **First-generation** (can cause orthostatic hypotension and dizziness, which may be potentiated by sildenafil [*Viagra*], vardenafil [*LEVITRA*], and perhaps tadalafil [*Cialis*])
    - Terazosin▲ [T: 1, 2, 5, 10]: increase dosage as tolerated: days 1–3, 1 mg/d hs; days 4–7, 2 mg; days 8–14, 5 mg; day 15 and beyond, 10 mg. Avoid use as antihypertensive or in patients with syncope.[BC]
    - Doxazosin▲ [T: 1, 2, 4, 8]: start 0.5 mg with max of 16 mg/d. Avoid use as antihypertensive or in patients with syncope.[BC]
  - **Second-generation** (less likely to cause hypotension or syncope, also benefits hematuria; more likely to cause ejaculatory dysfunction)
    - Tamsulosin▲ [T: 0.4]: 0.4 mg 30 min after the same meal each day and increase to 0.8 mg if no response in 2–4 wk; decreases ejaculate volume; increases risk of retinal detachment, lost lens or lens fragment, or endophthalmitis if taken within 14 d before cataract surgery
    - Silodosin *(Rapaflo)* [C: 4, 8]: 8 mg/d or 4 mg/d in moderate kidney impairment; not recommended in severe kidney or liver impairment, may have more sexual AEs (decreased ejaculate volume; retrograde ejaculation in ~30%)
    - Alfuzosin ER▲ [T: 10]: 10 mg after the same meal every day
- **5-α Reductase Inhibitors** (reduce prostate size and are more effective with large [>30 g] glands; do not use in the absence of prostate enlargement; tx for 6–12 mo may be needed before symptoms improve) may help prostate-related bleeding and can decrease libido, ejaculation, and erectile function. Both finasteride and dutasteride reduce the incidence of prostate cancer but may lead to higher incidence of high-grade tumors in later years. Increased risk of depression and self-harm.

- ∘ Finasteride▲ [T: 5]: 5 mg/d
- ∘ Dutasteride▲ [C: 0.5]: 0.5 mg/d
- **Antimuscarinic agents** (bladder relaxants) may have additional benefit beyond α_1-blockers on urinary frequency and urgency (**Table 70**) but use with caution if PVR >250–300 mL.
- **Phosphodiesterase-5 (PDE5) Inhibitors (Table 123)** may improve symptoms of BPH/LUTS in men with or without erectile dysfunction but do not improve flow rates. Do not use daily if CrCl <30 mL/min/1.73 m². Tadalafil *(CIALIS)* 5 mg taken at the same time daily has been approved for BPH.

Surgical Management: Indicated if recurrent UTI, recurrent or persistent gross hematuria, bladder stones, hydronephrosis, or renal insufficiency are clearly secondary to BPH or as indicated by severe symptoms (AUA score >16), patient preference, or ineffectiveness of medical tx. For men with moderate symptoms (AUA scores 8–15), surgical tx is more effective than watchful waiting, but the latter is a reasonable alternative.

Surgical options include:

Large Prostate

- Transurethral resection of the prostate (TURP), increasingly bipolar is used because of safety; standard tx, best long-term outcome data; 1% risk of UI and no increased risk of sexual dysfunction.
- Open prostatectomy for large glands (>50 g), usually longer hospital stay and more blood loss
- Transurethral plasma vaporization of the prostate ("button" procedure) is associated with less bleeding and hyponatremia (TURP syndrome) but higher rates of postoperative irritative voiding symptoms, dysuria, urinary retention, recatheterization, and repeat surgery. Also no tissue available for pathology.
- Laser photoselective vaporization (PVP) or laser enucleation (HoLEP, ThuLEP) using laser as a knife

Small Prostate with Bladder Outlet Obstruction

- Transurethral incision of the prostate (TUIP), which is limited to prostates with estimated resected tissue weight (if done by TURP) of ≤30 g. Lower rates of ejaculatory dysfunction.
- Transurethral (TUMT) or transrectal microwave thermotherapy (TRMT) is the least operator-dependent but has inconsistent results; lower rates of retrograde ejaculation compared to TURP.

High-Risk Patients

- Laser photoselective vaporization (PVP); effects on symptoms have been maintained for up to 2 y with complication rates similar to TURP
- Transurethral radiofrequency ablation is less effective than TURP but may be an option for men with substantial comorbidity who are poor surgical candidates.
- Convective water-vapor energy ablation (WAVE) 50% reduction in IPSS scores by 3 mo, sustained at 12 and 36 mo and preserves sexual function
- Radiofrequency ablation
- TUIP
- Prostatic urethral lift (sutures that hold the prostate away from the urethra) has evidence for up to 5 y) benefit and preserves sexual function. 14% require surgical retreatment within 5 y.
- Botulinum toxin and prostatic arterial embolization may be effective but require further study before these can be recommended.

PROSTATE CANCER

USPSTF recommends that for men aged 55–69, periodic PSA-based screening should be an individual decision; recommends against PSA-based screening in men aged ≥70

Evaluation

Predicting the extent of disease:

- PSA (p 294)
- Biopsy (Gleason primary and secondary grade)
- Digital rectal examination
- Family hx (diagnosis <60 y; BCRA2 mutation or Lynch syndrome)
- If life expectancy ≤5 y and asymptomatic, workup only if high or very high risk (**Table 105**)
- Bone scan if unfavorable intermediate, high, very high (**Table 105**)
- CT or MRI abdomen and pelvis if intermediate, high, or very high or symptomatic, and nomogram-predicted probability of lymph-node involvement >10%

Do not perform PET, CT, and radionuclide bone scan in the staging of early prostate cancer at low risk of metastasis.[CW]

Consider molecular testing in men who are potential candidates for active surveillance and have low-risk or favorable intermediate-risk disease with a life expectancy >10 y.

Histology

- Gleason score ≤6 has low 15- to 20-y morbidity and mortality; watchful waiting is usually appropriate.
- Gleason score ≥7, higher PSA and younger age are associated with higher morbidity and mortality; best tx strategy (surgery, radiation tx, ADT, etc) is not known.

Grading system that incorporates Gleason score

- Grade group 1 (Gleason score 3+3)
- Grade group 2 (Gleason score 3+4)
- Grade group 3 (Gleason score 4+3)
- Grade group 4 (Gleason score 4+4, 3+5, or 5+3)
- Grade group 5 (Gleason score 4+5, 5+4, or 5+5)

Staging

T1 = Clinically inapparent tumor, neither palpable nor visible by imaging

    a. Incidental finding <5% of tissue

    b. Incidental finding >5% of tissue

    c. Identified by needle biopsy (eg, because of increased PSA)

T2 = Tumor confined within prostate

    a. <1/2 of 1 lobe

    b. >1 lobe

    c. Both lobes

T3 = Tumor extends through the prostate capsule

    a. Unilateral or bilateral extracapsular extension

    b. Invading seminal vesicle

T4 = Tumor is fixed or invades adjacent structures other than seminal vesicles

N = Regional nodes indicating Stage IV disease

M = Distal metastasis indicating Stage IV disease

Treatment

Don't treat low-risk clinically localized prostate cancer without discussing active surveillance as part of the shared decision-making process.[CW]

Modalities

- Radical prostatectomy reduces short- and long-term overall and disease-specific mortality, metastasis, and local progression compared with watchful waiting in men aged <65 with early disease, regardless of histology and PSA, including those who are at low risk. UI and sexual dysfunction are more common compared to EBRT and may gradually improve but not back to baseline. Irritative urinary symptoms are less than radiation tx or active surveillance.
- Radiation tx may cause transient PSA increase that does not reflect cancer recurrence. Bloody stools after 12 mo are more common compared to prostatectomy.
  - EBRT is associated with acute worsening of urinary and bowel obstructive symptoms but tend to resolve over 24 mo.
  - Brachytherapy (radioactive seed implantation) has greater effect on prostate than EBRT.
- Proton-beam tx should not be recommended outside of a prospective clinical trial or registry.[CW]
- Hormonal tx is reserved for locally advanced or metastatic disease.
  - Monotx can be either bilateral orchiectomy or a GnRH agonist.
  - Combined androgen blockade (GnRH agonist plus antiandrogen) is used to avoid "flare" phenomenon (ie, increased symptoms early in tx), but survival benefit is uncertain and side effects are greater than with monotx.

Table 105. Options for the Initial Treatment of Prostate Cancer

Early Cancer[1]		Treatment Modality							
Risk	Definition	Expected Survival[2]	Obs[3]	AS[4]	RP	PLND	EBRT	BRT	ADT
Very low	T1c, Gleason score <6, <3 positive biopsy cores, <50% cancer in each core, PSA <10 ng/mL, and PSA density 0.15 ng/mL	≥20 y		+	+	+/-	+	+	Short term
		10–20 y		+					
		<10 y	+						
Low	Stage T1 *or* T2a, Gleason score ≤6, PSA <10 ng/mL	≥10 y		+	+	+/-	+	+	
		<10 y	+						
Intermediate	Stage T2b–c *or* PSA 10–20 ng/mL *or* Gleason score 7	≥10 y		+	+	+/-	+	+	+/- Short term
	Favorable if <50% of biopsy cores are positive	<10y	+				+	+	
	Unfavorable if ≥50% of biopsy cores are positive	≥10 y			+	+/-		+	+/- Short term
		<10 y	+				+	+	+/- Short term

(cont.)

Table 105. Initial Treatment of Prostate Cancer (cont.)

Early Cancer[1]		Treatment Modality							
Risk	Definition	Expected Survival[2]	Obs[3]	AS[4]	RP	PLND	EBRT	BRT	ADT
High	T3a *or* Gleason score 8–10, PSA >20 ng/mL and >5 y survival (if PSA ≤2.5, poor response to hormonal tx)				+	+	+	+/-	+
Very high	T3b–T4, > 4 cores with Gleason score 8–10 (tx if >5 y survival)				+	+	+	+/-	+
Metastasis									
Regional							+[3]		with EBRT or alone[5]
Distant									+

ADT = androgen deprivation tx; AS = active surveillance; BRT = brachytherapy; DRE = digital rectal exam; EBRT = external beam radiation tx; Obs = observation; PLND = pelvic node dissection accompanying RP; RP = radical prostatectomy

[1] Options based on aggressiveness risk of cancer (National Comprehensive Cancer Network nccn.org/professionals/physician_gls/f_guidelines.asp#prostate)

[2] Based on age and other clinical prognostic characteristics

[3] PSA ≥q6mo, DRE ≥q12mo, prostate biopsy ≥q12mo. Tx if progression, defined as rise in PSA, or Gleason 4 or 5 on biopsy, or cancer is found in greater number of biopsies or involves greater extent of biopsy.

[4] Monitoring the course of disease with the expectation to deliver palliative tx for the development of symptoms or change in exam or PSA levels that suggest symptoms are imminent.

[5] May be given with abiraterone and prednisone.

Therapy for Metastatic Bone Disease

In men receiving long-term ADT or HT for cancer and in those with bone metastasis, zoledronic acid 5 mg IV annually or denosumab 120 mg SC q4wk reduces the proportion of patients with skeletal-related events or fracture.

Therapy for Castration-recurrent Metastatic Disease

• Maintain castrate levels of testosterone and chemotherapy (docetaxel works best if lymph node–only disease) or autologous cellular immunotherapy. (nccn.org/professionals/physician_gls/f_guidelines.asp#prostate)

Therapy for PSA-only Recurrence (no evidence of other disease)

• If after radical prostatectomy, EBRT ± ADT or observation.
• If after radiation tx, ADT or observation.

Therapy for Relapse Without Evidence of Metastasis

• Sequential hormonal manipulations are often used first:
  ◦ Withdrawal of antiandrogen may induce remission.
  ◦ Patients often respond when changed to a 2nd antiandrogen.
  ◦ When antiandrogens no longer control disease, adrenal suppression with aminoglutethimide or ketoconazole and hydrocortisone replacement may be effective.

Monitoring

After surgery or radiation tx, PSA should be <0.1 ng/mL or undetectable. Monitor PSA q6–12mo for 5 y (q3mo if high risk), then every year. Digital rectal exam yearly but may be omitted if PSA undetectable. If nodal or metastatic disease, physical exam and PSA q3–6 mo. If undetectable PSA after radical prostatectomy and subsequent detectable PSA that increases on ≥2 determinations, workup for distant metastasis. A PSA doubling time of 3–12 mo in the absence of clinical recurrence indicates a higher risk of the development of systemic disease and cancer-specific death.

Late Complications of Prostate Cancer

- Cardiovascular disease (controversial) due to effects of ADT on cardiac risk factors (obesity, lipids, decreased insulin sensitivity)
- GI, especially proctitis, from radiation
- Urinary frequency, urgency, stress incontinence, dysuria, stricture, retention, hematuria
- Erectile dysfunction, orgasmic dysfunction, penile fibrosis
- Hypogonadism (consider replacement if in remission)
- DM
- Osteoporosis as a result of ADT and RT
- Secondary malignancies in field of radiation (bladder, rectal)
- Psychosocial (fatigue, depression)

Table 106. Common Medications for Prostate Cancer Therapy

Class, Medication	Dosage	Metabolism	Adverse Events/ Comments
GnRH Agonists	*Class AEs:* certain symptoms (urinary obstruction, spinal cord compression, bone pain) may be exacerbated early in tx; risk is less when combined with antiandrogens		
Goserelin acetate implant *(Zoladex)*	3.6 mg SC q28d or 10.8 mg q3mo	(L, K)	Hot flushes (60%), breast swelling, libido change, impotence, nausea
Leuprolide acetate▲	7.5 mg IM qmo or 22.5 mg q3mo or 30 mg q4mo	Unknown	Hot flushes (60%), edema (12%), pain (7%), nausea, vomiting, impotence, dyspnea, asthenia (all 5%), thrombosis, PE, MI (all 1%); headache as high as 32%
Triptorelin *(Trelstar Depot, Trelstar LA)*	Depot: 37.5 mg q28d IM LA: 11.25 mg q84d	(L, K)	Hot flushes, ↑ glucose, ↓ Hb ↓ RBC, ↑ alkaline phosphatase ↑ ALT or AST, skeletal pain, ↑ BUN
Histrelin acetate *(Vantas)*	50-mg SC implant q12mo	(L)	Hot flushes, fatigue, headaches, nausea, mild renal impairment
Antiandrogens (most often used in combination with GnRH agonists)	*Class AEs:* nausea, hot flushes, breast pain, gynecomastia, hematuria, diarrhea, liver enzyme elevations, galactorrhea		
Bicalutamide▲	50 mg/d po [T: 50]	(L, K)	
Flutamide▲	250 mg po q8h [C: 125]	(K)	Greatest GI toxicity in the class; severe liver dysfunction reported
Nilutamide *(Nilandron)*	300 mg/d po for 30 d, then 150 mg/d po [T: 50]	(L, K)	Delayed light adaptation

(cont.)

Table 106. Common Medications for Prostate Cancer Therapy (cont.)			
Class, Medication	**Dosage**	**Metabolism**	**Adverse Events/Comments**
Abiraterone acetate *(Zytiga)*	Up to 1000 mg/d	(L)	Given with prednisone 5 mg/d or q12h
GnRH Antagonist			
Degarelix *(Firmagon)*	240 mg SC, then 80 mg SC q28d	(L 70–80%) (K 20–30%)	Prolonged QT interval, hot flushes, weight gain, fatigue, ↑AST and ALT

PROSTATITIS

Definition

Acute or chronic inflammation of the prostate secondary to bacterial (usually Gram-negative organisms) and nonbacterial causes

Symptoms and Diagnosis

Acute: fever; chills; dysuria; obstructive symptoms; tender, tense, or boggy on examination (examination should be minimal to avoid bacteremia); Gram stain and culture of urine (usually caused by Gram-negative organisms)

Chronic: recurrent UTIs, especially with same organism; obstructive or irritative symptoms with voiding, perineal pain (may include chronic pelvic pain syndrome). Examination often indicates hypertrophy, tenderness, edema, or nodularity, but may be normal. Compare 1st void or midstream urine with prostatic secretion or postmassage urine: bacterial if leukocytosis and bacteria in expressed sample (typically caused by Gram-negative organisms, especially *E coli*), nonbacterial if sample sterile with leukocytosis

Treatment (Table 77)

Antibiotic tx should be based on Gram stain and culture. Begin tx for acute prostatitis empirically to cover likely organisms (Gram-negative) while culture is pending. If occurs after transrectal prostate biopsy, more likely to be due to drug-resistant organisms. Do not insert Foley catheter in acute prostatitis. If urinary retention, consult a urologist.

Acute prostatitis (recommend tx for 6 wk)
• Co-trimoxazole[ABC] DS 1 po q12h, *or*
• Ciprofloxacin[ABC] 500 mg po or 400 mg IV q12h, *or*
• Ofloxacin[A] 400 mg po 1×, then 300 mg q12h, *or*
• 3rd-generation cephalosporin or aminoglycoside IV
• If patient is toxic, combine aminoglycoside with fluoroquinolone.

Chronic prostatitis (fluoroquinolones have good penetration of inflamed prostate and are generally considered 1st choice for initial and recurrent infections)
• Co-trimoxazole[ABC] DS 1 po q12h × 2–4 mo, *or*
• Ciprofloxacin[ABC] 500 mg po q12h × at least 6 wk, *or*
• Levofloxacin 500 mg po q24h × at least 6 wk, *or*
• Ofloxacin[A] 200 mg q12h × 3 mo
• If resistant to other antibiotics, fosfomycin at high dosages, doxycycline, or both.

α-blockers may help chronic prostatitis in combination with antibiotics. Less consistent benefits have been demonstrated with anti-inflammatory agents and finasteride.

DIFFERENTIAL DIAGNOSIS
- Bipolar affective disorder
- Delirium
- Dementia
- Medications/drugs: eg, antiparkinsonian agents, anticholinergics, benzodiazepines or alcohol (including withdrawal), stimulants, corticosteroids, cardiac medications (eg, digitalis), opioid analgesics
- Late-life delusional (paranoid) disorder
- Major depression
- Physical disorders: hypo- or hyperglycemia, hypo- or hyperthyroidism, sodium or potassium imbalance, Cushing syndrome, Parkinson disease, B_{12} deficiency, sleep deprivation, AIDS
- Pain, untreated
- Schizophrenia
- Structural brain lesions: tumor or stroke
- Seizure disorder: eg, temporal lobe

Risk Factors for Psychotic Symptoms in Older Adults: chronic bed rest, cognitive impairment, female sex, sensory impairment, social isolation

MANAGEMENT
- Establish a trusting therapeutic relationship with the patient; focus on empathizing with the distress that symptoms cause rather than reality orientation.
- Encourage patients to maintain significant, supportive relationships.
- Alleviate underlying physical causes.
- Address identifiable psychosocial triggers.
- Before using an antipsychotic to treat behavioral symptoms of dementia, carefully assess for possible psychotic features (ie, delusions and hallucinations) and if psychotic symptoms are severe, frightening, or may affect safety.
- Parkinson disease psychosis: Pimavanserin *(Nuplazid)*, an inverse agonist at the 5HT2A receptor, has been specifically approved. Same warning for risk of QTc prolongation as for antipsychotics (**Table 90**).
- For *DSM5*, rate presence and severity (most severe in last 7 d) of psychotic symptoms (eg, hallucinations, delusions, disorganized speech) on a 5-point scale ranging from 0 (not present) to 4 (present and severe).
- Aripiprazole, olanzapine, quetiapine, risperidone[▲] are 1st choice because of fewer AEs (TD extremely high in older adults taking 1st-generation antipsychotics). See **Table 108** and **Table 109** for AEs of 2nd-generation antipsychotics.
- Caution if hx of falls and fractures.[BC]
- All antipsychotics are associated with increased mortality in older adults.[BC]

Table 107. Representative Medications for Treatment of Psychosis

Class, Medication	Dosage[1]	Formulations	Comments (Metabolism)
Second-generation Antipsychotics			Avoid for behavioral problems of dementia
✓Aripiprazole *(Abilify)*	2–5 (1) initially; max 30/d	T: 2, 5, 10, 15, 20, 30 ODT: 10, 15 IM: 9.75 mg/1.3 mL S: 1 mg/mL	Wait 2 wk between dosage changes (CYP2D6, -3A4) (L)
(Ability Maintena)	300–400 q30d	Long-acting IM: 441 mg/1.6 mL	Deltoid or gluteal injection. Ensure adequate muscle mass. Adjust dose for CYP2D6 and -3A4 interactions. Not for complications of dementia.
Aripiprazole lauroxil *(Aristada)*	400–6620 q30d; 882 q4–6wk 1064 q2mo	Long-acting IM: 441 mg/1.6 mL; 662 mg/2.4 mL; 882 mg/3.2 mL; 1064 mg/3.4 mL	441-mg deltoid or gluteal injection; 662-mg, 882-mg, and 1064-mg gluteal-only injections. Ensure adequate muscle mass. Adjust dose for CYP2D6 and -3A4 interactions. Not for complications of dementia.
Asenapine *(Saphris)*	5–10 mg q12h	SL: 5, 10	Do not swallow (L)
Clozapine▲	25–150 (1)	T: 25, 100 ODT: 12.5, 25, 100	May be useful for parkinsonism and TD; significant risk of neutropenia and agranulocytosis; weekly CBCs × 6 mo, then biweekly (L)
Iloperidone *(Fanapt)*	Initial: 1 mg q12h, increase by ≤2 mg q12h daily to 6–12 mg q12h; max 24 mg/d	T: 1, 2, 4, 6, 8, 10, 12	Very limited geriatric data (CYP2D6), inhibits 2C19 and 3A4 (L)
Lurasidone *(Latuda)*	40 mg	T: 40–80	Very limited geriatric data Dose should not exceed 40 mg/d in renal impairment (CrCl <50)
✓Olanzapine▲	2.5–10 (1)	T: 2.5, 5, 7.5, 10, 15, 20 ODT: 5, 10, 15, 20 IM: 5 mg/mL	Weight gain (L)
Paliperidone *(Invega)*	3–12 (1)	T: ER 3, 6, 9	CrCl 51–80, max 6 mg/d; CrCl ≤50, max 3 mg/d; very limited geriatric data (K)
✓Quetiapine▲	25–800 (1–2)	T: 25, 100, 200, 300 T: ER 50, 150, 200, 300, 400	Ophthalmic examination recommended q6mo (L, K)

(cont.)

Table 107. Representative Medications for Treatment of Psychosis (cont.)

Class, Medication	Dosage[1]	Formulations	Comments (Metabolism)
✓Risperidone▲	0.25–1 (1–2)	T: 0.25, 0.5, 1, 2, 3, 4 ODT: 0.5, 1, 2, 3, 4 S: 1 mg/mL IM long-acting: 25, 37.5, and 50 mg/2 mL	Dose-related EPS; IM not for acute tx; do not exceed 6 mg (L, K)
Ziprasidone▲	20–80 (1–2)	C▲: 20, 40, 60, 80 IM: 20 mg/mL	May increase QTc; very limited geriatric data (L)
Low Potency First Generation			
Thioridazine▲	25–200 (1–3)	T: 10, 15, 25, 50, 100, 150, 200 S: 30 mg/mL	Substantial anticholinergic effects, orthostasis, QTc prolongation, sedation, TD; for acute use only. Avoid. [BC] (L, K)
Intermediate Potency First Generation			
Perphenazine▲	2–32 (1–2)	T: 2, 4, 8, 16	Risk of TD with long-term use. Avoid.[BC] (L, K)
High Potency First Generation			Avoid.[BC]
Haloperidol▲	0.5–2 (1–3); depot 25–200 mg IM q4wk	T: 0.5, 1, 2, 5, 10, 20 S: conc 2 mg/mL Inj: 5 mg/mL (lactate)	EPS, TD; for acute use only (L, K) Depot form is for chronic use; monitor for TD and D/C if signs appear
Fluphenazine	1–2.5 mg/d (max 5 mg/d) (1)	T: 1, 2.5, 5, 10 S: conc 5 mg/mL IM: 2.5 mg/mL (decanoate)	EPS, TD, akathisia (L, K)

✓ = preferred for treating older adults but does not imply low risk; mortality may be increased in patients with dementia.

[1]Total mg/d (frequency/d)

CrCl unit = mL/min/1.73 m^2

Table 108. Adverse Events of Preferred Second-generation Antipsychotics

AE	Aripiprazole	Olanzapine	Quetiapine	Risperidone
Cardiovascular				
Hypotension	?	+	+++	+
QTc prolongation[1]	0	++	++	++
Endocrine/Metabolic				
Weight gain	+	+++	++	++
DM	?	+++	++	++
Hypertriglyceridemia	0	+	0	?
Hyperprolactinemia	0	+	0	+++

(cont.)

Table 108. Adverse Events of Preferred Second-generation Antipsychotics (cont.)

AE	Aripiprazole	Olanzapine	Quetiapine	Risperidone
Gastrointestinal				
Nausea, vomiting, constipation	0	0	?	?
Neurologic				
EPS	+	+	+	+++
Seizures	?	?	?	ND
Sedation	+	++	++	+
Systemic				
Anticholinergic	0	++	+	0
Neuroleptic malignant syndrome	ND	ND	ND	+

ND = no data; ? = unpredictable effect; 0 = no effect; + = mild effect; ++ = moderate effect; +++ = severe effect

[1] QTc upper limit of normal = 440 millisec

Table 109. Management of Adverse Events of Antipsychotic Medications

AE	Treatment	Comment
Drug-induced parkinsonism	Reduce dosage or change drug or drug class	Often dose related; avoid anticholinergic agents[BC]
Akathisia (motor restlessness)	Consider adding β-blocker (eg, propranolol[▲] 20–40 mg/d) or low-dose benzodiazepine (eg, lorazepam[▲] 0.5 mg q12h)	Also seen with 2nd-generation antipsychotics; more likely with traditional agents
Hypotension	Slow titration; reduce dosage; change drug class	More common with low-potency agents
Sedation	Reduce dosage; give hs; change drug class	More common with low-potency agents
TD	Stop drug (if possible); consider 2nd-generation antipsychotic (eg, aripiprazole, quetiapine) with lower potential for EPS	Increased risk in older adults; may be irreversible

Note: Periodic (q4mo) reevaluation of antipsychotic dosage and ongoing need is important (see CMS guidance on unnecessary drugs in the nursing home: cms.gov/transmittals/downloads/R22SOMA.pdf). Older adults are particularly sensitive to AEs of antipsychotic drugs. They are also at higher risk of developing TD. Periodic use of an AE scale such as the AIMS is highly recommended.

Tardive Dyskinesia

TD, a polymorphous, hyperkinetic movement disorder, is commonly orofacial but can be truncal and in severe cases can be disabling. Caused by exposure to dopamine-receptor antagonists, especially 1st-generation antipsychotics, risk increases after age 65. Postmenopausal women at highest risk. AIMS is the gold standard for monitoring (cqaimh. org/pdf/tool_aims.pdf).

Valbenazine *(Ingrezza)* is a VMAT2 inhibitor recently approved to treat patients with TD. 40 mg 1×/d for 1 wk, then 80 mg 1×/d, no dosage adjustment for age. SAEs: somnolence, QTC prolongation. Drug interactions: MAOIs, strong CYP3A4 and -2D6 inhibitors, digoxin.

COUGH

Among the most common presenting symptoms in office practice; consider likely diagnosis based on duration of symptoms and treat the specific disorder (**Table 110**). **Table 111** lists agents sometimes used in symptomatic management of cough.

Table 110. Diagnosis and Treatment of Cough by Duration of Symptoms	
Cause	**Preferred Treatment**
Acute cough: duration up to 3 wk	
The common cold, acute rhinosinusitis	Sinus irrigation or nasal ipratropium (*Atrovent NS 0.06%*, **Table 114**). Not recommended: sedating antihistamines (dry mouth, urinary retention, confusion); oral pseudoephedrine[BC] (HTN, tachycardia, urinary retention). Don't routinely treat uncomplicated rhinosinusitis or bronchitis with antibiotics.[CW]
Acute bronchitis	Criteria for antibiotics: Illness >1 wk; high-risk patients; HF, COPD, asthma; Antibiotic choice: amoxicillin, doxycycline, erythromycin for 5 d; depending on local resistance patterns 3rd generation cephalosporin or macrolide Criteria for bronchodilators: troublesome cough, bronchospasm, wheezing, FEV_1 <80% Criteria for antitussives: (**Table 111**) cough causing discomfort
Allergic rhinitis	p 309
Bacterial sinusitis	Oxymetazoline[▲] nasal spr × 5 d; antibiotic against *Haemophilus influenzae* and streptococcal pneumonia (eg, amoxicillin-clavulanate or doxycycline) × 5–7 d.
Pertussis	Macrolide or trimethoprim-sulfa antibiotic × 2 wk
Other: pneumonia, HF, asthma, COPD exacerbation	Pneumonia, p 172; HF, p 48; asthma, p 316; COPD, p 312
Subacute cough: duration 3–8 wk	
Postinfectious	Inhaled ipratropium; systemic steroids tapered over 2–3 wk; if protracted, dextromethorphan with codeine; use bronchodilators if there is bronchospasm (**Table 114**)
Subacute bacterial sinusitis	As for acute bacterial sinusitis, but treat for 3 wk
Asthma	p 316
Pertussis	Macrolide or trimethoprim-sulfa antibiotic × 2 wk; may need to treat as above for postinfectious cough
Chronic cough: duration >8 wk	(25% of patients have more than 1 cause requiring concurrent tx); See Stepwise Approach, p 307
Perennial/allergic rhinitis	p 309. Tx for 2–4 wk for reduction/resolution
Chronic bacterial sinusitis (suspect if purulent sputum)	Same as for subacute bacterial sinusitis but also cover mouth anaerobes × 3 wk; may need follow-up course of nasal steroids
Asthma or cough-variant asthma	p 316. Tx for 6–8 wk for reduction/resolution
Other: ACEIs, smoking, reflux esophagitis, occupational exposure	Stop ACEI, smoking (cough may persist for 4 wk); treat reflux for up to 3 mo for reduction/resolution using a PPI q12h
Aspiration	Dysphagia, p 131. Evaluate with modified barium swallow

(cont.)

Table 110. Diagnosis and Treatment of Cough by Duration of Symptoms (cont.)	
Cause	**Preferred Treatment**
Sleep apnea	May present as cough that is also present at night (see Sleep chapter, p 341)
Eosinophilic bronchitis	Eosinophils in sputum, but no reversible airway obstruction on spirometry; treat with inhaled glucocorticoids (p 310) for 3–4 wk
External ear disease	Tx according to etiology
Bronchiectasis (purulent sputum)	Cyclic antibiotics often needed
Pulmonary fibrosis/Sarcoidosis	Pulmonary consultation
Idiopathic refractory cough	See Stepwise Approach, below

Stepwise Approach to Evaluating Chronic Cough

- Step 1: Hx and physical exam, medication review, red flags (hemoptysis or weight loss); obtain CXR, spirometry. If CXR and spirometry are normal, common causes are perennial/allergic rhinitis, reflux, cough-variant asthma.
- Step 2: Assess bronchial hyperresponsiveness with methacholine challenge, sputum eosinophil count (cough-variant asthma).
- Step 3: Consider rarer causes: refer to otolaryngologist for nasendoscopy; high-resolution chest CT (pulmonary fibrosis); bronchoscopy; refer to cough clinic.
- Step 4: Consider neuromodulatory tx for idiopathic refractory chronic cough.
  - Speech and language tx
  - Pharmacotherapy: low-dose slow-release morphine sulfate 5 mg po 2×/d, or gabapentin or pregabalin titrated to effect (Reduce gabapentin/pregabalin dose if CrCl <60 mL/min/1.73 m[2,BC]). Amitriptyline[BC] 10 mg po hs is superior to codeine + guaifenesin.

Management

- Do not suppress cough in stable COPD.
- For symptomatic relief of acute or subacute cough, see **Table 111**.

Table 111. Antitussives and Protussives		
Medication	**Dosage and Formulations**	**Adverse Events (Metabolism)**
Benzonatate[▲1]	100 mg po q8h (max: 600 mg/d) C: 100, 200	CNS stimulation or depression, headache, dizziness, hallucination, constipation (L)
Dextromethorphan[▲1]	10–30 mL po q4–8h C: 30 S: 10 mg/5 mL	Mild drowsiness, fatigue; interacts with SSRIs and SNRIs; combination may cause serotonin syndrome (L)
Guaifenesin[▲2]	5–20 mL po q4h S: 100 mg/5 mL	None at low dosages; high dosages cause nausea, vomiting, diarrhea, drowsiness, abdominal pain (L)
Codeine phosphate/ Guaifenesin[▲3]	S: 10 mg/5 mL/100 mg/5 mL; 10 mg/5 mL/300 mg/5 mL T: 10 mg/300 mg	Sedation, constipation (L)
Hydrocodone/ Homatropine[▲1]	5 mL po q4–6h S: 5 mg/5 mL/1.5 mg/mL T: 5 mg/1.5 mg	Sedation, constipation, confusion (L)

[1] Antitussive, inconsistent evidence of benefit.

[2] Protussive (increases secretions); in common use although evidence of effectiveness is lacking.

[3] Antitussive and protussive

DYSPNEA

Definition

A subjective experience of breathing discomfort that consists of qualitatively distinct sensations that vary in intensity (ATS).

- **Acute dyspnea** develops over hours to days; almost always due to MI, PE, acute COPD or asthma exacerbation, pneumonia
- **Chronic dyspnea**: when symptoms present for >4–8 wk

Considerations in Chronic Dyspnea

- Age >65: occurs in 17% at rest at least occasionally; in 38% when hurrying on level ground or on slight hill
- Hx: consider if level of dyspnea is appropriate to level of exertion (vs suggests pathology)
  ∘ Consider age, peers, usual activities, level of fitness
  ∘ Ask, "What activities have you stopped doing?"
- Associated symptoms: cough, sputum, wheezing, chest pain, orthopnea, paroxysmal nocturnal dyspnea

Evaluation

Hx and physical examination should suggest organ system; then evaluate for cause (**Table 112**). Also check for anemia and hypothyroidism.

- Exertional dyspnea that develops after walking 50–100 ft suggests HFpEF or pulmonary hypertension.
- Exercise-induced asthma begins about 3 min into exercise and peaks at 10–15 min.
- Intermittent dyspnea suggests asthma or PEs; dyspnea of HF waxes and wanes but has some baseline level of symptoms.

Table 112. Diagnosis of Dyspnea		
Suspected System	**Diagnostic Strategy**	**Diagnosis**
Cardiac	Chest radiograph, ECG, echocardiogram, radionuclide imaging, BNP or NT-proBNP (p 49)	Ischemic or other form of heart disease
Lung	Spirometry	Asthma, COPD, or restriction
	Diffusing capacity	Emphysema or interstitial lung disease
	Echocardiogram	Pulmonary HTN
Respiratory muscle dysfunction	Inspiratory and expiratory mouth pressures	Neuromuscular disease (eg, myasthenia gravis)
Deconditioning/obesity vs psychological disorders	Cardiopulmonary exercise test	Deconditioning shows decreased maximal oxygen consumption but normal cardiorespiratory exercise responses.

Therapy

Nonpharmacologic

- Exercise reduces dyspnea and improves fitness in almost all older adults regardless of cause; physical conditioning reduces dyspnea during ADLs and exercise, and is primary tx for deconditioning.
  ∘ Use low-impact, indoor activity
  ∘ Base intensity on HR or symptom of dyspnea
  ∘ Recommend 20–30 min on most days

- Indications for pulmonary rehabilitation include the following:
  - Dyspnea during rest or exertion
  - Hypoxemia, hypercapnia
  - Reduced exercise tolerance or a decline in ADLs
  - Worsening dyspnea and a reduced but stable exercise tolerance level
  - Pre- or postoperative lung resection, transplantation, or volume reduction
  - Chronic respiratory failure and the need to initiate mechanical ventilation
  - Ventilator dependence
  - Increasing need for emergency department visits, hospitalization, and unscheduled office visits

Pharmacologic: See specific diseases elsewhere in this chapter.

ALLERGIC RHINITIS

Description

- The most common atopic disorder; may be seasonal, episodic or perennial; in older adults, most often perennial.
- Symptoms include rhinorrhea, sneezing, and irritated eyes (Allergic Conjunctivitis, p 120), nose, and mucous membranes; the presence of at least 2 of these symptoms suggests allergic rhinitis.
- Postnasal drip, mainly from chronic rhinitis, is the most common cause of chronic cough.

Therapy

Nonpharmacologic: Avoid allergens, eliminate pets and their dander, dehumidify to reduce molds; saline and sodium bicarbonate nasal irrigation (eg, *SinuCleanse*) are helpful as primary or adjunctive tx; reduce outdoor exposures during pollen season; reduce house dust mites by encasing pillows and mattresses. Arachnocides reduce mites.

Pharmacologic: Target tx to symptoms and on whether symptoms are seasonal or perennial; **Table 113** and **Table 114.**

Stepped tx: For mild or intermittent symptoms, begin with an oral 2nd-generation antihistamine or nasal steroid; for moderate or severe symptoms, begin maximum dose of a nasal steroid; if symptoms uncontrolled, add a nasal or an oral antihistamine; if still uncontrolled, add or substitute a leukotriene modifier for one of the other agents.

Refractory symptoms: Consider other causes of chronic rhinosinusitis, refer to otolaryngologist; refer to allergist/immunologist for immunotherapy; consider omalizumab **(Table 120)** or a short course of oral steroids.

Ocular symptoms: Oral H_1 antihistamine or topical ophthalmic H_1 antihistamine are drugs of choice (allergic conjunctivitis, p 120 and **Table 113**).

Table 113. Choosing Medication for Allergic Rhinitis or Conjunctivitis

Medication or Class	Rhinitis	Sneezing	Pruritus	Congestion	Eye Symptoms
Nasal steroids[1]	+++	+++	++	++	++
Ipratropium, nasal[1]	++	0	0	0	0
Antihistamines[2,3]	++	++	++	+	+++
Pseudoephedrine[BC]	0	0	0	++++	0
Phenylephrine nasal[4]	0	0	0	+++	0
Cromolyn, nasal[3]	+	+	+	+	0
Leukotriene modifiers	+	+	+	+	++

0 = drug is not effective; the number of "+'s" grades the drug's effectiveness.

[1] Effective in seasonal, perennial, and vasomotor rhinitis.

[2] Better in seasonal than in perennial rhinitis; nasal, ocular, and oral forms; ocular form effective only for eye symptoms, but nasal form may help ocular symptoms.

[3] Start before allergy season.

[4] Topical tx rapid in onset but results in rebound if used for more than a few days; enhances effectiveness of nasal steroids and improves sleep during severe attacks.

Table 114. Medications for Allergic Rhinitis

Type, Medication	Geriatric Dosage	Formulations	Adverse Events/Comments
H1-Receptor Antagonists or Antihistamines		*Class AEs:* bitter taste, nasal burning, sneezing (nasal preparations); eye burning, stinging, injection (ocular preparations) (K, L)	
Oral			
Cetirizine[▲OTC]	5 mg/d (max)	T: 5, 10▲ syr: 5 mg/5 mL	Sedating at recommended doses; lower dose; avoid in dry eye (K)
✓Desloratadine *(Clarinex)*	5 mg/d	T: 5	
✓Fexofenadine[▲OTC,1]	60 mg po q12h; q24h if CrCl <40	T▲: 30, 60, 180; C: 60 ODT: 30 S▲: 30/5 mL	Least sedating in the class; fruit juice reduces absorption, so take 4 h before or 1–2 h after ingestion of juice
Levocetirizine *(Xyzal)*	2.5 mg/d po if CrCl 50–80; q48h if CrCl 30–50; 2×/wk if CrCl 10–30. Not recommended if CrCl <10.	T: 5 mg S: 0.5 mg/mL	Somnolence, pharyngitis, fatigue
✓Loratadine[▲OTC,1]	5–10 mg/d	T: 10; rapid disintegrating tab 10 mg; syr 1 mg/mL	Avoid in dry eye

(cont.)

Table 114. Medications for Allergic Rhinitis (cont.)

Type, Medication	Geriatric Dosage	Formulations	Adverse Events/Comments
Nasal			
✓Azelastine▲	1–2 spr q12h[2]	137 mcg/actuation, 0.15%	Rhinitis, headache, dyspnea
✓Olopadine *(Patanase)*	2 spr q12h[2]	0.6%	Epistaxis
Decongestant			
Pseudoephedrine▲ [BC] (also in combination preparations[OTC])	60 mg po q4–6h	T: 30, 60 SR: 120 S: elixir 30 mg/5 mL	Arrhythmia, insomnia[BC], anxiety, restlessness, elevated BP, urinary retention in men Oral use not recommended.[BC]
Phenylephrine▲ (has replaced pseudoephedrine in many combination products[OTC])	10–20 mg po q4–6h 2–3 spr/gtt each nares q4h prn	T: 10 SR: 10, 20 S: 7.5–10 mg/5 mL 0.25, 0.5, 1.0% spr and gtts	Bradycardia, hypertension, MI, HF, insomnia[BC] In oral combination products, not more effective than placebo Use for >3 d causes rhinitis medicamentosa
Nasal Steroids		*Class AEs:* nasal burning, sneezing, bleeding; septal perforation (rare); fungal overgrowth (rare); ulceration; increased IOP	
Second generation (systemic bioavailability <1% or undetectable)			
✓Fluticasone propionate▲[OTC]	2 spr/d[2] or 1 spr 2×/d 1 spr/d[2] maintenance	120 spr	
Fluticasone furoate[OTC] *(Flonase Sensimist)*	2 spr/d[2], 1 spr/d maintenance	60, 120 spr	
Mometasone *(Nasonex)*	2 spr/d[2]	120 spr	
Ciclesonide *(Omnaris) (Zetonna)*	2 spr/d[2] 1 spr/d[2]	250 spr	
First generation (systemic bioavailability 10–50%)			
Beclomethasone *(Beconase AQ) (Qnasl)*	1–2 spr q12h[2] 2 spr/d[2]	80 spr	*Same as Class AEs* **plus** systemic ADEs from absorbed steroids
Triamcinolone *(Nasacort Allergy 24* [OTC]*, Nasacort AQ)*	2 spr/d2	100 spr	
Budesonide▲[OTC]	1 spr/d[2]	200 spr	
Flunisolide▲	2 spr 2×/d[2]	200 spr	
Mast Cell Stabilizer			
Cromolyn▲[OTC]	1 spr q6–8h[2]; begin 1–2 wk before exposure to allergen	2%, 4%	Nasal irritation, headache, itching of throat
Leukotriene Modifiers (p 320)			Act synergistically with antihistamines

(cont.)

Table 114. Medications for Allergic Rhinitis (cont.)			
Type, Medication	**Geriatric Dosage**	**Formulations**	**Adverse Events/Comments**
Other			
Ipratropium▲	2 spr q6–12h[2]	0.03, 0.06%[3] sol	Epistaxis, nasal irritation, dry nose and mouth, pharyngeal irritation Caution: Do not spray in eyes, may increase IOP
Fluticasone: Azelastine (*Dymista*)	2 spr/d[2]	137 mcg–50 mcg/ actuation	May improve adherence when both are required

✓ = preferred for treating older adults; [BC] Avoid; CrCl unit of measure = mL/min/1.73 m[2].

[1] *Allegra-D* and *Claritin-D*, also available as *Allegra-D 24 Hour* and *Claritin-D 24 Hour*, are not recommended; all contain pseudoephedrine. Contraindicated in narrow angle glaucoma, urinary retention, MAOI use within 14 d, severe HTN, or CAD. May cause headache, nausea, insomnia.

[2] Spr per nares

[3] Use 0.06% for tx of viral upper respiratory infection.

CHRONIC OBSTRUCTIVE PULMONARY DISEASE

Diagnosis

Consider COPD if any of these factors are present in an individual over age 40. The greater the number of factors, the more likely is the diagnosis. 10% of people aged >65 are affected.

• **Dyspnea:** that is progressive, worse with exercise, and persistent
• **Chronic cough:** with or without sputum production
• **Hx of exposure to risk factors:** tobacco smoke, smoke from heating fuels, occupational dust, and chemicals
• **Family hx of COPD** (if positive, check α1 antitrypsin level)

Spirometry is required to establish a diagnosis. Assess airflow limitation based on spirometry measures after bronchodilators. COPD is diagnosed when FEV_1/FVC <0.70 or perhaps 0.65 (in patients over age 65) or FEV_1/FEV_6 <0.70 in patients over age 65 or those with severe disease.

Therapy

• Should be based on 3 factors: symptoms, airflow limitation, and frequency of exacerbations
• Assess **symptoms** using quantitative scale, eg, The Modified Medical Research Council Dyspnea Scale (MMRC) shown below:
  0 "I only get breathless with strenuous exercise"
  1 "I get short of breath when hurrying on the level or walking up a slight hill"
  2 "I walk slower than people of the same age on the level because of breathlessness or have to stop for breath when walking at my own pace on the level"
  3 "I stopped for breath after walking about 100 yards or after a few minutes on the level"
  4 "I am too breathless to leave the house" or "I am breathless when dressing"

MMRC 0–1, indicates fewer symptoms; MMRC ≥2, indicates more symptoms

- Then determine stage of **airflow limitation** by FEV_1 after bronchodilators in patients with FEV_1/FVC <0.7:

Gold Stage	Stage	% predicted
1	Mild	$FEV_1 \geq 80\%$
2	Moderate	$50\% FEV_1 < 80\%$
3	Severe	$30\% FEV_1 < 50\%$
4	Very Severe	$FEV_1 < 30\%$

- Finally, classify frequency of **exacerbations** as follows: low risk ≤1 exacerbation/y and no hospitalization, high risk ≥2 exacerbations/y or ≥1 exacerbation/y with ≥1 hospitalizations.
- Use **Table 115** to classify patients by type which determines tx.

Table 115. Combined Assessment of COPD				
		Risk: based on highest risk from either spirometry or exacerbation		
Patient Type	Characteristic	Spirometric Classification	Exacerbations per year	Symptom Score (mMRC)
A	low risk, fewer symptoms	mild/moderate	≤1	Low 0–1
B	low risk, more symptoms	mild/moderate	≤1	High ≥2
C	high risk, fewer symptoms	severe/very severe	≥2 or ≥1 with ≥1 hospitalization	Low 0–1
D	high risk, more symptoms	severe/very severe	≥2 or ≥1 with ≥1 hospitalization	High ≥2

Source: Adapted from goldcopd.org.

- The goals of pharmacologic and nonpharmacologic tx are to minimize both symptoms and exacerbations and improve quality of life. The degree of airflow limitation should not be the sole determinant of tx.

Pharmacotherapy

General Approach
- Smoking cessation is essential at any age (p 352).
- All get as needed short-acting bronchodilators (β-agonist [SABA] or anticholinergic); the combination of the 2 gives greater acute relief.
- If patient is on a long-acting anticholinergic, use SABA for acute relief.
- Many patients prefer 1×/d inhaled anticholinergic to 2×/d long-acting β-agonist (LABA).
- Mucolytic tx is not recommended in stable COPD. Consider for patients with chronic productive cough; continue if reduced cough and sputum during a trial. Example tx: guaifenesin▲ long-acting 600 mg po q12h.
- Pulmonary rehab for all patients, especially Gold types B–D. Patients at all stages benefit from exercise training, ie, increased exercise tolerance results in decreased dyspnea and fatigue (p 293). Adding nutritional support promotes weight gain and fat-free mass.
- O_2 for all patients with chronic hypoxia (**Table 118**)

Stepped Approach: Add agents when symptoms or exacerbations are inadequately controlled; D/C medication if no improvement. Assess improvement in symptoms, ADLs, exercise capacity, rapidity of symptom relief (**Table 110**) Long-term tx with long-acting anticholinergics (eg, tiotropium), LABAs, and inhaled steroids (combined with LABA or LAMA) slows the loss of FEV_1 and reduces the number of exacerbations and/or hospitalization. For acute exacerbations, see **Table 117**.

	Table 116. Pharmacotherapy for Stable COPD[1]		
Patient Group	**First Choice**	**Second Choice**	**Alternate Choice[2]**
A	SAMA prn **or** SABA prn	LAMA **or** LABA	Theophylline[3]
B[4]	LAMA **or** LABA	LAMA + LABA	SABA **and/or** SAMA **or** Theophylline[3]
C[4]	LAMA + SABA prn	LAMA + LABA **or** ICS[5] + LAMA	PDE4 inhibitor +SABA **and/or** SAMA **or** Theophylline[3] Consider surgical tx
D[4]	LABA + LAMA **or** ICS[5] + LABA (if asthma COPD overlap)	ICS[5] + LABA + LAMA **or** ICS[5] + LABA + PDE4 inhibitor **or** LAMA + PDE4 inhibitor	Theophylline[3] Add chronic tx with a macrolide Consider stopping ICS

ICS = inhaled corticosteroids; LABA = long-acting β_2-agonist; LAMA = long-acting muscarinic receptor antagonist; SABA = short-acting β_2-agonist: SAMA = short-acting antimuscarinic.

Source: Adapted from goldcopd.org.

[1] Medications are mentioned in alphabetical order; not necessarily in order of preference.

[2] Medications in this column can be used alone or in combination with other options in the First and Second Choice columns.

[3] Avoid in insomia[BC]; caution in patients taking other medications that interact.

[4] Also SABA prn and pulmonary rehab

[5] Consider osteoporosis prophylaxis.

Table 117. Outpatient Management of COPD Exacerbation

Stage and Evaluation	Treatment
COPD Exacerbation	
(Assess cardinal symptoms: increased dyspnea, sputum volume, and sputum purulence; check oximetry)	
Mild exacerbation (1 cardinal symptom; no resting dyspnea or respiratory distress; able to perform ADLs)	Increase dosage and/or frequency of SABA or SABA + SAMA with spacer or by nebulizer; no antibiotics; monitor for worsening
Moderate or severe exacerbation (2 or 3 cardinal symptoms; assess pulse oximetry; obtain CBC, CXR, ECG, ABG [if acute or acute on chronic hypercapnia]; consider BNP and D-dimer and rapid flu test or other respiratory virus)	**Add steroid** (eg, prednisone 40 mg po qd for 5 d) **Start antibiotic:** if <3 mo antibiotic exposure, use alternative class. Base choice on whether COPD is complicated or uncomplicated (see below) **Titrate O$_2$** to 88–92% sat; if new O$_2$ requirement consider hospital stay Nutritional supplement
• **Uncomplicated COPD** (age <65; FEV1 >50%, <2 exacerbations/y, no cardiac diagnosis)	Macrolide (azithromycin, clarithromycin) or cephalosporin (cefuroxime, cefpodoxime, cefdinir) or doxycycline or TMX/Sulfa
• **Complicated COPD** (1 or more of: age >65, FEV1 <50%, ≥2 exacerbations/y, cardiac diagnosis)	Fluoroquinolone (moxifloxacin, levofloxacin) or amoxicillin-clavulanate If at risk for pseudomonas, use ciprofloxacin and obtain sputum culture.

Other Considerations for Patients with COPD

- Anxiety or major depression: seen in up to 40% of patients and should be treated.
- Palliative and end-of-life care. Offer discussion of these issues for patients with severe COPD. In particular, if the patient should become critically ill, verify that ICU care is consistent with goals of care and if the patient is willing to accept the burdens of such care.

Long-term Oxygen Therapy: For indications, see **Table 118**. Assess patients with FEV$_1$ <30%, cyanosis, edema, HF, resting O$_2$ saturation <92%.

Table 118. Indications for Long-term Oxygen Therapy [1,2]

PaO$_2$ Level	SaO$_2$ Level	Other
≤55 mmHg	≤88%	>15 h/d for benefit[1], greater if 20 h/d[3]
55–59 mmHg	≥89%	Signs of tissue hypoxia (eg, cor pulmonale by ECG, HF, hematocrit >55%); or nocturnal desaturation, sats <90% for >30% of the time
≥60 mmHg	≥90%	Desaturation with exercise Desaturation with sleep apnea not corrected by CPAP

[1] Titrate O$_2$ saturation to ~90%.

[2] For patients recently discharged home on supplemental oxygen after hospitalization for acute illness, don't renew oxygen without reassessing need.[CW]

[3] Improves survival, hemodynamics, polycythemia, exercise capacity, lung mechanics, and cognition.

Source: goldcopd.org

ASTHMA

Definition

- A heterogeneous disease usually characterized by airway inflammation. It is defined by the hx of respiratory symptoms such as wheezing, shortness of breath, chest tightness, and cough that vary over time and intensity together with variable airflow limitation on spirometry.

Diagnosis in Older Adults

- Half of older people with asthma have not been diagnosed.
- Atopy and nocturnal symptoms are *less* common.
- Diagnosis is based on symptoms and requires spirometry.[cw]
  - Aging causes a decline in lung function through reduction in both respiratory muscle function and elastic recoil that produces a pattern of irreversible fixed obstruction; this effect is greater in less active persons.
  - Aging reduces FEV_1/FVC and may result in the overdiagnosis of COPD. This results in the misdiagnosis of COPD in some older adults with asthma.
  - Suspect asthma in the presence of any of these symptoms: wheezing, cough, shortness of breath, chest tightness, or when these symptoms are brought on by viral illness.
  - If FEV_1/FVC is ≤0.65 and the diffusing capacity of carbon dioxide is reduced, COPD is likely. The diffusing capacity of carbon dioxide is normal in asthma.
  - If a SABA does not reverse airflow obstruction during pulmonary function tests (asthma is not excluded), do one of the following:
    - Perform bronchial provocative testing (induce obstruction), **or**
    - Repeat testing after 2 wk of oral steroids to determine if obstruction seen in the initial test is reversible. *Note:* The component of age-related irreversible obstruction will persist.
  - More than half of people aged >65 with reversible airflow obstruction have both COPD and asthma ("overlap" syndrome); inhaled glucocorticoids must be part of tx.

Additional Considerations

- Age of onset: Some older adults have had asthma from a young age; others develop asthma for the first time after age 65. Second peak in incidence after age 65; 5–10% after age 65 are affected and account for two-thirds of asthma deaths.
- Those with long-standing asthma develop fixed obstruction (reduced FEV_1/FVC that is not reversed by bronchodilators) as an effect of both the disease and aging.
- Cough is a common presentation for asthma in those aged >65.
- Symptoms may be confused with those of HF, COPD, GERD, or chronic aspiration.
- Typical triggers: aeroallergens, irritants (eg, smoke, paint, household aerosols), viral upper respiratory infection, GERD, allergic rhinitis, metabisulfate ingestion (eg, wine, beer, food preservatives), medications (eg, ASA, NSAIDs, β-blockers).
- About 95% of patients with asthma also have perennial rhinitis and tx of both improves asthma outcomes.

Therapy

Nonpharmacologic

Avoid triggers; educate patients on disease management. Peak flow meters are less helpful in monitoring older adults; aging decreases peak flow and increases variability.

Pharmacologic

Good evidence on best tx for older adults with asthma is lacking because most clinical trials exclude people aged >65 and those with comorbidities or a hx of smoking >10 pack-years.

Stepped approach:

- The **number of the following symptoms** that were present in **the last 4 wk** determines the level of symptom control:
  - Daytime symptoms >2×/wk?
  - Limitations of activities due to asthma?
  - Nighttime waking due to asthma?
  - Reliever needed more than 2×/wk?
- Asthma is "Well controlled" if 0 (zero) symptoms, "Not well controlled" with 1–2 symptoms, and "Very poorly controlled" with 3–4 symptoms.
- Any exacerbation should prompt review of maintenance tx to ensure that it is adequate.
- By definition, an exacerbation in any week makes that an uncontrolled asthma week.
- If control is not achieved, step up, but first review medication technique, adherence, and avoidance of triggers (**Table 119**).
- When symptoms are controlled for 3 mo, try stepwise reduction, eg, step down from 2×/d ICS and LABA combination to 1×/d.
- LABAs should not be used unless given in combination with an ICS. LABAs as monotx are associated with increased mortality and are contraindicated as monotx.

Table 119. Asthma Therapy for Older Adults

Step[1]	Preferred	Other Controller Options
Step 1	Inhaled SABA prn	Consider ICS
Step 2	Inhaled SABA prn +Low-dose ICS	LTRA or low-dose theophylline[2, BC]
Step 3	Inhaled SABA prn + Low-dose ICS + LABA (consider specialist consultation)	Medium-/high-dose ICS **or** low-dose ICS + LTRA **or** SR theophylline[2, BC]
Step 4	(Consult asthma specialist) Inhaled SABA prn + Medium-dose ICS + LABA	High-dose ICS + either LTRA **or** SR theophylline[2,BC] Tiotropium mist inhaler is add-on for those with hx of exacerbations
Step 5	(Consult asthma specialist) Inhaled SABA prn +High-dose ICS + LABA	**and** consider omalizumab for patients with allergies
Step 6	(Consult asthma specialist) Inhaled SABA prn + High-dose ICS + LABA + po systemic glucocorticoid	**and** consider omalizumab for patients with allergies

ICS = inhaled corticosteroid; LABA = long-acting β-agonist; LTRA = leukotriene modifier; SABA = short-acting β-agonist.

[1] Go to next step if symptoms not controlled; prn SABA at all steps. After 3 mo of stability, try reduction but do not stop ICS.

[2] Many drug interactions with theophylline limit its use in older people; CNS stimulant.[BC]

Source: Adapted from ginasthma.org.

Therapy of Acute Exacerbations in Primary Care

- **Assess severity.**
  - **Mild to moderate attacks**
    - **Symptoms/signs:** Talks in phrases, prefers sitting to lying, not agitated, RR increased, HR 100–120; O_2 sats 90–95%
    - **Treatment:** Begin SABA 4–10 puffs by metered-dose inhaler (MDI) or nebulizer with ipratropium q20min × 1 h, then 2–4 puffs q3–4h for 24–48 h. Prednisolone 1 mg/kg; oxygen to keep sats 93–95%. Monitor hourly for worsening. Ready for home discharge when not needing SABA, O_2 sats >94% on room air, and home resources adequate. Continue prednisolone for 5–7 d. Step up controller tx; check inhaler technique and adherence.
  - **Severe attack or life-threatening attacks**
    - **Symptoms and signs:** speaks in words, sits hunched forward, agitated, uses accessory muscles, HR >120, O_2 sats <90%. **Life threatening:** drowsy, confused, or silent chest.
    - **Therapy:** Urgent transfer to hospital. While waiting: inhaled SABA and ipratropium, O_2, systemic steroids.

DELIVERY DEVICES FOR ASTHMA AND COPD

All of these devices have 10–14 steps to achieve correct drug delivery; all patients should be observed initially and periodically for adequacy of technique.

Metered-dose inhalers (MDIs): prescribed as number of puffs. Spacers (require a separate prescription) improve drug delivery and should be used for essentially all older patients. Use separate spacers for steroids. Wash spacer monthly.

Potential errors in use: failure to shake canister before use; difficulty depressing canister

Dry powder inhalers (DPIs): prescribed as caps or inhalations; require moderate to high inspiratory flow. DPIs are not used correctly by 40% of people aged >60 and 60% of those aged >80. Instructions should be repeated and reinforced for proper use and effective tx.

Potential errors in use: Ellipta: forget to open cover until it clicks. *Diskus:* dose counter is difficult to read. *HandiHaler* and *Neohaler:* difficulty removing capsules from foil; greater number of steps.

Soft mist inhalers (SMIs): prescribed as inhalations. Less dependent on inspiratory flow rates. Drug delivery to lung is similar to MDI with spacer, however proper technique can be complex for patients.

Potential errors in use: difficulty in twisting inhaler

Nebulizers: prescribed as milligrams or milliliters of solution. Consider for patients with disabling or distressing breathlessness on maximal tx with inhalers. Often the best choice for patients with cognitive impairment or when patients cannot manage SMIs, DPIs, or MDIs. Caution when patients with glaucoma use nebulized antimuscarinics; the mask should fit well or a T-type delivery device should be used. Ultrasonic and jet nebulizers are available; the latter can be used with supplemental oxygen.

Table 120. Asthma and COPD Medications

Medication Class/Agent [Delivery Device]	Dosage	Adverse Events (Metabolism, Excretion)
Short-acting Antimuscarinics (SAMAs)		
✓ Ipratropium *(Atrovent)* [MDI, nebulizer]	2–puffs q6h or 0.5 mg by nebulizer▲ q6h	Dry mouth, urinary retention, possible increase in cardiovascular mortality (lung, poorly absorbed; F)
Long-acting Antimuscarinics (LAMAs)		
Aclidinium *(Tudorza Pressair)* [DPI]	1 inhalation (400 mcg) q12h	Bronchospasm, nasopharyngitis, cough, diarrhea, and drug-related AEs seen with ipratropium (lung, poorly absorbed; F)
Tiotropium *(Spiriva)* [DPI]	1 inhalation cap (18 mcg) daily (inhale 2× from cap)	Same as ipratropium except good data on cardiovascular safety (14% K, 86% F)
(Spiriva Respimat Spray) [SMI (1.25, 2.5)]	2 inhalations (5 mcg) q24h for COPD 2 inhalations (2.5 mcg) q24h for asthma	
Umeclidinium *(Incruse Ellipta)* [DPI]	1 inhalation (62.5 mcg)/d	Nasopharyngitis, upper respiratory infection, cough, arthralgia, AF <1% in trials
Glycopyrrolate *(Seebri Neohaler)* [DPI]	1 inhalation (15.6 mcg) q12h	Upper respiratory infection, nasopharyngitis (K)
Short-acting β 2-Agonists (SABAs)[1]	*Class AEs:* tremor, nervousness, headache, palpitations, tachycardia, cough, hypokalemia. *Caution:* use half-doses in patients with known or suspected coronary disease. (L)	
✓ Albuterol *(Ventolin, Proventil, ProAir)* [MDI]	2 puffs q4–6h, max 12 puffs/d	
[nebulizer]	1.25, 2.5, 5 mg by nebulizer q6h▲	
(ProAir RespiClick) [DPI]	1–2 inhalation q4–6h, max 12 inhalation/d	
Levalbuterol *(Xopenex)* [nebulizer, MDI]	0.31, 0.63, 1.25 mg q6–8h by nebulizer; inhaler 2 puffs q4–6h	No advantage over racemic albuterol (intestine, L)
Long-acting β-Agonists (LABA)	*Class AEs:* tremor, nervousness, headache, palpitations, tachycardia, cough, hypokalemia; do not use in Asthma without an inhaled steroid.	
Arformoterol *(Brovana)* [nebulizer]	2 mL q12h by nebulizer	*Caution:* use half-doses in patients with known or suspected coronary disease; not for acute exacerbation.
✓ Salmeterol *(Serevent Diskus)* [DPI]	1 cap q12h; 50 mcg/cap	
✓ Formoterol *(Foradil)* [DPI, nebulizer]	1 cap q12h; 20 mcg/2 mL q12h per nebulizer	Onset of action 1–3 min (L, K)

(cont.)

Table 120. Asthma and COPD Medications (cont.)

Medication Class/Agent [Delivery Device]	Dosage	Adverse Events (Metabolism, Excretion)
Indacaterol *(Arcapta)* [DPI]	1 cap q24h (75 mcg/cap)	Greater bronchodilator effect than other LABAs, also greater risk of cough after inhalation, HTN
Olodaterol *(Striverdi Respimat)* [SMI]	2 inhalations q24h	Pharyngitis
Corticosteroids: Inhaled	*Class AEs:* nausea, vomiting, diarrhea, abdominal pain; oropharyngeal thrush; dysphonia; dosages >1 mg/d may cause adrenal suppression, reduce calcium absorption and bone density, and cause bruising (L)	
✓ Beclomethasone *(QVAR)* [MDI]	2–4 puffs q6–12h [40, 80 mcg/puff, max 640 mcg/d]	
✓ Budesonide▲ [DPI, nebulizer]	180–720 mcg q12h [90, 180 mcg/inhalation] 0.25, 0.5, 1.0 mg/2 mL q12h	
Ciclesonide *(Alvesco)* [SMI]	80–320 mcg q12h [80, 160 mcg/inhalation]	
✓ Flunisolide *(Aerospan)* [SMI]	80–320 mcg q12h [80 mcg/inhalation]	
✓ Fluticasone propionate *(Flovent Diskus)* [DPI]	88–880 mcg q12h [50, 100, 250 mcg/puff]	
✓ Fluticasone furoate (*Arnuity Ellipta*) [DPI]	1 inhalation/d [100, 200 mcg/inhalation]	
Mometasone *(Asmanex HFA)* [SMI]	1–2 inhalation q12h [100, 200 mcg]	
(Asmanex Twisthaler) [DPI]	1 inhalation q12h [110, 220 mcg/inhalation]	
Corticosteroids: Oral		
Prednisone▲	20 mg po q12h [T: 1, 2.5, 5, 10, 20, 50; elixir 5 mg/5 mL]	Leukocytosis, thrombocytosis, sodium retention, euphoria, depression, hallucination, cognitive dysfunction; other effects with long-term use (L)
Methylxanthines Long-acting theophyllines▲ BC		*Class AEs:* atrial arrhythmias, seizures, increased gastric acid secretion, ulcer, reflux, diuresis; clearance ↓ by 30% after age 65; initial dosage ≤400 mg/d, titrate using blood levels; 16-fold greater risk of life-threatening events or death after age 75 at comparable blood levels (L)
(eg, *Theo-Dur, Slo-Bid*)	100–200 mg po q12h [T: 100, 200, 300, 450]	
(eg, *Theo-24*)	400 mg/d po [C: 100, 200, 300, T: 400, 600]	
Leukotriene Modifiers (LTRAs)		
✓ Montelukast▲	10 mg po in AM [T: 10; ChT: 4, 5]	Headache, drowsiness, fatigue, dyspepsia (L)

(cont.)

Table 120. Asthma and COPD Medications (cont.)

Medication Class/Agent [Delivery Device]	Dosage	Adverse Events (Metabolism, Excretion)
Zafirlukast▲	20 mg po q12h 1 h ac or 2 h pc [T: 10, 20]	Headache, somnolence, dizziness, nausea, diarrhea, abdominal pain, fever; monitor LFTs; monitor coumarin anticoagulants and LFTs; (L, reduced by 50% if age >65)
Zileuton-CR▲	1200 mg po q12h [T: 600]	Dizziness, insomnia, nausea, abdominal pain, abnormal LFTs, myalgia; monitor coumarin anticoagulants; other drug interactions; inhibits synthesis of leukotrienes less studied, least preferred in the class (L)
PDE4 Inhibitor		
Roflumilast (Daliresp)	500 mcg/d po, for use in severe COPD (FEV$_1$ <50%) associated with chronic bronchitis but not emphysema [T: 500 mcg]	Weight loss, nausea, headache, back pain, influenza, insomnia; do not use if acute bronchospasm or moderate or greater liver impairment; caution in patients with depression (suicidality); inhibits CYP3A4 and -1A2 (eg, erythromycin) (L)
Combination: Long-acting β-Agonists + Inhaled Corticosteroids		
Vilanterol-Fluticasone (Breo Ellipta) [DPI]	1 inhalation q24h (25 mcg/100 mcg)	Same as LABAs and ICSs
✓Budesonide-Formoterol (Symbicort) [MDI]	2 inhalations q12h (80 mcg, 160 mcg/4.5 mcg)	Same as individual agents (L, K)
✓Formoterol-Mometasone (Dulera) [MDI]	1–2 inhalations (5 mcg/100, 200 mcg per inhalation)	Nasopharyngitis, sinusitis, headache
✓Salmeterol-Fluticasone (Advair Diskus) [DPI]	1 inhalation q12h (50 mcg/100, 250, or 500 mcg/cap)	approved for asthma and COPD
(Advair HFA) [MDI]	1 inhalation q12h (21 mcg/45,115, 230 mcg)	approved for asthma
Salmeterol-Fluticasone (Teva Pharmaceuticals) [DPI]	1 inhalation q12h (14 mcg/55, 115, 232 mcg)	approved for asthma
(AirDuo RespiClick) [DPI]	1 inhalation q12h (14 mcg/55, 113, 232 mcg)	approved for asthma
Combination: Long-acting β-Agonists + Long-Acting Anticholinergics		
Tiotropium-Olodaterol (Stiolto Respimat) [SMI]	2 inhalations q24h (2.5/2.5 mcg per inhalation)	Same as LABAs and tiotropium (L, K)
Umeclidinium-Vilanterol (Anoro Ellipta) [DPI]	1 inhalation q24h (62.5 mcg/25 mcg)	Same as LABAs; see also Umeclidinium. Not for use in asthma. (L, K)

(cont.)

Table 120. Asthma and COPD Medications (cont.)

Medication Class/Agent [Delivery Device]	Dosage	Adverse Events (Metabolism, Excretion)
Glycopyrrolate-Indacaterol *(Utibron Neohaler)* [DPI]	1 inhalation q12h (15.6 mcg/27.5 mcg)	Same as LABAs and glycopyrrolate (K, L)
Other Medications and Combinations		
✓ Albuterol-Ipratropium▲ [nebulizer]	3 mg/0.5 mg by nebulizer q6h	Same as individual agents (L, K)
✓ *(Combivent Respimat)* [SMI]	100 mcg/20 mcg 1 inhalation q6h (not to exceed 6 inhalations in 24 h)	
Cromolyn sodium▲ [nebulizer]	2 mL (10 mg/mL), 5 mL (20 mg/mL) q6h	Cough, throat irritation (L, K)
Omalizumab *(Xolair)* [injection]	150–375 mg SC q2–4wk based on body weight and pre-tx IgE level	Malignancy, rare anaphylaxis; half-life 26 d (L, bile)
Fluticasone furoate-umeclidinium-vilanterol *(Trelegy Ellipta)* [DPI]	100 mcg/62.5 mcg/25 mcg 1 inhalation daily	Same as individual agents

✓ = preferred for treating older adults

[1] Older nonselective β_2-agonists such as isoproterenol, metaproterenol, or epinephrine are not recommended and are more toxic.

RESTRICTIVE LUNG DISEASE (RLD)

- Up to 11% of people over age 75 meet criteria for RLD. In old age, RLD is often due to disorders outside of the lung itself. RLD can be disabling, progressive, and sometimes treatable.
- RLD is more likely to produce ADL disability (RR = 9.0; 95% CI: 3.1–26.6) than is moderate COPD (RR = 2.3; 95% CI: 0.7–4.5).
- These disorders are characterized by reduced total lung capacity (TLC). However, TLC is not part of routine pulmonary function tests (PFTs). In practice, FVC is used as a surrogate for TLC.

Diagnosis and Staging

- Patients present with exertional dyspnea, which often has insidious onset. PFTs show decreased lung volumes (FVC <80% of the lower limit of normal [LLN]), an FEV_1/FVC ratio >85–90%, and flow volume curve shows a complex profile.
- Disease severity is based on the degree of reduction of FVC; FVC 60–80% of LLN = mild, 50–60% = moderate, <50% = severe.

Differential Diagnosis

The many disorders that cause RLD can be grouped as shown in **Table 121** along with differentiating characteristics and some common causes in the older population.

Table 121. **Common Causes of Restrictive Lung Diseases in Older Adults**		
Category (Mechanism)	**Differentiating PFT Findings**	**Common Causes**
Intrinsic lung diseases (inflammation or scarring of the lung tissue)	Abnormal DLCO	Idiopathic pulmonary fibrosis Postinflammatory lung fibrosis Radiation Drug induced Connective tissue diseases (RA, etc) Chronic HF
Extrinsic disorders (mechanical compression of lungs or limitation of expansion)	Normal DLCO	Kyphosis/Kyphoscoliosis Obesity
Neuromuscular disorders (decreased ability of the respiratory muscles to inflate/deflate lungs)	Normal DLCO Reduced maximal inspiratory and/or expiratory pressures	ALS Thyroid and adrenal disorders Vitamin D deficiency Postpolio syndrome
CNS disorders	Normal DLCO	Parkinson disease Multisystemic atrophy Progressive supranuclear palsy Multiple sclerosis

DLCO = diffusing capacity of the lung for carbon monoxide.

Therapy

Follows the underlying cause. Because many of these disorders are outside of the lung itself, diagnosis and management often falls to geriatric healthcare providers.

CHANGES IN SEXUAL FUNCTION WITH AGING

Men

- Between age 60–70, 50–80% of men engage in any sexual activity, and that decreases to 15–20% for those aged ≥80.
- Factors influencing decreased activity include poor health, social issues, partner availability, decreased libido, and ED (see below).
- Changes in the sexual response cycle with age include:
  - *Excitement phase:* delay in erection, decreased tensing of the scrotal sac, loss of testicular elevation
  - *Plateau phase:* prolonged time in phase, reduced pre-ejaculatory secretion
  - *Orgasm* is reduced in intensity and duration.
  - *Refractory period* between erections is prolonged.

Women

- Between age 75–85, 17% of women report sexual activity, and of those, over half report sexual activity 2–3×/mo.
- Among women with a spouse or other partner, factors reported to reduced sexual activity include partner's or their own physical health problems.
- Changes in the sexual response cycle after menopause and which are attributed to decline in estrogen include:
  - *Excitement phase:* clitoris requires longer direct stimulation, reduced and delayed vaginal lubrication.
  - *Plateau phase:* less expansion and congestion of the vagina
  - *Orgasm:* fewer and weaker contractions, but multiple orgasm can occur.
  - *Resolution phase:* vascular congestion lost more rapidly

A reliable resource to assist older men and women in addressing these changes can be found at aarp.org/home-family/sex-intimacy/

IMPOTENCE (ERECTILE DYSFUNCTION OR ED)

Definition

Inability to achieve sufficient erection for intercourse. Prevalence nearly 70% by age 70.

Causes

Often multifactorial; >50% of cases arterial, venous, or mixed vascular cause (**Table 122**).

Table 122. Causes of Erectile Dysfunction (ED) in Older Men

Causes (in order of frequency)	Associated Findings/Risk Factors	Onset
Vascular	Vascular risk factors; femoral bruits; poor pedal pulses. Venous vascular disease suggested by penile plaques (Peyronie disease).	Gradual
Neuropathic	DM; hx of pelvic trauma, surgery, irradiation; spinal injury or surgery; Parkinson disease, multiple sclerosis; alcoholism; loss of bulbocavernosus reflex or orthostatic BP changes	Gradual
Drug induced (p 329)	Loss of sleep-associated erections	Sudden
Psychogenic, including bereavement	Sleep-associated erections or erections with masturbation are intact	Sudden
Hypogonadism[1]	Decreased libido >ED; low T, small testes, gynecomastia; 1/3 of patients with type 2 DM have low T.	Gradual
Other Endocrine	Hyper-/hypocortisolism, hyper-/hypothyroidism, hyperprolactinemia	Gradual

[1] Don't prescribe testosterone (T) for men with ED and normal T levels.[CW]

Therapy

An at-home trial of a PDE5 inhibitor (**Table 123**) is both diagnostic of ED and therapeutic for the common causes of ED (vascular, neuropathic, mixed); these agents are also effective for ED after most prostate cancer tx and in DM-2. Alternate tx (devices, injections) are included in **Table 123**.

Table 123. Management of Erectile Dysfunction

Therapy	Dose	Formulation	Comments
PDE5 Inhibitors	*All Agents*: Effective in 60–70% of men with ED of various etiologies. Contraindicated with use of nitrates and nonischemic optic neuropathy. PDE5 inhibitors potentiate the hypotensive effects of α-blockers. Potent CYP3A4 inhibitors reduce metabolism of all PDE5 inhibitors and increase risk of toxicity. *Common tx-related AEs*: headache, flushing, rhinitis, dyspepsia *Other tx-related AEs*: priapism, low-back pain, possibly nonarteritic anterior ischemic optic neuropathy Start lowest dose and titrate prn. *All should be taken on an empty stomach to maximize absorption.*		
Avanafil *(Stendra)*	start 50 mg 30 min before sexual activity	50, 100, 200	
Sildenafil▲	start 25 mg 1 h before sexual activity	20, 25, 50, 100	*Other AEs*: increased sensitivity to light, blurred vision, bluish discoloration of vision; 20-mg tabs least expensive option
Vardenafil *(LEVITRA)*	start 2.5 mg 1 h before sexual activity	2.5, 5, 10, 20	*Other AEs*: Avoid using in congenital or acquired QT prolongation and in patients taking class IA or III antiarrhythmics.

(cont.)

Table 123. **Management of Erectile Dysfunction (cont.)**			
Therapy	**Dose**	**Formulation**	**Comments**
Tadalafil *(Cialis)*	start 5 mg 30–60 min before sexual activity; lasts 24 h	2.5, 5, 10, 20	*Other AEs*: myalgia, pain in limbs; 2.5 mg/d may be as effective as taking higher doses prn.
Devices			
Vacuum tumescence devices (eg, *Osbon-Erec Aid*)	N/A	N/A	*Rare*: ecchymosis, reduced ejaculation, coolness of penile tip. Good acceptance in older population; intercourse successful in 70–90% of cases.
Penile prosthesis	N/A	N/A	*Complications*: infection, mechanical failure, penile fibrosis
Prostaglandin E			
Alprostadil[1]	Intracavernosal 5–40 mcg *or* intraurethral 125–1000 mcg	Intracavernosal: 5, 10, 20, 40 mcg *or* intraurethral: 125, 250, 500, 1000 mcg	*Risks*: hypotension, bruising, bleeding, priapism; erection >4 h requires emergency tx; intraurethral safer and more acceptable. Rarely used since PDE5 inhibitors became available. 50% of patients stop tx within 1 y due to discomfort or inconvenience.

[1] Also used in *Trimix*, a compounded injectable formulation that also includes phentolamine and papaverine

Diagnosis of Hypogonadism in Middle-aged and Older Men

• Hypogonadism is more closely associated with libido than with ED.
• Diagnose T deficiency only in men with consistent symptoms and unequivocally low T levels.
• Morning total T level <320 ng/dL (11 nmol/L) that remains <320 ng/dL on repeat testing and a free T level of <640 pg/dL (<220 pmol/L) using a reliable assay suggests deficiency.
• When total T is near the lower limit of normal or when sex hormone–binding globulin is altered, obtain a free (bioavailable) T level using either equilibrium dialysis or by estimating it using an accurate formula.
• Ask the following questions from the European Male Aging Study Sexual Function Questionnaire. If the answer to **all 3 questions** is the response in **bold**, hypogonadism is likely present.
  ○ How often did you think about sex? This includes times of just being interested in sex, day dreaming, or fantasizing about sex, as well as times when you wanted to have sex.
    ▪ **2 or 3 times or less in the last month**
    ▪ Once/wk or more often
  ○ It is common for men to experience erectile problems. This may mean that one is not always able to get or keep an erection that is rigid enough for satisfactory activity (including sexual intercourse and masturbation). In the last *month*, are you:
    ▪ Always able to keep an erection that would be good enough for sexual intercourse, or usually able to get and keep an erection that would be good enough for sexual intercourse
    ▪ **Sometimes or never able to get and keep an erection that would be good enough for sexual intercourse**

- How frequently do you awaken with full erection?
  - **Once in the last month or less often**
  - 2 or 3 times or more often in the last month

Therapy for Hypogonadism

- Prescribe T only when there is clear evidence of moderate to severe deficiency.[CW, BC]
- The T trials of men aged ≥65 with unequivocally low T levels (<275 pmol/L) and either low libido, mobility limitations, mild anemia, and/or low vitality, treated for 1 y with normalization of T levels produced results shown in **Table 124**:

Table 124. Effects of Normalizing Testosterone in Men Over 65 with Low Libido, Mobility Limitations, and/or Low Vitality

Parameter	Effect	Comment
Libido, sexual activity, erectile function	↑	
Cognition	No change	Tested in those with age-associated cognitive impairment
Hemoglobin	↑	By 1 g in those with anemia of unknown cause
CAD plaque	↑	
BMD	↑	More in spine than hip
Physical function and mood	↑	Slight

- Testosterone possibly increases cardiovascular events in men with cardiovascular risk.
- Testosterone is not recommended with breast or prostate cancer, prostate nodule or induration, PSA >3 ng/dL, or significant prostate obstructive symptoms.
- Testosterone is not recommended if hematocrit >50%, untreated sleep apnea, or HF.
- Monitor AEs and response q3mo. *AEs:* polycythemia, fluid retention, liver dysfunction.
- During tx, check serum T concentration and adjust dose to achieve concentration in midrange of normal; check midway between injections (except undecanoate, check before next injection); all other preparations check manufacturer's recommendation for monitoring levels and adjusting dose.
- Probably effective in the tx of opioid-induced androgen deficiency.

Table 125. Management of Hypogonadism with Testosterone Replacement

Testosterone Preparation	Starting Dose	Formulation
Injectable		
Testosterone enanthate▲	50–200 mg IM q2–4wk	200 mg/mL
Testosterone cypionate▲	50–400 mg IMq2–4wk	100, 200 mg/mL
Testosterone undecanoate (Aveed)	750 mg IM at 0 and 4 wk then q10 wk	250 mg/mL
Transdermal		
Androderm	4 mg/d	2, 4 mg/24-h pch
AndroGel metered-dose pump▲	4 pumps/d 2 pumps/d	1%: 12.5 mg/pump 1.62%: 20.25 mg/pump

(cont.)

Table 125. Management of Hypogonadism with Testosterone Replacement (cont.)		
Testosterone Preparation	**Starting Dose**	**Formulation**
AndroGel transdermal gel▲	50 mg qd	1%: 25, 50 mg/pk
	40.5 mg qd	1.6%: 20.25, 40.5 mg/pk
Fortesta	4 spr/d	60-g canister (10 mg/spr)
Testim	1 tube/d	5-g tube (50-mg)
Buccal		
Striant	1 tab q12h	T: 30 mg
Intranasal		
Natesto	1 pump each nares 3×/d	5.5 mg/pump

FEMALE SEXUAL DYSFUNCTION

Definition: a sexual problem that is persistent or recurrent and causes distress or interpersonal problems; cause is often multifactorial.

Evaluation
• Ask about problems (eg, changes in libido, partner's function, and health issues).
• Ask about absence or significantly reduced sexual interest/arousal.
• Screen for depression.
• Ask about incontinence.
• When dyspareunia is reported, perform pelvic examination for vulvovaginitis, vaginal atrophy, conization (decreased distensibility and narrowing of the vaginal canal), scarring, pelvic floor hypertonus (vaginismus), pelvic inflammatory disease, cystocele, and rectocele.
• Factors aggravating dyspareunia:
  ◦ Anticholinergic medications (vaginal dryness)
  ◦ Gynecologic tumors
  ◦ Interstitial cystitis
  ◦ Myalgia from overexertion during Kegel exercises
  ◦ Pelvic fractures
  ◦ Retroverted uterus
  ◦ Sacral nerve root compression
  ◦ Vaginal atrophy from estrogen deprivation
  ◦ Osteoarthritis
  ◦ Vulvar or vaginal infection

Management

Dyspareunia: pain with intercourse
• Identify and treat clinical pathology.
• In a randomized trial of women (mean age 61), water-soluble lubricants were as effective as topical vaginal estrogens for dyspareunia and other vulvovaginal symptoms (itching, dryness, irritation).
• Water-soluble lubricants (eg, *KY Jelly*, *Replens*) are highly effective as monotx for dyspareunia and are recommended as 1st-line tx by the American College of Gynecology.

- If dyspareunia is uncontrolled by lubricants and vaginal atrophic changes are present, topical estrogens (**Table 126**) can be considered; these produce minimal systemic levels when used 2–3×/wk.
- Moderate to severe atrophic vaginitis may also be treated with the selective estrogen-receptor modulator, ospemifene 60 mg orally 1×/d with food for the shortest duration necessary; in women with a uterus, consider concomitant progestin tx. Contraindications: stroke, MI, DVT, or PE, estrogen-dependent neoplasia, and genital bleeding.
- For pelvic floor hypertonicity (vaginal muscle spasm), trial cessation of intercourse and gradual vaginal dilation or pelvic PT

Other Therapies

- Counseling for one or both partners; sex and couples therapy are often helpful.
- Treat urinary and or fecal incontinence (see Incontinence chapter).
- The OTC botanical massage oil *Zestra* appears to improve desire and arousal in women with mixed desire/interest/arousal/orgasm disorders but can cause vaginal burning.
- Studies of sildenafil have not consistently shown effectiveness.
- Flibanserin (*Addyi*, a postsynaptic 5-HT1A agonist 5-HT2A antagonist) 100 mg qhs studied only in premenopausal women; dizziness was the most common AE (also somnolence, nausea, fatigue).
- Testosterone added to estrogen (with or without progesterone) improves desire, arousal, and orgasmic response in most studies (not approved in the US).

Table 126. Topical Estrogens Without Systemic Effects

Estrogen	Dosage
Estrogen cream *(Premarin, Ogen, Estrace)*	Use minimum dose (0.5 g[1] for *Premarin*, 2 g[2] for *Ogen* and *Estrace*) daily × 2 wk, then 2–3×/wk thereafter
Estradiol vaginal ring *(Estring)*	Insert intravaginally and change q90d
Estradiol vaginal tablets *(Vagifem)*	Insert 25 mcg intravaginally daily × 2 wk, then 2×/wk

[1] A dime-sized amount is an easy way to describe to patients.

[2] About 4 times the dime-sized amount is needed.

DRUG-INDUCED SEXUAL DYSFUNCTION

Agents Associated with Sexual Dysfunction in Both Men and Women

The following drugs and drug classes are believed to sometimes cause sexual dysfunction. In cases of suspected drug-induced sexual dysfunction, improvement after drug withdrawal provides the best evidence for the adverse effect. Tx with a drug from an alternative class to treat an underlying condition may be necessary.

- Antidepressants: SSRIs (see below) reduce libido and delay orgasm; lithium causes ED, MAOIs may cause ED or anorgasmia.
- Antipsychotics: olanzapine produces less loss of libido/ED than risperidone, clozapine, and oral and depot 1st-generation agents.
- Antihypertensives: any agent may cause ED related to reduced genital blood flow.
  - Spironolactone has antiandrogen effect.
  - Centrally acting sympatholytics (eg, clonidine) produce relatively high rates of sexual dysfunction (ED and loss of libido).
  - Peripherally acting sympatholytics, eg, reserpine (ED and loss of libido).
- Digoxin: possibly related to reduced T levels
- Lipid-lowering agents: fibrates (gynecomastia and ED) and many statins (eg, lovastatin, pravastatin, simvastatin, atorvastatin) are the subject of case reports of both ED and

gynecomastia. Statins affect the substrate for sex hormones and have been shown to reduce total and sometimes also bioavailable T.

- Acid-suppressing drugs: The H2RAs cimetidine and, more rarely, ranitidine cause gynecomastia. Famotidine has caused hyperprolactinemia and galactorrhea. The PPI omeprazole has caused gynecomastia.
- Metoclopramide: induces hyperprolactinemia
- Anticonvulsants: phenobarbital, phenytoin, carbamazepine, primidone; all increase metabolism of androgen.
- Anticholinergics and antihistamines produce vaginal dryness.
- Alcohol: high dosages reduce libido.
- Opioids: reduce libido and produce anorgasmia related to reduced T levels.

Management of SSRI-Induced Sexual Dysfunction

- Wait for tolerance to develop (4–6 mo of tx may be needed).
- Pharmacologic management:
  - For escitalopram and sertraline (not other SSRIs), reducing dosage or "drug holidays" (skip or reduce weekend dose) may help, but may result in relapse and nonadherence.
  - In both men and women, sildenafil 50–100 mg po improved sexual function in prospective, parallel-group, randomized, double-blind, placebo-controlled clinical trials.
  - Consider change in tx to bupropion, mirtazapine, nefazodone, or vilazodone.
  - Adding bupropion to SSRI reduces sexual dysfunction.

CHRONIC WOUND ASSESSMENT AND TREATMENT

Wound Assessment

Evaluation of chronic wounds should include the following (**Table 127** for wound characteristics specific to ulcer type):

- Location
- Wound size and shape: length, width, depth, stage (pressure ulcer), grade (diabetic foot ulcer), wound edges
- Wound bed: color, presence of slough, necrotic tissue, granulation tissue, epithelial tissue, undermining or tunneling
  - Note warmth, capillary refill, and presence of pulses, edema, anasarca, and lymphedema
  - Darkly pigmented skin may appear blue, purple, or just darker and misinterpret Stage 1 pressure ulcers, deep-tissue pressure injury, and other dermatitis. Palpate for temperature and consistency.
- Exudate: purulent vs nonpurulent (serous, serosanguineous)
- Periwound skin and soft tissue: warmth, erythema, induration
  - also presence of pulses, edema, anasarca, lymphedema
- Presence of pain at rest and with wound care procedures
- Signs of wound infection:
  - Worsening wound (increased necrotic tissue, drainage, enlargement, purulence)
  - Foul odor
  - Purulent exudate
  - Surrounding erythema
  - Increasing pain
  - Local swelling, warmth

Table 127. Typical Wound Characteristics by Ulcer Type

	Arterial	Diabetic	Pressure	Venous
Location	Distal location, areas of trauma	Plantar surface of foot, especially over metatarsal heads, toes, and heel	Over bony prominences (eg, trochanter, coccyx, ankle)	Gaiter area, particularly medial malleolus
Size and shape	Shallow, well-defined borders	Wound margins with callus	Variable length, width, depth depending on stage (staging system, p 335)	Edges may be irregular with depth limited to dermis or shallow subcutaneous tissue
Wound bed	Pale or necrotic	Granular tissue unless PAD present	Varies from bright red, shallow crater to deeper crater with slough and necrotic tissue; tunneling and undermining	Ruddy red; yellow slough may be present; undermining or tunneling uncommon

(cont.)

	Arterial	**Diabetic**	**Pressure**	**Venous**
Exudate	Minimal amount due to poor blood flow	Variable amount; serous unless infection present	May be purulent, becoming serous as healing progresses; foul odor with infection	Copious; serous unless infection present
Surrounding skin	Halo of erythema or slight fluctuance indicates infection	Normal; may be calloused	May be distinct, diffuse, rolled under; erythema, edema, induration if infected	May appear macerated, crusted, or scaly; presence of stasis dermatitis, hyperpigmentation
Pain	Cramping or constant deep aching	Variable intensity; none with advanced neuropathy	Painful, unless sensory function impaired or with deep, extensive tissue necrosis	Variable; may be severe, dull, aching, or bursting in character

Table 127. Typical Wound Characteristics by Ulcer Type (cont.)

- Swab culture of wound surface exudates is of no value in diagnosing infection due to wound contamination. Educate staff not to collect cultures of wound slough or pus; encourage use of Levine's technique.
  - Levine's technique (cleanse with NS followed by rotating a swab over a 1-cm square area of viable wound tissue [not necrotic] with sufficient pressure to express fluid from the wound tissue beneath the wound surface)

Principles of Wound Treatment
- Establish wound care goals, considering advance directives and patient's values and preferences to determine tx
- Address pain, nutrition, underlying illnesses
- Remove debris and necrosis
  - Remove debris from wound surface.
    - Cleanse using NS or Lactated Ringer's with each dressing change. Avoid antiseptics because of cytotoxicity.
    - Irrigate using 4–15 psi to cleanse adherent debris. Use 8 mmHg pressure (19-gauge catheter and 35-mL syringe) when wound is deep, tunneled, or undermined.
    - Clostridial collagenase ointment along with negative-pressure wound tx improves speed of debridement and rate of wound closure.
  - Remove necrotic tissue. Consider combining autolytic or topical enzyme debridement methods with sharp debridement to facilitate more rapid removal of necrotic tissue, by experienced clinician or licensed podiatrist.
    - Sharp debridement
    - Autolytic methods (eg, moisture-retaining dressings or hydrogels)
    - Mechanical (eg, hydrotherapy, irrigation)
    - Biological (maggot debridement tx)
    - Chemical (eg, topical enzymes such as collagenase)
- Pack dead space (tunnels, undermining) loosely with moistened gauze dressings or strips of calcium alginate.
- Control pain associated with wound care procedures by offering pain medication 30 min before procedure. Choose least painful tx option.
  - Use complementary approaches, such as massage, touch, high-intensity TENS

- Gauze-based negative-pressure wound tx (NPWT), rather than foam, less painful in older adults, those with bone and tendon exposition wounds.
- Topical lidocaine gel
- For moderate to severe pain not managed by oral medications or with dose-limiting AEs, topical opioids may be used, eg, mixture of 10 mg MS injectable combined with 8 g of neutral water-based gel applied 2×/d. Can titrate up to 10 mg MS injectable with 5 g neutral water-based gel applied 2–3×/d. Caution in ulcers with large surface area because of the risk of systemic absorption.

- Control bacterial burden/infection.
  - Monitor for signs of infection. Odor dependent on microbe present. Gram negative and anaerobic foul odor; Pseudomonas sweet. Cellulitis may be present and systemic signs of infection.
  - Treat infected wounds by addressing underlying condition and protecting wound from contamination.
  - Control odor with silver, charcoal, chlorophyllin dressings, cadexomer iodine.
  - Debride all necrotic tissue (*except* in lower extremity with arterial insufficiency).
  - If infection is suspected, assess type and quantity of bacteria by validated quantitative swab or tissue biopsy. Suspect infection if epithelialization from margin is not progressing within 2 wk of debridement and initiation of offloading (use of cast, splint, or special shoe to shift pressure from wound to surrounding support structure).
  - For ulcers with ≥1 million CFU/g of tissue or any tissue level of β-hemolytic streptococci, use a topical antimicrobial (eg, dressings with bioavailable silver, cadexomer iodine at concentrations up to 0.45%; p 337). Limit duration of use of topical antimicrobials to avoid cytotoxicity or bacterial resistance.
  - Consider 2-wk trial of topical antibiotic for clean ulcers that are not healing after 2–4 wk optimal care, including mupirocin, neomycin, polymyxin B, and bacitracin; antibiotic spectrum should include Gram-negative, Gram-positive, and anaerobic organisms. Topical antifungals include imidazole, triazole, and thiazole compounds.
  - Use systemic antibiotics if obvious signs of localized infection, cellulitis, osteomyelitis, or systemic inflammatory response (**Table 127**).

Table 128. Empiric Antibiotic Therapy to Treat Infections in Chronic Wounds

Severity of Infection	Clinical Features	Medication Options	Duration of Treatment
Mild	Superficial, localized signs of inflammation/infection, without signs of a systemic response or osteomyelitis, and ambulatory management planned	Cephalexin Clindamycin Amoxicillin/clavulanate Clindamycin plus ciprofloxacin, moxifloxacin, or linezolid (for MRSA)	2 wk
Moderate	Superficial to deep-tissue involvement, a systemic response, no osteomyelitis, and either planned ambulatory or inpatient management	Clindamycin plus ciprofloxacin Clindamycin po plus ceftriaxone Vancomycin (for MRSA) Linezolid (for MRSA)	2–4 wk
Severe	Deep tissue with a systemic response, presence of osteomyelitis, or is life-/limb-threatening, and requires inpatient care	Clindamycin po plus ceftriaxone Piperacillin/tazobactam Clindamycin po plus gentamicin Imipenem Meropenem Vancomycin (for MRSA) Linezolid (for MRSA)	2–12 wk (Bone and joint involvement requires prolonged oral tx after IV tx completed.)

- Treat cellulitis surrounding ulcer with a systemic Gram-positive bactericidal antibiotic (cellulitis, p 94) unless Gram-negative organisms are suspected and require aggressive IV tx.
  - If osteomyelitis is suspected, evaluate with X-ray, CT, MRI, or bone biopsy.
  - Referral for surgical evaluation if warranted.
- Provide moist wound environment and control exudates using appropriate dressings
- Local Wound Care. Select dressings appropriate to wound type and characteristics (**Table 129**). *Note*: Wound care products are classified by the FDA as medical devices (ie, exempt from the requirement to demonstrate efficacy), so little evidence-based support. Choices based on product availability, insurance coverage, cost, rationale for product type.
- Healable wounds use normal saline, potable water, or commercially available wound cleansers. Goal: moisture balance and exudate adsorption.
- Nonhealable/palliative wounds use povidone iodine, chlorhexidine, or polyhexamethylene biguanide (PHMB). Goal: moisture reduction and colonization management.

Table 129. Recommended Dressings by Wound Characteristics

Product	Superficial Skin Disruption	Eschar	Exudate	Granulating/ Epithelializing	Fibrinous Wound bed/ Slough	Deep Wounds	Colonized/ Infected
Alginates			+			+	
Collagen			+				
Foams			+				
Gauze packing (with saline)			+			+	
Hydrocolloids		+		+	+	+	
Hydrogels		+		+	+		
Hydrofibers			+			+	
Polymeric membrane dressings	+	+	+	+		+	
Protease lowering dressings					+		
Silver/Iodide							+
Transparent films	+						

- Adjunctive tx to support wound healing process
  - Negative-pressure wound tx
    - Indications: Stage 3 and 4 pressure ulcers, neuropathic ulcers, venous ulcers, dehisced incisions with trapping of 3rd-space fluid around wound
    - Contraindications: Presence of *any* nonviable, necrotic tissue in wound; untreated osteomyelitis; malignancy in or surrounding wound
    - Avoid use in frail older patients on anticoagulants
    - Guidelines for use:
      - Dressing change regimen: 48 h after placement, then every other day
      - Specialized training in application and monitoring of tx essential for successful outcome
  - Electrical stimulation may be an option to stimulate healing. Refer to wound specialist.

- ◦ Ultrasound
  - ▪ Low frequency (22.5–35 kHz) ultrasound applied in contact rapidly debrides wound surface with minimal discomfort
  - ▪ Promotes healing with and without antibiotics in small clinical studies; larger RCTs needed.
  - ◦ Hyperbaric oxygen
- • Prevent further injury
  - ◦ Use pressure-reducing mattresses or chair cushions and float the heels (pillows under the calf and knee) and device to keep covers off toes
  - ◦ Reposition q2h and avoid any pressure on the wound
  - ◦ Manage moisture from incontinence (eg, *ultra-absorbent* underpads)
- • Support repair process
  - ◦ Protein (1.25–1.5 g/kg/d) and calories (30–35/kg/d) unless contraindicated because of impaired renal function
  - ◦ Correct deficiencies of vitamin C and zinc if suspected
  - ◦ Arginine-containing nutritional supplements (4.5 g/d)
  - ◦ Avoid exposure to cold; vasoconstriction reduces blood flow to wound
  - ◦ Avoid smoking to prevent vasoconstriction that reduces blood flow to wound
  - ◦ Ensure adequate hydration with oral or parenteral fluids
- • If ulcer does not show signs of healing over 2-wk period of optimal tx, reevaluate wound management strategies and factors affecting healing.

PRESSURE INJURY

Definition

Localized damage to skin and/or underlying soft tissue usually over a bony prominence or related to a medical or other device. The injury can present as intact skin or an open ulcer and may be painful. The injury occurs as a result of intense or prolonged pressure or pressure in combination with shear. The tolerance of soft tissue for pressure and shear may also be affected by microclimate, nutrition, perfusion, comorbidities, and condition of the soft tissue (National Pressure Ulcer Advisory Panel; www.npuap.org).

Wound Assessment

- • See Chronic Wound Assessment (p 331). Early identification—with at least weekly assessment—is important to healing.
- • Look for pressure ulcers under area subjected to constant pressure (ie, bony prominences, orthopedic devices)
- • Consistent measurement is important for evaluating tx effectiveness. Use centimeter ruler for length and width and cotton-tipped swab to measure depth, tunneling, and undermining.
- • Determine extent of tissue injury by using Pressure Ulcer Staging System. Illustrations available at www.npuap.org/resources/educational-and-clinical-resources/pressure-injury-staging-illustrations:
  - ◦ **Stage 1 Pressure Injury** (nonblanchable erythema of intact skin): Intact skin with a localized area of nonblanchable erythema, which may appear differently in darkly pigmented skin. Presence of blanchable erythema or changes in sensation, temperature, or firmness may precede visual changes. Color changes do not include purple or maroon discoloration; these may indicate deep-tissue pressure injury (see below).
  - ◦ **Stage 2 Pressure Injury:** partial-thickness skin loss with exposed dermis only or clear blisters

- **Stage 3 Pressure Injury:** full-thickness skin loss, may have necrotic tissue, but not into muscle or bone
- **Stage 4 Pressure Injury:** full-thickness loss of skin and tissue with exposed or palpable bone, tendon, or muscle
- **Unstageable Pressure Injury:** obscured full-thickness skin and tissue loss prevents visualization of anatomic involvement.
- **Deep-Tissue Pressure Injury** (persistent nonblanchable deep red, maroon, or purple discoloration): Sacrum and heel are the most and 2nd most common areas, respectively, for deep-tissue pressure injuries. May appear as blood-filled blister with tissue consistency changes.
- **Medical Device–related Pressure Injury**: Injuries resulting from the use of devices designed and applied for diagnostic or tx purposes (eg, catheters, oxygen tubing). The resultant pressure injury generally conforms to the pattern or shape of the device and should be staged using the staging system.
- **Mucosal Membrane**: Injury found on mucous membranes with hx of a medical device in use at the location of injury. Due to the anatomy of the tissue, these injuries cannot be staged.

Management

Refer to Principles of Wound Treatment, p 331

Surgical referral may be warranted for Stage 4 pressure ulcers and for severely undermined or tunneled wounds.

Local Wound Care: Common Dressings for Pressure Ulcer Treatment

(Ordered by use in Pressure Ulcer Stage)

Transparent film

Indications and Use: Stages 1 and 2 protection from friction, superficial scrape, autolytic debridement of slough; apply skin prep to intact skin to protect from adhesive

Contraindications: Draining ulcers, suspicion of skin infection or fungus

Composites (2 or more physically distinct dressing products combined as a single dressing)

Indications and Use: Stages 1, 2, 3, and 4; light, moderate, or heavy exudate; conform to skin surface shape; designed with adhesive border; easy application and removal; dressing change frequency dependent on wound type (follow package insert)

Contraindications: Caution with fragile skin; adhesive may injure skin; some types may be contraindicated with Stage 4 ulcers (refer to package insert); may not maintain moist wound environment

Hydrogel sheets

Indications and Use: Stage 2; needs to be held in place with topper dressing

Contraindications: Avoid use in macerated areas; wounds with moderate to heavy exudate

Foam

Indications and Use: Stages 2 and 3, light to moderate exudate; leave in place 3–5 d, can apply as window to secure transparent film

Contraindications: Excessive exudate; dry, crusted wound; dry eschar; periwound maceration likely if not changed appropriately

Hydrocolloids

Indications and Use: Stages 2 and 3; light to moderate drainage; reduces wound pain; autolytic debridement of slough; preventive for high-risk friction areas; leave in place 3–7 d; can apply as window to secure transparent film or under-taping; can apply over alginate to control drainage; must control maceration; apply skin prep to intact skin to protect from adhesive

Contraindications: Fragile skin; infected ulcers; heavily draining wounds, sinus tracts

Collagen

Indications and Use: Stage 3 and selected Stage 4 (refer to package insert); light, moderate, or heavy exudate; chronic, nonhealing ulcers; nonadherent, absorbent, biodegradable gel; accommodates to wound surface; may be combined with topical agents; change dressing q1–3d

Contraindications: Sensitivity to collagen or bovine products; avoid use with necrotic ulcers; rehydration may be needed

Gauze packing▲ (moistened with saline)

Indications and Use: Stages 3 and 4; moderate to heavy exudate; wounds with depth, especially those with tunnels, undermining; must be remoistened at least q4h to maintain moist wound environment

Contraindications: May macerate periwound skin; may be painful to remove; can traumatize tissue when removed

Calcium alginate

Indications and Use: Stages 3 and 4; excessive drainage; sinus tracts, tunnels, or cavities; apply dressing within wound borders; must use skin prep to protect periwound skin; requires secondary dressing; change q24–48h

Contraindications: Dry or minimally draining wound; dry eschar; superficial wounds with maceration; may produce odor during dressing change; can macerate periwound skin

Silver

Indications and Use: Silver can be added to any dressing as bacteriostatic. It increases cost and has unknown efficacy. Consider in infected ulcers; highly colonized ulcers; antimicrobial.

Contraindications: Sensitivity to silver; avoid use with topical medications; inactivates enzymatic debriding agents; avoid use with heavily draining wounds; may cause periwound maceration; signs of systemic side effects, especially erythema multiforme; fungal proliferation.

ARTERIAL ULCERS

Definition

Any lesion caused by severe tissue ischemia secondary to atherosclerosis and progressive arterial occlusion

Wound Assessment (See PAD p 67)

- See Chronic Wound Assessment (p 331). Most often located in distal areas of lower extremities, including toes, and the tops and outside edges of the foot. Typically pale wound bed with minimal exudate.

- Wound healing unlikely if ABI <0.5. Exercise caution when relying only on the ABI due to high prevalence of hardened arteries that artifactually give normal or supranormal readings. Diminished or absent distal pulses, pale skin, slow capillary refill are common.
- Assess circulation using noninvasive tests such as pulse volume recording (PVR), toe pressures, and transcutaneous oxygen readings.

Management (also PAD, p 67, Diabetes, p 104, Chronic Heart Failure, p 48, and Renal Failure, p 193)

Protect from Injury

- Avoid compression of arterial wounds when ABI is <0.8.
- Avoid friction and pressure by using lamb's wool or foam between toes.
- Float the heels (pillows under the calf and knee) and use suitable device to keep covers off toes.
- Use positioning devices to avoid pressure on feet (eg, heel protectors).

Local Wound Care

Tx dictated by adequacy of perfusion and status of wound bed:
- Avoid debridement of necrotic tissue until perfusion status is determined.
- Assess vascular perfusion and refer for surgical intervention if consistent with overall goals of care.
- If wound is infected, revascularization procedures, surgical removal of necrotic tissue, and systemic antibiotics are tx of choice.
- Topical antibiotics should not be used solely to treat infected ischemic wounds and may cause sensitivity reactions.
- If wound is uninfected and dry eschar is present, maintain dry intact eschar as a barrier to bacteria. Application of an antiseptic may decrease bacterial burden on wound surface although evidence is lacking.
- If wound is uninfected and soft slough and necrotic tissue are present, apply moisture-retaining dressings that allow frequent inspection of wound for signs of infection.

DIABETIC (NEUROPATHIC FOOT) ULCERS
Definition

Any lesion on the plantar surface of the foot caused by neuropathy and repetitive pressure on foot.

Wound Assessment

- See Chronic Wound Assessment (p 331). Usually occur in repetitive stress areas and often painless. Covered with fibrotic tissue or callus and may penetrate to bone.
- Assess for specific DM-related signs of infection:
  ○ Sudden increase in blood glucose
  ○ Wound can be probed to the bone—highly sensitive indicator of osteomyelitis
  ○ Exclude gross arterial disease by assessment for palpable pedal pulses, a transcutaneous oxygen pressure of >30 mmHg, or normal Doppler-derived wave form.
- Determine grade of ulcer (Wagner Classification). Do not use National Pressure Ulcer Advisory Panel (NPUAP) staging system.
  Grade 0: Preulcerative lesions; healed ulcers present; bony deformity present
  Grade 1: Superficial ulcer without subcutaneous tissue involvement
  Grade 2: Penetration through subcutaneous tissue
  Grade 3: Osteitis, abscess, or osteomyelitis
  Grade 4: Gangrene of digit
  Grade 5: Gangrene of foot requiring disarticulation

Management (also Diabetes, p 104)

Local Wound Care

In addition to recommendations under Chronic Wound Treatment (p 331):

- Debride devitalized tissue and callus: surgical debridement is method of choice for effective, rapid removal of nonviable tissue
- Avoid occlusive dressings to reduce risk of wound infection
- Offload pressure and stress from foot
  - Avoidance of pressure on foot essential to management of diabetic foot ulcer
  - Use orthotic that redistributes weight on plantar surface of foot when ambulating (eg, total contact cast, *DH Offloading Walker*)
- If ulcer does not reduce in size by ≥50% after 4 wk of tx, reassess tx and consider alternative options (eg, NPWT, growth factor tx, skin substitutes, extracellular matrix, hyperbaric oxygen tx).
  - Skin substitutes *(Apligraf, Dermagraft)* containing growth factors present in the skin may stimulate healing and decrease time to wound closure. Wound must be granular to be effective.
  - Hyperbaric oxygen tx effective in promoting healing of complicated chronic diabetic foot ulcers is covered by Medicare and some insurance companies. Caution in patients with HF, advanced COPD, and those treated with anticancer drugs. Tx applied in chamber for 1.5–2 h/d for 20–40 d.

VENOUS ULCERS

Definition

Any lesion caused by venous insufficiency precipitated by venous HTN

Wound Assessment

- See Chronic Wound Assessment (p 331). Ulcer typically superficial with a moist pink-to-red bed and irregular edges. Edema, induration, and loss of hair are common. Skin is often darkened with variable drainage, depending on the presence of infection and edema.
- Assess lower-extremity edema.
- Assess pedal pulses to exclude ischemic ulcers (see Leg Edema in Cardiovascular chapter p 52).

Management (See Leg Edema, Cardiovascular p 52)

Compression Therapy

- Essential component of venous ulcer tx decreases healing time and pain
- Therapeutic level of compression is 30–40 mmHg at ankle, decreasing toward knee
- Types of compression tx:
  - Static compression device
    - Layered compression wraps *(PROFORE, PROGUIDE)*
    - Short-stretch wraps *(Comprilan)*
    - Paste-containing bandages *(Unna's boot)*
      - Preferable for actively ambulating patient; support compression of calf muscle "pump"
  - Dynamic compression devices (indicated when static compression not feasible)
    - Pneumatic compression device (intermittent pneumatic pumps)
    - Powered devices that propel venous blood upward when applied to lower leg

◦ Compression tx for long-term maintenance
    ▪ Therapeutic compression stockings *(Jobst, Juzo, Sigvaris, Mediven Strumpf, Therapress Duo)*

Local Wound Care

In addition to recommendations under Chronic Wound Treatment (p 331):
- Use exudate-absorbing dressings (eg, calcium alginate dressings, foam dressings). *Note:* A recent review indicates no benefit of alginate dressing over hydrocolloid or plain nonadherent dressings.
- Use skin sealant to protect skin around wound from exudates.
- Infected venous ulcers should be treated with systemic antibiotics because of the development of resistant organisms with topical antibiotics.
- Refer to a wound specialist for the use of skin substitutes (eg, *Apligraf, Dermagraft, GammaGraft*) containing growth factors present in skin may decrease wound healing time and decrease pain. Wound must be granular to be effective.

SKIN TEAR

Definition

Separation of skin layers resulting from shearing, friction, or blunt trauma (eg, wheelchair injuries, falls, transfer injury, tape removal)

Assessment

See Chronic Wound Assessment (p 331). Can be partial thickness or full thickness and appear as either a small linear split in the skin or peeled back skin. Use International Skin Tear Advisory Panel (ISTAP) classification system. Type 1: skin tear without tissue loss; Type 2: partial loss of skin tear flap; Type 3: complete loss of epidermal flap.

Management

- Preserve skin flap and protect surrounding tissue; encourage healing and prevent infection.
- Control bleeding with pressure and elevation of limb.
- Cleanse wound with warm tap water or saline.
- Approximate flap with gentle unfolding and smoothing over the wound.
- Use atraumatic dressing to keep flap in place. Leave for several days for flap to adhere to the wound bed.
- Monitor for signs of infection. If flap becomes necrotic, refer to a wound care specialist.

CLASSIFICATION

- Circadian rhythm disorders (eg, jet lag)
- **Insomnia** (difficulty initiating or maintaining sleep, or poor quality sleep). *Note:* Phase advance (reduced sleep during early morning and peak sleepiness earlier in the evening) are normal aspects of aging and do not need to be treated.
- Parasomnias (disorders of arousal, partial arousal, and sleep stage transition)
- Hypersomnia of central origin (eg, narcolepsy)
- **Sleep-related breathing disorders** (central and obstructive sleep apnea and sleep-related hypoventilation-hypoxia syndromes)
- **Sleep-related movement disorders** (eg, RLS, periodic limb movement disorder)

Bolded disorders are covered here. Others are covered in *JAGS* 2009;57:761–789.

INSOMNIA

Risk Factors and Aggravating Factors

Treatable Associated Medical and Psychiatric Conditions: adjustment disorders, anxiety, bereavement, cough, depression, dyspnea (cardiac or pulmonary), GERD, nocturia, pain, paresthesias, Parkinson disease, stress, stroke

Medications That Cause or Aggravate Sleep Problems: alcohol, antidepressants, β-blockers, bronchodilators, caffeine, clonidine, corticosteroids, diuretics, L-dopa, methyldopa, nicotine, phenytoin, progesterone, quinidine, reserpine, sedatives, sympathomimetics including decongestants

Management

Avoid polysomnography unless symptoms suggest a comorbid sleep disorder.[CW] For most patients, behavioral tx should be initial tx. Don't use benzodiazepines or other sedative hypnotics as 1st choice for insomnia.[CW] Despite benefits of hypnotics on sleep quality, total sleep time, and frequency of nighttime awakening, these are small compared to the risk of cognitive or psychomotor AEs. Combined behavioral tx and pharmacotherapy is more effective than either alone.

- Sleep improvements are better sustained over time with behavioral tx, including discontinuing pharmacotherapy after acute tx.

Nonpharmacologic

- Stimulus control
  Measures recommended to improve sleep hygiene:
  ○ During the daytime:
    ▪ Get out of bed at the same time each morning regardless of how much you slept the night before.
    ▪ Exercise daily but not within 2 h of bedtime.
    ▪ Get adequate exposure to bright light during the day.
    ▪ Decrease or eliminate naps, unless necessary part of sleeping schedule.
    ▪ Limit or eliminate alcohol, caffeine, and nicotine, especially before bedtime.
  ○ At bedtime:
    ▪ If hungry, have a light snack before bed (unless there are symptoms of GERD or it is otherwise medically contraindicated), but avoid heavy meals at bedtime.

- Don't use bedtime as worry time. Write down worries for next day and then don't think about them.
- Sleep only in your bedroom.
- Control nighttime environment, ie, comfortable temperature, quiet, dark.
  - Wear comfortable bedclothes.
  - If it helps, use soothing noise (eg, a fan or other appliance, a "white noise" machine, or an app such as *myNoise* or *White Noise Free Sleep Sounds*).
  - Remove or cover the clock.
  - No television watching in the bedroom.
  - Avoid reading e-books or tablets with light-emitting device. Uvex Skyper safety eyewear eliminates almost all blue light. Standard Kindle doesn't emit light.
- Maintain a regular sleeping time, but don't go to bed unless sleepy.
- Develop a sleep ritual (eg, hot bath 90 min before bedtime followed by preparing for bed for 20–30 min, followed by 30–40 min of relaxation, meditation, or reading).
- If unable to fall asleep within 15–20 min, get out of bed and perform soothing activity, such as listening to soft music or reading (but avoid exposure to bright light or computer screens).
- CBT for insomnia (CBT-I) combines multiple behavioral approaches (eg, sleep restriction, stimulus control, cognitive tx); Face-to-face may be more effective but can be delivered effectively either by telephone or via the Internet (CBT-I Coach App, CBTforInsomnia.com). CBT-I is likely to be most effective option for maintaining long-term improvement regardless of initial tx.
- Sleep restriction: reduce time in bed to estimated total sleep time (minimum 5 h) and increase by 15 min/wk when ratio of time asleep to time in bed is ≥90%. During the period of sleep restriction, daytime sleepiness may be increased and reaction time may be slower. Effect size is comparable to CBT.
- Relaxation techniques—physical (progressive muscle relaxation, biofeedback); mental (imagery training, mindfulness meditation, hypnosis)
- Bright light: 10,000 lux for 30 min/d upon awakening for difficulty initiating sleep; 2500 lux for 2 h/d in evening for difficulty maintaining sleep

Pharmacologic—Meta-analysis indicates improved sleep quality, total sleep time, and less frequent awakenings, but 2–5× increase in AEs.

Principles of Prescribing Medications for Sleep Disorders

- Combine with behavior tx rather than give medication alone.
- Use lowest effective dose.
- All increase risk of falls. Zolpidem is also associated with traumatic brain injury and hip fractures due to falls.
- Do not use OTC antihistamines to treat insomnia in older adults.
- For patients with anxiety at bedtime, consider SSRIs or buspirone.
- For sleep-onset insomnia, use a shorter-acting agent (eg, zolpidem, zaleplon, or suvorexant). For sleep-maintenance insomnia, use a longer-acting agent (eg, eszopiclone, zolpidem ER, doxepin).
- Prescribe medications for short-term use (no more than 3–4 wk) or use intermittent dosing (2–4×/wk).
- D/C medication gradually. See Deprescribing (p 19) and deprescribing.org .
- Be alert for rebound insomnia after discontinuation.

- For patients with AD, reducing insomnia risk factors and behavioral approaches are 1st-line tx. In clinical trials, melatonin or ramelteon have not been beneficial; trazodone confers only modest benefit.

Table 130. Useful Medications for Sleep Disorders in Older Adult

Class, Medication	Usual Dose	Formulations	Half-life	Comments (Metabolism, Excretion)
Antidepressant, sedating				
Trazodone▲	25–50 mg	T: 50, 100, 150, 300	12 h	Moderate orthostatic effects; effective for insomnia with or without depression (L)
Doxepin *(Silenor)*	3 mg	T: 3, 6	15.3 h	May cause next-day sedation; many potential drug interactions
Benzodiazepines, intermediate-acting [1,BC]				May impair next-day performance, including driving; may cause aggressive behavior
Estazolam▲	0.5–1 mg	T: 1, 2	12–18 h	Rapidly absorbed, effective in initiating sleep; slightly active metabolites that may accumulate (K)
Lorazepam▲	0.25–2 mg	T: 0.5, 1, 2	8–12 h	Effective in initiating and maintaining sleep; associated with falls, memory loss, rebound insomnia (K)
Temazepam▲	7.5–15 mg	C: 7.5, 15, 30	8–10 h[2]	Daytime drowsiness may occur with repeated use; effective for sleep maintenance; delayed onset of effect (K)
Nonbenzodiazepines [1,BC]				May impair next-day performance, including driving; may increase the risk of infections
Eszopiclone▲	1 mg	T: 1, 2, 3	5–6 h	CYP3A4 interactions; avoid administration with high-fat meal; not for tx of anxiety (L)
Zaleplon▲	5 mg	C: 5, 10	1 h	Avoid taking with alcohol or food (L)
Zolpidem▲	5 mg	T: 5, 10	1.5–4.5 h[3]	CYP3A4 interactions; confusion and agitation may occur but are rare (L)
(Edluar)	5 mg	T: 5, 10 (sl)	2.8 h	
(Ambien CR)	6.25 mg	T: 6.25, 12.5	1.6–5.5 h	Do not divide, crush, or chew. Avoid driving the day after taking.
(Zolpimist)	5 mg	Spr: 5 mg/spr	2–3 h	Spray over tongue; absorption more rapid
(Intermezzo)	1.75 mg	SL: 1.75, 3.5	2.4 h	SL: For middle-of-the-night insomnia
Orexin Receptor Agonist				
Suvorexant *(Belsomra)*	10–20 mg	T: 5, 10, 15, 20	12 h	Metabolized by CYP34A; can impair next-day driving and cause REM-sleep behavior disorder
Hormone and Hormone Receptor Agonists				
Melatonin▲	0.3–5 mg	Various	1 h	May be best taken 3–5 h before bedtime; not regulated by FDA

(cont.)

Class, Medication	Usual Dose	Formulations	Half-life	Comments (Metabolism, Excretion)
Ramelteon *(Rozerem)*	8 mg within 30 min of bedtime	T: 8	Ramelteon: 1–2.6 h; active metabolite: 2–5 h	Do not administer with or immediately after high-fat meal (L, K)
Tasimelteon *(Hetlioz)*	20 mg hs	T: 20		Indicated for non-24-h sleep-wake disturbance; very expensive (L)

¹ May cause severe allergic reactions and complex sleep-related behavioral disturbances

² Can be as long as 30 h in older adults

³ 3 h in older adults; 10 h in those with hepatic cirrhosis

SLEEP APNEA

Definition

Repeated episodes of apnea (cessation of airflow for ≥10 sec) or hypopnea (transient reduction [≥30% decrease in thoracoabdominal movement or airflow and with ≥4% oxygen desaturation, or an arousal] of airflow for ≥10 sec) during sleep with excessive daytime sleepiness or altered cardiopulmonary function. Predicts future strokes and cognitive impairment. HF (in men), and all-cause mortality (if severe).

Classification

Obstructive (OSA) (90% of cases): Airflow cessation as a result of upper airway closure in spite of adequate respiratory muscle effort. Older persons are more likely to have airway collapsibility as a cause.
• Mild Apnea-Hypopnea Index (AHI): 5–15
• Moderate: AHI 15–30
• Severe: AHI: >30

Central (CSA): Cessation of respiratory effort

Mixed: Features of both obstructive and central

Associated Risk Factors

Family hx, increased neck circumference, male sex, Asian ethnicity, hx of hypothyroidism (in women), obesity, smoking, upper airway structural abnormalities (eg, soft palate, tonsils), HTN, HF, atrial fibrillation, stroke, chronic lung diseases, including asthma, polycythemia, GERD

Clinical Features

Excessive daytime sleepiness, loud snoring, choking or gasping on awakening, morning headache, nocturia

Evaluation

• Epworth Sleepiness Scale (umms.org/midtown/health-services/sleep-disorders/patient-information/sleepiness) is useful for documenting and monitoring daytime sleepiness.
• Full night's sleep study (polysomnography) in sleep laboratory is indicated for those who habitually snore and either report daytime sleepiness or have observed apnea.

- "Out-of-center" sleep testing can be used if high pretest probability of moderate to severe OSA but should not be used if patients have comorbid conditions (eg, HF) that predispose to a sleep-related breathing disorder or another sleep disorder.
- Results are reported as AHI, which is the number of episodes of apneas and hypopneas per hour of sleep.
- Medicare reimbursement threshold for CPAP based on a minimum of 2 h sleep by polysomnography is AHI (1) ≥15 or (2) ≥5 and ≤14 with documented symptoms of excessive daytime sleepiness, impaired cognition, mood disorders, or insomnia, or documented HTN, ischemic heart disease, or hx of stroke.
- No need for retitration if asymptomatic, adherent patients with stable weight.[CW]

Management

Nonpharmacologic

- Patient education including information about increased risk of motor vehicle crashes
- Weight loss (eg, through very low-calorie diets, bariatric surgery) with active lifestyle counseling is effective in mild and moderate OSA but does not normalize OSA parameters. Benefit is less in severe OSA.
- Avoidance of alcohol or sedatives
- Lying in lateral rather than supine position (if normalization of AHI in nonsupine position is confirmed by sleep study) but usually not sufficient as sole tx; may be facilitated by soft foam ball in a backpack or devices that use vibratory feedback.
- Exercise (eg, 150 min/wk [4 d/wk]): moderate-intensity aerobic exercise, even in the absence of weight loss, can improve symptoms.
- Oral appliances that keep the tongue in an anterior position during sleep or keep the mandible forward; less effective than CPAP in reducing AHI score but may be better tolerated. Generally used in mild to moderate OSA (AHI <30) for patients who do not want CPAP.
- For moderate sleep apnea (>15 and <30 AHI), Positive airway pressure (PAP) or oropharyngeal exercises, including tongue, soft palate, and lateral pharyngeal wall, performed daily improves symptoms and reduces AHI score.
- PAP is initial tx for clinically important sleep apnea (eg, AHI ≥30 events/h). PAP may also improve HTN and the metabolic syndrome associated with OSA. PAP can be delivered through several modes:
  - Continuous (CPAP) by nasal mask, nasal prongs, or mask that covers the nose and mouth is the simplest and most effective at reducing AHI. A short course (14 d) of eszopiclone may facilitate adherence when initiating CPAP.
  - Bilevel (BPAP) uses 2 present (inspiratory and expiratory) levels of pressure.
  - Autotitrating (APAP) changes PAP in response to change in air flow, circuit pressure, or vibratory snore.
  - Nasal (NPAP) *(Provent)* is a 1-way valve inserted into each nostril that creates resistance during exhalation.
- Bariatric surgery improves but does not cure moderate or severe OSA.

Pharmacologic (should not be used as primary tx)

- Modafinil *(Provigil)* 200 mg qam for excessive daytime sleepiness (CYP3A4 inducer and CYP2C19 inhibitor) [T: 100, 200]; use in addition to (not instead of) CPAP. High rate of AEs.
- Small studies suggest potential benefit of dronabinol but causes somnolence; more trials are needed. AASM recommends against the use of this or medical cannabis.

Surgical
- Palatal implants (for mild to moderate OSA)
- Tracheostomy (indicated for patients with severe apnea who cannot tolerate positive pressure or when other interventions are ineffective)
- Uvulopalatopharyngoplasty (curative in fewer than 50% of cases). Less invasive alternatives include laser-assisted uvulopalatoplasty, radiofrequency ablation, and maxillomandibular advancement. All decrease the AHI but have not been demonstrated to be superior to medical management.
- Hypoglossal nerve stimulation with an implantable neurostimulator device (*Inspire, Sleep Therapy System*). FDA eligibility criteria include: moderate or severe OSA, predominantly obstructive events, CPAP failure or intolerance, and no anatomical findings that would compromise performance of the device.
- Maxillofacial surgery (rare cases)

SLEEP-RELATED MOVEMENT DISORDERS
Nocturnal Leg Cramps
- Must have muscle contraction, occur during time in bed, and be relieved by forceful stretching of affected muscles
- Most are idiopathic but may be due to hypocalcemia, extracellular volume depletion, neurologic disorders (eg, Parkinson disease, myopathies, neuropathies), lower extremity structural abnormalities, prolonged sitting, or working on concrete flooring.

Nonpharmacologic Treatment
- Treat acute cramps by:
  - Forcefully stretching affected muscle (eg, dorsiflexion of foot with knee extended to relieve calf cramp).
  - Walking or jiggling leg followed by elevating the leg.
  - Ice massage.
- Prevent recurrent leg cramps
  - Daily stretching exercises (eg, feet flat on floor, legs straight, lean forward, arms above head on wall, and hold 10–30 sec up to 5×/night)
- Avoid dehydration.

Pharmacologic Treatment
- Despite evidence of effectiveness, quinine is not recommended for nocturnal leg cramps because of the potential for serious AEs.
- Magnesium oxide is ineffective.
- Small studies have supported the use of vitamin B complex, verapamil, and diltiazem. Gabapentin has been used but with little evidence to support its effectiveness.

Restless Legs Syndrome (RLS; the majority will also have periodic limb movement disorder)

Diagnostic Criteria
- A compelling urge to move the limbs, usually associated with paresthesias or dysesthesias
- Motor restlessness (eg, floor pacing, tossing and turning in bed, rubbing legs)
- Vague discomfort, usually bilateral, most commonly in calves
- Symptoms occur while awake and are exacerbated by rest, especially at night
- Symptoms relieved by movement—jerking, stretching, or shaking of limbs; pacing

Secondary Causes: Iron deficiency, spinal cord and peripheral nerve lesions, uremia, DM, Parkinson disease, venous insufficiency, medications/drugs (eg, TCAs, SSRIs, lithium, dopamine antagonists, caffeine)

Don't use polysomnography to diagnose RLS unless clinical history is ambiguous and documentation of periodic leg movements is necessary.[CW]

Nonpharmacologic Treatment

• Sleep hygiene measures (p 341)
• Avoid alcohol, caffeine, nicotine.
• Rub limbs.
• Use hot or cold baths, whirlpools.
• Complementary and alternative tx (eg, transcutaneous direct current stimulation, acupuncture, pneumatic compression devices, yoga)
• Vibrating pad *(Relaxis)* available by prescription only (FDA approved)

Pharmacologic Treatment

• Exclude or treat iron deficiency (treat if ferritin <75 mcg/L), peripheral neuropathy.
• If possible, avoid SSRIs, TCAs, lithium, and dopamine antagonists.

Start at low dosage, increase as needed. AASM recommendations:

• Standard medications (best benefit/burden and higher quality of evidence): Dopamine agonists pramipexole (begin at 0.125 mg/d; most will require ≤0.5 mg/d but some require up to 1 mg/d) or ropinirole (begin at 0.25 mg/d; most will require 2 mg/d, and some will require 4 mg/d) 1 h before time of usual onset of symptoms (**Table 91**).
• Guideline medications (less favorable benefit/burden or lower quality of evidence)
  ○ Carbidopa-levodopa *(Sinemet)* 25/100 mg, 1–2 h before bedtime. Begin at 1/2 tab and can increase to 2 tab max. Symptom augmentation may develop earlier in the day (eg, afternoon instead of evening) and may be more severe with carbidopa-levodopa; tx may require reducing dosage or switching to dopamine agonist
  ○ Gabapentin ER formulation, gabapentin enacarbil *(Horizant)* [T: 600] 600 mg daily at 5 PM, has been FDA approved for RLS; reduce dose when CrCl <60 mL/min/1.73 m^2.[BC]
  ○ Pregabalin *(Lyrica)* [C: 25, 50, 75, 100, 150, 200, 225, 300] begin 150 mg/d but may need 300 mg/d; less augmentation compared to pramipexole; reduce dose when CrCl <60 mL/min/1.73 m^2.[BC]
  ○ Low-dose opioids
  ○ Cabergoline *(Dostinex)* [T: 0.5] beginning 0.25 mg 2×/wk; may also be effective but has potential for causing valvular heart disease.
• Optional medications (lower quality of evidence): carbamazepine (**Table 92**), clonidine, and for patients with low ferritin levels, iron supplementation.
• If refractory, can use combination tx.
• If augmentation (symptoms worsen with long-term tx, earlier onset of symptoms, shorter symptom latency with rest, shorter drug effect, spread to trunk or arms), switch tx regimen.
• If symptoms are intermittent, can use dopamine agonist or L-dopa prn.
• Rotigotine *(Neupro)* transdermal 1 mg/24 h daily to max 3 mg/24 h may be effective for very severe RLS.

Periodic Limb Movement Disorder (a minority will also have RLS)

Diagnostic Criteria

• Insomnia or excessive sleepiness

- Repetitive, highly stereotyped limb muscle movements (eg, extension of big toes with partial flexion of ankle, knee, and sometimes hip) that occur during non-REM sleep
- Polysomnographic monitoring showing >15 episodes of muscle contractions per hour and associated arousals or awakenings
- No evidence of a medical, mental, or other sleep disorder that can account for symptoms

Treatment: Indicated for clinically significant sleep disruption or frequent arousals documented on a sleep study.
- Nonpharmacologic: See sleep hygiene measures, p 341.
- Pharmacologic: See RLS, Pharmacologic Treatment, above. Pramipexole may be more effective than pregabalin.

Rapid Eye Movement (REM) Sleep Behavior Disorder
- Loss of atonia during REM sleep (ranging from simple limb twitches to acting out dreams), exaggeration of features of REM sleep (eg, nightmares), and intrusion of aspects of REM sleep into wakefulness (eg, sleep paralysis)
- High risk (80–90%) of developing neurodegenerative disorder (eg, Parkinson disease, multisystem atrophy, Lewy body dementia); conversion rate is approximately 50% every 10 y. Higher risk if subtle motor dysfunction, abnormal color vision, olfactory dysfunction.
- Can rarely be caused by antidepressant medications and pontine lesions.

Evaluation: If needed, in-laboratory video polysomnography

Nonpharmacologic Treatment: change sleeping environment to reduce risk of injury

Pharmacologic Treatment: high-dose melatonin 3–15 mg or clonazepam 0.25–1 mg hs; if associated with Parkinson disease, L-dopa, or pramipexole

SLEEP DISORDERS IN LONG-TERM CARE FACILITIES
Risk Factors
- Medical and medication factors (Insomnia, p 341)
- Environmental factors (eg, little physical activity, infrequent daytime bright light exposure, extended periods in bed, nighttime noise and light interruptions)

Nonpharmacologic Treatment
- Morning bright light tx
- Exercise (eg, stationary bicycle, tai chi) and physical activity
- Reduction of nighttime noise and light interruptions
- Maintain a consistent schedule of meals and activities
- Multicomponent interventions combining the above and a bedtime routine
- Match roommates based on nighttime routine (eg, incontinence care, turnings)
- Preliminary evidence for lavender oil aromatherapy, chamomile extract

SCOPE OF THE PROBLEM

- *Alcohol:*
  - Misuse/abuse is the primary substance use disorder in people aged ≥50.
  - Higher blood concentrations per amount consumed is due to decreased lean body mass and total body water.
  - Many medical conditions (eg, dementia, HTN) interact with alcohol.
  - Many drugs interact with alcohol: APAP, anesthetics, antihypertensives, antihistamines, antipsychotics, narcotic analgesics, NSAIDs, sedatives, antidepressants, anticonvulsant medications, nitrates, β-blockers, oral hypoglycemic agents, anticoagulants.
  - Baby boomers are likely to maintain higher alcohol consumption.
- *Illicit drugs:* Baby boomers have more frequent use of illicit drugs, particularly marijuana and cocaine, than the current cohort of older people.
- *Smoking:* 10% of people aged >65 (12% of men, 8% of women) are current smokers.
- *Prescription drug misuse/dependence:* is an important problem in the older population; in particular, opioids and benzodiazepines are a growing problem.

DSM-5 SUBSTANCE USE AND ADDICTIVE DISORDERS

Evaluation and Classification

DSM-5 consolidates substance abuse with substance dependence and addresses each substance-related disorder (alcohol, opioid, tobacco, and sedative, hypnotic, anxiolytic) as a separate disorder but uses 11 overarching criteria (see below) for diagnosis. The number of criteria met determines the severity of the disorder.

DSM-5 Criteria/Symptoms for Substance Use Disorders

- Continuing to use a substance despite negative consequences.
- Repeated inability to carry out roles (at work, home) on account of use.
- Recurrent use in physically hazardous situations.
- Continued use despite recurrent/persistent social/interpersonal problems during use.
- Tolerance, needing increased dose to achieve effect/diminished effect with same amount.
- Withdrawal syndrome or use of the drug to avoid withdrawal.
- Using more substance or using for a longer period than intended.
- Persistent desire to cut down use or unsuccessful attempts to control use.
- Spending a lot of time obtaining, using, or recovering from use.
- Stopping/reducing important occupational, social, or recreational activities due to use.
- Craving or strong desire to use.

DSM-5 Criteria for Diagnosis and Classification of Substance-related Disorder

Two or more symptoms (above) indicate a substance-related disorder; severity is determined by the number of symptoms.
- Mild use disorder: 2–3 symptoms
- Moderate use disorder: 4–5 symptoms
- Severe use disorder: 6 or more symptoms

ALCOHOL USE DISORDERS (AUDs)
Evaluation and Classification

AUDs are often missed in older adults because of reduced social and occupational functioning; signs more often include poor self-care, malnutrition, and medical illness. Because these disorders occur along a spectrum, it is recommended that all adults are screened for use with validated questionnaires that include the following:

• How many days per week?
• How many drinks on those days?
• Maximal intake on any one day?
• What type (ie, beer, wine, or liquor)?
• What is in "a drink"?

Hazardous or At-Risk Drinking

• Will probably eventually cause harm
• No current alcohol problems
• The National Institute on Alcohol Abuse and Alcoholism (NIAAA) defines at-risk drinking for men as 15 or more drinks/wk or 5 or more on one occasion and for women and anyone aged >65 as >7 drinks/wk or >3 drinks on one occasion.
• A standard drink is 12 oz beer, 5 oz of wine, or 1.5 oz of 80-proof liquor.

DSM-5 Criteria for AUDs (see above DSM-5 Substance-related and Addictive Disorders)

Alcohol Misuse Screening: CAGE questionnaire has been validated in the older population.

C Have you ever felt you should **C**ut down?
A Does others' criticism of your drinking **A**nnoy you?
G Have you ever felt **G**uilty about drinking?
E Have you ever had an "**E**ye opener" to steady your nerves or get rid of a hangover?
(Positive response to any suggests problem drinking.)

AUDIT-C

The Alcohol Use Disorders Identification Test Consumption Questions (AUDIT-C) identifies patients along the spectrum of unhealthy alcohol use. It can be self-administered, takes as little as 1–2 min via interview. Scoring (as shown) can also be linked to management (**Table 131**).

Table 131. AUDIT-C

	Question	0 points	1 point	2 points	3 points	4 points
Scoring	1. How often did you have a drink containing alcohol in the past year?	Never	Monthly or less	2–4×/mo	2–3×/wk	≥4×/wk
	2. On days in the past year when you drank alcohol how many drinks did you typically drink?	1 or 2	3 or 4	5–6	7–9	10 or more
	3. How often do you have 6 or more drinks on an occasion in the past year?	Never	Less than monthly	Monthly	Weekly	Daily or Almost daily
Management	Total Score =	0–3	4–5	6–7	8–9	10–12
	Health Promotion	✓				
	Brief Intervention		✓	✓		
	Pharmacotherapy			+/-	✓	
	Psychosocial interventions			+/-	+/-	
	Specialty care management				+/-	✓

Management of Alcohol Use Disorders

Brief Interventions

- *Primary care intervention*—effective for at-risk alcohol use; educate patient on effects of current drinking, point out current AEs, specify safe drinking limits (<7 drinks/wk, <3 on any 1 occasion). Patients who cannot moderate should abstain.
- Medicare pays for annual screening and up to 4 brief counseling sessions for patients with at-risk drinking who are not yet experiencing adverse effects to their mental or emotional health. No copay or deductible when provided by a primary care provider who accepts assignment.
- The NIAAA provides an online resource: *Helping Patients Who Drink Too Much: A Clinician's Guide* (niaaa.nih.gov/guide).

Pharmacotherapy (is probably underutilized.)

- **First line**
  - Naltrexone▲ 25 mg × 2 d po, then 50 mg/d [T: 50]; Depot naltrexone *(Vivitrol)* 380 mg IM monthly; monitor LFTs, avoid in kidney failure, hepatitis, cirrhosis, and with opioid use; ~10% get nausea, headache (L, K). Risk of injection site abscess with depot naltrexone.
  - Acamprosate *(Campral)* 666 mg q8h po, reduce dosage to 333 mg q8h if CrCl 30–50 mL/min/1.73 m^2 or weight <132 lb (60 kg) [T: 333]; contraindicated if CrCl <30 mL/min/1.73 m^2; diarrhea is most common drug-related AE (K). Large US trials have not shown efficacy.
- **Second line**
  - Topiramate▲ 300 mg/d po is effective at reducing relapse. The magnitude of the effect is equal to naltrexone. Drug-related AEs: cognitive impairment, paresthesias, weight loss, dizziness, depression.
  - SSRIs and other antidepressants reduce intake when alcohol dependence and depression co-occur; more favorable in later onset AUDs and with high psychosocial morbidity.
- The duration of drug tx should be at least 3 mo, or up to 12 mo, which is the period when relapse is highest.
- Combining these agents does not improve effectiveness.

- If significant depression persists after 1 wk of abstinence, tx for depression improves outcomes.
- Disulfiram *(Antabuse)* has limited if any use in older people due to the possible serious (even lethal) consequences when consumed with alcohol.

Psychosocial Interventions

- Have proven benefit for at-risk drinking through the spectrum of AUDs and include:
  - Motivational Interviewing—a counseling technique for eliciting behavior change by exploring and resolving the patient's ambivalence about change
  - Cognitive-behavioral therapy (CBT)
  - Contingency management: creates a system of incentives for sustained abstinence and/or tx adherence.
  - Self-help groups (eg, Alcoholics Anonymous)
- Therapeutic communities either inpatient or outpatient

Acute Alcohol Withdrawal

- Symptoms begin 6–24 h after last alcohol and are treated with as-needed benzodiazepines (p 75).
- Symptoms and signs: tremors, agitation, nausea, sweating, vomiting, hallucinations, insomnia, tachycardia, hypertension, delirium, seizures
- Assess severity of withdrawal symptoms using a validated instrument (Clinical Institute Withdrawal Assessment for Alcohol Scale-revised [CIWA-Ar] or the Short Alcohol Withdrawal Scale [SAWS]).
- Severity of symptoms dictate whether inpatient or outpatient management is appropriate.

TOBACCO USE DISORDERS AND SMOKING CESSATION

Approach

What Health Providers Should Do

Ask about tobacco use at every visit. **Advise** all users to quit. **Assess** willingness to quit. **Assist** the patient with a quit plan, education, pharmacotherapy.

Making the Decision to Quit

Patients are more likely to stop smoking if they believe they could get a smoking-related disease and can make an honest attempt at quitting, that the benefits of quitting outweigh the benefits of continued smoking, or if they know someone who has had health problems as a result of smoking.

Setting a Quit Date and Deciding on a Plan

Pick a specific day within the next month (gives time to develop a plan). Will pharmacotherapy be used? Discuss available supports (eg, class, counseling, quit line). On quit day, get rid of all cigarettes and related items.

Treatment

Pharmacotherapy (Table 132)

- Doubles or triples quit rates compared to placebo.
- Combining different agents (eg, nicotine pch + ad lib gum, varenicline +14 mg pch, bupropion with pch, SSRI/SNRI + nicotine pch) improves long-term abstinence.
- Optimal duration of tx may be 3–6 mo.

- Nicotine replacement is contraindicated with recent MI, uncontrolled high BP, arrhythmias, severe angina, gastric ulcer. May not be needed if patient smokes fewer than 10 cigarettes/d.
- E-cigarettes have some data on safety and suggest modest short-term effectiveness, but insufficient data on long-term abstinence. E-cigarettes are probably safer than continuing to smoke. FDA regulates as a tobacco product.
- Varenicline in trials achieved the highest quit rate of any single agent; slightly increased risk of neuropsychiatric disturbance in persons with hx of these disorders.

Table 132. Pharmacotherapy for Tobacco Abuse

Drug	Dosage	Formulations	Comments (Metabolism, Excretion)
Tobacco Abuse			
Bupropion SR▲	150 mg q12h × 7–12 wk	SR: 100, 150	Contraindicated with seizure disorders, stroke, brain tumor, brain surgery (L)
Varenicline *(Chantix)* [1]	0.5 mg × 3 d, 0.5 mg q12h × 4 d, then 1 mg q12h × 12–24 wk or longer	0.5, 1	Start 7 d before quit date. AEs: nausea, vivid dreams, constipation, depression, small increased risk of cardiovascular events (L, K); reduce dosage if CrCl <30 mL/min/1.73 m²
Nicotine Replacement			
Transdermal patches▲	15, 21, 22, 25 mg/d × 4–8 wk 10, 11, 14, 15 mg/d × 2–6 wk 5, 7, 10, 11 mg/d × 2–8 wk	5, 7, 11, 14, 15, 21, 22	Apply to clean, nonhairy skin on upper torso, rotate sites; start 10–15 mg/d with CVD or body weight <100 lb or if smoking <10 cigarettes/d (L)
Polacrilex gum▲ (eg, *Nicorette*)	9–12 pieces/d	2, 4	Chew 1 piece when urge to smoke; usual 10–12/d, max 30/d; 4 mg if smoking >21 cigarettes/d (L)
Nasal spray *(Nicotrol NS)*	1 spr each nostril q30–60min	0.5 mg/spr	Do not exceed 5 applications/h or 40 in 24 h; use should not exceed 3 mo (L)
Inhaler *(Nicotrol Inhaler)*	6–16 cartridges/d	4 mg delivered/cartridge	Max 16 cartridges/d with gradual reduction after 6–12 wk (L)
Lozenge▲	1 po prn	2, 4	Do not exceed 20/d; do not bite or chew; wean over 12 wk

[1] Partial nicotine agonist that eases withdrawal and blocks effects of nicotine if patients resume smoking.

Psychological

- Avoid people and places where tempted to smoke.
- Alter habits: (1) switch to juices or water instead of alcohol or coffee, (2) take a walk instead of a coffee break, (3) use oral substitutions (eg, sugarless gum or hard candy).
- Effective interventions include advice from healthcare provider to quit, self-help materials, proactive telephone counseling, group counseling, individual counseling, intra-treatment social support (from a clinician), extra-treatment social support (family, friends, coworkers, and smoke-free home).
- Programs that include counseling in person or by telephone increase quit rates by 10–25% when combined with pharmacotherapy.

- Medicare pays for 4 counseling episodes per attempt to quit; up to 2 attempts/y. Up to 8 face-to-face visits/y focused on counseling for smoking cessation CPT codes 99406 (≤10 min) 99407 (>10 min). Codes apply to both asymptomatic patients and those with a smoking-related health condition.

Maintaining Smoking Cessation: Use the same methods that helped during withdrawal; long-term nicotine replacement reduces relapse.

PRESCRIPTION DRUG USE DISORDERS

Diagnosis of Prescription Medication-Related Use Disorders—see DSM-5 criteria to classify degree of misuse (p 350); prescription misuse and abuse in older people may be as high as 11%. Risk factors include female sex, social isolation, depression, and mental health problems.

Common Prescription Medications Associated with Use Disorders

According to the National Institute on Drug Abuse, the following 3 classes most commonly:
- Opioids—usually prescribed to treat pain
- CNS depressants—used to treat anxiety and sleep disorders
- Stimulants—prescribed to treat attention deficit hyperactivity disorder and narcolepsy

Adverse Events

- Benzodiazepines: falls, mobility and ADL disability, cognitive impairment, motor vehicle accidents, pressure ulcers, UI
- Nonbenzodiazepine sedatives: anxiety, depression, nervousness, hallucinations, dizziness, headache, sleep-related behavioral disturbances
- Opioids: falls and fractures
- If there is a hx or current IV drug abuse, check for hepatitis C infection.

Assessing for Risk of Medication Misuse/Abuse

- Patient education on avoiding misuse is enhanced by a standard patient-prescriber agreement (eg, https://www.tirfremsaccess.com/TirfUI/rems/pdf/ppaf-form.pdf).
- General risk factors include use of a psychoactive drug with abuse potential, use of other substances (alcohol, tobacco, etc), female sex, possibly social isolation, and hx of mental health disorder.
- Persons with a substance abuse hx are more likely to misuse opioids.
- Screen for risk of opioid misuse/abuse with the Opioid Risk Tool; this instrument differentiates low-risk from high-risk patients.

Detection of Medication Misuse/Abuse

- Detection relies on clinical judgment; monitor at-risk patients when prescribing benzodiazepines, stimulants, and opioid analgesics.
- Observe for behavior that may suggest nonadherence to prescribed medication schedule (eg, early fill request, frequent lost prescriptions).
- Record any suspicious drug-seeking or other aberrant behaviors observed or reported by others, along with actions taken.
- Document evaluation process, rationale for long-term tx, and periodic review of patient status.
- Ask about purchases of medication over the Internet. Controlled substances can readily be purchased through illegitimate Internet-based pharmacies.

Treatment for Prescription Drug Abuse/Misuse/Dependence

- Opioids
  - May need to undergo medically supervised detoxification
  - Gradual tapering of opioids is necessary (Adjustment of Dosage, p 266).
  - Behavioral tx, usually combined with medications (buprenorphine/naloxone), *is* effective.
  - Opioid abuse-deterrent products (eg, *Embeda*) may reduce diversion. These agents do not have street value because they release naltrexone if not used as intended.
- CNS depressants or stimulants (general rules)
  - Primary provider encouragement to reduce use
  - Short-term substitution of other medications (eg, trazodone) for sleep
  - Gradual slow tapering of the drug
- Benzodiazepine dependence
  - Studies show supervised gradual withdrawal to be most effective.
  - CBT is directed at the symptom for which the benzodiazepine was originally prescribed, most often insomnia or anxiety; for sleep-specific CBT, see p 342; may be less effective in older adults.
  - An effective program (EMPOWER) uses patient education on adverse effects and very gradual withdrawal guided by symptoms over 4 mo to >1 y (see deprescribing.org).

Medical Marijuana

- Effects of short-term use: impaired short-term memory (learning), impaired coordination (eg, reduced driving skills), altered judgment; in high doses, paranoia and psychosis
- Effects of long-term use: addiction (about 9% of users overall), cognitive impairment, decreased life satisfaction and attainment, chronic bronchitis, and psychosis
- Marijuana (cannabis sativa) contains 60 cannabinoids, 2 of which, tetrahydrocannabinol (THC) and cannabidiol (CBD), have been considered for medicinal uses. CBD is considered to have therapeutic effects, while THC is responsible for most adverse effects. Purified and synthetic preparations of THC, CBD, and several other cannabinoids are under study for many chronic conditions (**Table 133**). All remain illegal under federal law and are not FDA regulated except for agents specifically approved (nabilone, dronabinol, *Epidiolex*).
- Marijuana remains a federally designated Schedule I controlled substance. About half of states have legalized medical marijuana. In those states, healthcare providers authorize use and that authorization has been viewed by federal courts as protected physician-patient communication. **Table 133** summarizes available evidence for conditions studied in randomized clinical trials.
- Beware of withdrawal symptoms (eg, when hospitalized). Symptoms: anxiety, headache, hypersomnia.
- Potential drug interactions: THC is a substrate for CYP2CP and CYP3A4.
- An appropriate candidate for medical marijuana should have:
  - A debilitating condition that has been studied in clinical trials (**Table 133**)
  - Failure to respond to standard first- and second-line tx
  - Failure to respond to an FDA-approved cannabinoid (nabilone 1–2mg po 2×/d, or dronabinol, p 263)
  - No active substance use or psychiatric disorder
  - Residence in a state with medical marijuana laws and meets those criteria
- The Federation of State Medical Boards recommends the following steps before authorizing marijuana use to ease the symptoms caused by a debilitating medical condition:
  - Advise about other options for managing the condition

- Determination that the patient may benefit from the authorization of marijuana
- Advise about the potential risks of the medical use of marijuana to include:
  - The variability of quality and concentration of marijuana (low-THC/high-CBD preparations are preferred for beneficial effects and fewer adverse CNS effects)
  - The risk of cannabis use disorder
  - AEs, exacerbation of psychotic disorder, adverse cognitive effects for children and young adults, and other risks, including falls or fractures. All more likely with high-THC preparations.
  - Use of marijuana during pregnancy or breastfeeding
  - The need to safeguard all marijuana and marijuana-infused products from children and pets or domestic animals
  - The need to notify the patient that the marijuana is for the patient's use only and the marijuana should not be donated or otherwise supplied to another individual
- Document authorization for use in the EMR as specified in state law.
- Additional diagnostic evaluations or other planned tx
- A specific duration for the marijuana authorization for a period no longer than 12 mo
- A specific ongoing tx plan as medically appropriate

Table 133. Medical Reasons Why Adult Patients May Want to Use Cannabis or Cannabinoids and Evidence for Effectiveness or Ineffectiveness

Condition	Substance Studied		Strength of Evidence	Notes
	Cannabis	Cannabinoids (THC, CBD)		
Chronic pain	+		E, Substantial	
Nausea, vomiting		+ oral formulations	E, Substantial	During chemotherapy[1]
MS spasticity		+ oral formulations	E, Substantial	Patient-reported symptoms
Short-term sleep outcomes		+ primarily nabiximols	E, Moderate	In OSA, chronic pain, MS
Poor appetite/ weight loss	+	+	E, Limited	In HIV/AIDS
MS spasticity		+	E, Limited	Clinician-rated symptoms
Dementia symptoms		+	I, Limited	
Glaucoma		+	I, Limited	
Depression in chronic pain or MS		+ nabiximols, dronabinol, nabilone	I, Limited	

No or insufficient evidence to support or refute use in: cancer (glioma), cancer associated anorexia, anorexia nervosa, spasticity of spinal cord injury, symptoms of ALS, motor symptoms or dyskinesia of Parkinson disease, dystonia, abstinence from addictive substances

[1] Dronabinol is FDA approved for this indication. E = effective; I = ineffective; MS = multiple sclerosis; OSA = obstructive sleep apnea.

- For patients who tell you that they are already or will be starting to use CBD or THC:
  - Caution patients on the additive effects with their CNS active medications; drug interactions with warfarin, anticholinergics, alcohol, other highly protein-bound medications (glipizide, loop diuretics, statins).
  - No driving for 6 h after inhalation; for 8–9 h after edible ingestion
  - THC products:
    - Edibles: start 1/4 to 1/2 of a single serving; standard serving is 10 mg
    - Inhaled vaporized: avoid high-THC strains
  - CBD products: starting dose should not be more than 5–10 mg; potent inhibitor of CYP3A4, CYP2C19, CYP2D6.

Table 134. Adverse Effects of Cannabis

Acute	Chronic
Cardiovascular: tachycardia, hypertension palpitations	**Bone health**: reduced BMD
Respiratory: coughing, wheezing, increased sputum	**Respiratory:** chronic bronchitis, impaired alveolar macrophage activity
CNS: disorientation, sedation, dizziness, euphoria, dry mouth, slowed reaction time, impaired coordination, anxiety, psychosis	**CNS:** depression, impaired memory, attention, and decision making
	Endocrine: reduced testosterone

COMMON DISORDERS

Breast Cancer

- Screen with mammography (**Table 103**) until age 70–74, perhaps longer in women with life expectancy >10 y.**CW**

Evaluation of patients over age 65 with newly diagnosed breast cancer should consist of:

- Hx and physical exam
- Diagnostic bilateral mammography and ultrasound if indicated
- CBC, LFTs, serum alkaline phosphatase
- Assessment of:
  - life expectancy (**Table 7**, p 10)
  - comorbidity (eg, Charlson Index); calculators available online
  - function (ADL and IADL)
- Considering life expectancy, comorbidity, and functional status, discuss goals of care with the patient.
- If the goal of care is cure or life prolongation, the next steps in evaluation are resection of the tumor and possibly sentinel lymph node (SLN) biopsy.
- Older women with clinically negative axillary exams, small (<2-cm tumors), and who will be treated with adjuvant HT may be managed without axillary surgery. Don't perform axillary lymph node (ALN) dissection for clinical stage I and II without attempting SLN biopsy.**CW**
- If an SLN biopsy is positive, ALN dissection, radiation tx, or both, should be considered depending on whether mastectomy or lumpectomy is planned, the extent of the tumor, and plans for systemic tx. Older women are more likely to experience lymphedema after ALN dissection.
- Further evaluation depends on the stage of the disease as follows:
  - At Stage I and II, no additional evaluation for metastatic disease is needed.
    - Stage I (tumor ≤2 cm), negative nodes (N0), or no more than microscopic (0.2 cm) disease
    - Stage II (tumor >2 and ≤5 cm) with either N0 or N1; or tumor >5 cm and N0. N1 has more than microscopic disease, and mobile nodes (not matted or fixed).
  - At Stage III, patients need imaging for bone, liver, and pulmonary metastases.
    - Stage III (tumor >5 cm) or tumor of any size with fixed or matted lymph nodes on clinical exam or tumor of any size that extends directly to the chest wall or skin.
  - Stage IV is tumor with metastasis.
- Assess tumor biology
  - In women over age 65, 85% of tumors are positive for estrogen receptor (ER) and/or progesterone receptor (PR), which predicts response to adjuvant HT.
  - Among women over age 85, ER/PR expression shows a decreased frequency of PR and an increase in androgen receptor positivity.
  - HER2/*neu* overexpression is less common in the tumors of older women, but when present has the same adverse prognosis.
  - In patients with tumors that are ER-/PR-positive and HER2-negative and who could be candidates for chemotherapy, assessing the gene expression of the tumor by *Oncotype Dx* or *MammaPrint* can further assess the value of adding chemotherapy.
- Don't perform PET, CT, and radionuclide bone scans in staging early breast cancer at low risk for metastases.**CW**

- Patients with limited life expectancy and those who are too ill or frail to undergo surgery for the primary tumor, and whose tumors are ER-positive, can be offered tx with an aromatase inhibitor.

Monitoring Women with a History of Breast Cancer

- Hx, physical examination q3–6mo for 3 y, then every 6–12 mo for 2 y; pelvic examinations as appropriate for age and health status
- Increase surveillance for 2nd primary in breasts, ovaries, colon, and rectum
- Annual mammography

Oral Adjuvant Therapy for Breast Cancer

- Postmenopausal women with ER- or PR-positive tumors at high risk of recurrence (tumors >1 cm, or positive nodes) should be treated with oral adjuvant tx. Tx should be with an aromatase inhibitor (AI) for 5–10 y (**Table 135**).
- Long-term (>5 y) tx is associated with fractures and cardiovascular events.
- If an AI is discontinued in the 1st 5 y, it is reasonable to switch to tamoxifen for at least 2 y. For women who have completed 5 y of tamoxifen, an additional 5 y of AI is recommended.
- Obtain bone density before initiating tx with an AI and consider initiating a bisphosphonate (Osteoporosis p 247).
- Most patients treated with AIs will experience musculoskeletal side effects. Treat symptomatically (acetaminophen, exercise) or switch to alternate AI or tamoxifen.
- Obtain baseline and sequential lipid profiles.
- Treat dyspareunia with water-soluble lubricants (Sexual Dysfunction, p 328). However, low-dose vaginal estrogens can be used for intractable vaginal symptoms.

Table 135. Oral Agents for Breast Cancer Treatment

Class, Medication	Dosage and Formulations	Monitoring	Adverse Events, Interactions (Metabolism)
Antiestrogen Drugs			
Tamoxifen▲[1]	20 mg/d po T: 10, 20	Annual eye examination; endometrial cancer screening	Avoid fluoxetine, paroxetine, bupropion, duloxetine, and other potent CYPD26 inhibitors that reduce tamoxifen activity; ↑ risk of thrombosis (L)
Toremifene *(Fareston)*	60 mg/d po T: 60	CBC, Ca, LFTs, BUN, Cr	Drug interactions: CYP3A4–6 inhibitors and inducers; ↑ warfarin effect (L)
Aromatase Inhibitors			*Class AEs*: arthritis, arthralgia, bone pain, carpal tunnel, alteration in lipid profiles, sexual dysfunction, dyspareunia *Other AEs*: fatigue, sleep disorders, depression, asthenia, fracture, MI or ischemia, anemia, leukopenia, pancytopenia, hot flushes, fractures, vaginal bleeding (L)
Anastrozole▲	1 mg/d po T: 1	Periodic CBC, lipids, serum chemistry profile	
Exemestane▲	25 mg/d po T: 25	Periodic WBC count with differential, lipids, serum chemistry profile	
Letrozole▲	2.5 mg/d po T: 2.5	Periodic CBC, LFTs, TSH	Metabolized by CYP3A4, CYP2A6; strongly inhibits CYP2A6 and moderately inhibits CYP2C19

[1] Reduce dosage if CrCl <10 mL/min/1.73 m^2

Adjuvant Chemotherapy: Is used after resection. Reduces risk of recurrence and improves survival, especially when risk of recurrence is >10% at 10 y. Recurrence is reduced by 30–50% with greater benefit in ER-poor or -absent breast cancer.

Bisphosphonates: Are commonly used in postmenopausal women on other adjuvant tx for breast cancer. Five years of zoledronic acid improves invasive disease-free survival in postmenopausal but not premenopausal women.

Therapy for Metastatic Bone Disease: Pamidronate or zoledronic acid reduces morbidity and delays time to onset of bone symptoms.

Vulvar Diseases

Nonneoplastic

Patients often do not report symptoms (burning, itching) unless asked.

Table 136. Common Vulvar Dermatoses

Condition	Clinical Presentation and Distribution	Characteristics Used in Diagnosis	Treatment
Candida vulvovaginitis	Burning, itching, pain involving vulva, vagina, perineum	Classic "satellite" lesions surrounding areas of erythema	Topical antifungal,[1] plus topical steroid speeds relief of symptoms (eg, betamethasone dipropionate 0.05%, clotrimazole 1%); **Table 45**.
Contact dermatitis	Burning, itching over the hair-bearing cutaneous vulva and surrounding skin	Erythema in areas of contact with pads or skincare products, look for superimposed candida	Eliminate offending garment or skincare product
Lichen sclerosis[2]	Burning, itching, or asymptomatic involving the labia minora, majora, clitoral hood; may involve perianus in classic hourglass distribution	Circumscribed pallor, scarring may cause loss of labia minora, stenosis of introitus. Biopsy if diagnosis is in doubt, failure to respond to superpotency steroid, or any suspicious areas	Superpotency steroid (**Table 46**) q24h for 4 wk, then every other day ×4 wk, then 2–3×/wk for 4 wk and prn
Lichen simplex chronicus	Chronic or intermittent pruritus; often worse in evening or night over the hair-bearing cutaneous vulva	Epidermal thickening, lichenified papules and plaques, ill-demarcated erythema, linear excoriations, erosions	Eliminate all but hypoallergenic skincare products; break scratch-itch cycle with midpotency steroid daily for 4 wk (**Table 46**)
Lichen planus	Pain, burning of the labia minora and introitus; most have lesions on either skin, nails, or oral mucosa	Most commonly: bright erythema and erosions, surrounded by white reticulated rim, scarring, vaginal stenosis	Superpotency steroids (**Table 46**), but often not sufficient. Often add calcineurin inhibitors, oral steroids, etc
Psoriasis	Mild to severe pruritus; pain or burning involving hair-bearing cutaneous vulva, 95% have psoriatic lesions elsewhere	Classic plaque or inverse psoriasis (very red lesions that characteristically appear in body folds)	Topical steroids (**Table 46**), Vitamin D analogs; calcineurin inhibitors

[1]Severe cases may require oral fluconazole.

[2]Associated with a low risk of squamous cell cancer; examine the vulva at least yearly, biopsy all suspicious lesions. Ask patients to look at the skin and search for lumps or nonhealing sores monthly.

Neoplastic Vulvar Diseases

- VIN may be asymptomatic or may cause pruritus or dysuria; hypo- or hyperpigmented keratinized plaques; often multifocal; inspection ± colposcopy of the entire vulva with biopsy of most worrisome lesions; lesions graded on degree of atypia. Tx: surgical or laser ablative tx.
- Vulvar malignancy—Half of cases are in women aged >70; 80% are squamous cell, with melanoma, sarcoma, basal cell, and adenocarcinoma <20%; biopsy any suspicious lesion. Tx: vulvectomy, radical local excision, or 3-incision surgical techniques.

Postmenopausal Bleeding

Defined as bleeding after 1 y of amenorrhea:

- Exclude malignancy, identify source (vagina, cervix, vulva, uterus, bladder, bowel), treat symptoms.
- Examine genitalia, perineum, rectum.
- If endometrial source, use endometrial biopsy or vaginal probe ultrasound to assess endometrial thickness (<5 mm virtually excludes malignancy).
- D&C when endometrium not otherwise adequately assessed.
- Evaluation is needed for:
  - Women on combination continual estrogen and progesterone who bleed after 12 mo.
  - Women on cyclic replacement with bleeding at unexpected times (ie, bleeding other than during the 2nd wk of progesterone tx).
  - Women on unopposed estrogen who bleed at any time.

Vaginal Prolapse

- Child-bearing and other causes of increased intra-abdominal pressure weaken connective tissue and muscles supporting the genital organs, leading to prolapse.
- Symptoms include pelvic pressure, back pain, FI, UI, or difficulty evacuating the rectum. Symptoms may be present even with mild prolapse.
- The degree of prolapse and organs involved dictate tx; no tx if asymptomatic.
- Estrogen and Kegel exercises (p 164) may help in mild cases.
- Pessary or surgery indicated with increase in symptoms. Don't exclude pessaries as an option for prolapse.^{CW} Surgery needed for fourth-degree symptomatic prolapse.
- Precise anatomic defect(s) dictates the surgical approach. Surgical closure of the vagina (colpocleisis) is a simple option for frail patients who are not sexually active.
- A common classification (ACOG) for degrees of prolapse:
  - First degree—extension to midvagina
  - Second degree—approaching hymenal ring
  - Third degree—at hymenal ring
  - Fourth degree—beyond hymenal ring

HORMONE THERAPY

Symptoms Associated with the Postmenopausal State

- Hot flushes and night sweats
- Vaginal dryness and dyspareunia
- Sleep disturbances
- Depression
- Insufficient evidence exists to link the following commonly reported symptoms to the postmenopausal state: cognitive disturbances, fatigue, sexual dysfunction.

Therapy for Menopausal Symptoms

- Vasomotor and vaginal symptoms respond to estrogen[BC] in a dose-response fashion; start at low dosage (eg, oral conjugated or esterified estrogen 0.3 mg/d, which should be combined with medroxyprogesterone in women with an intact uterus), titrate to effect. Dyspareunia and vaginal dryness respond to topical estrogen (**Table 126** [Sexual Dysfunction chapter]).
- Conjugated estrogens 0.45 mg/bazedoxifene 20 mg *(Duavee)* po, qd treats menopausal symptoms without apparent drug-related AEs on breast or uterus. Long-term risk for thromboembolism and ischemic stroke uncertain.
- "Bioidentical hormone therapy" refers to the use of naturally occurring (rather than synthetic or animal-derived) forms of progesterone, estradiol, and estriol. These preparations are compounded by pharmacies and readily available over the Internet but are not FDA approved. The FDA and the Endocrine Society believe there is insufficient evidence to evaluate the safety and efficacy of these agents relative to FDA-approved HT.

Risk of Hormone Therapy

- Risks associated with HT use may vary based on the length of time between menopause and initiation of HT. For information on the risks and benefits of HT initiated within the 1st 5 y after menopause, see the position statement of the North American Menopause Society (www.menopause.org/docs/default-document-library/psht12.pdf).
- Initiation of HT within the 1st 6 y after menopause may reduce progression of subclinical atherosclerosis.
- Beginning HT in women 10 or more years after menopause is not recommended due to increase risk of MI, DVT, PE, stroke, kidney stones, dementia, and ovarian cancer.
- Older women can get hot flushes if estrogen is discontinued suddenly. Tapering (eg, q48h for 1–2 mo and then q72h for a few months) may be better tolerated.
- The fracture-protective effect from HT is lost rapidly after discontinuation; women at risk of fracture should be evaluated and treated with alternative tx (Osteoporosis, p 247).

Contraindications to Hormone Therapy

- Undiagnosed vaginal bleeding
- Thromboembolic disease
- Breast cancer
- Prior stroke or TIA
- Endometrial cancer more advanced than Stage 1
- Possibly gallbladder disease
- CHD

Intolerable Vasomotor Symptoms

- 10% of women continue with vasomotor symptoms 12 y after menopause.
- HT (estrogen[BC] and/or progesterone) is the most effective tx.
- Note contraindications above.
- Assess risk of VTE and CVD:
  - VTE risk increased by hx of VTE, malignancy/myeloproliferative disorder, leg immobilization, or both, smoking, and obesity
  - CVD risk increased by known CAD, PAD, AAA, carotid artery disease, DM, or risk factors that confer a 10-y risk of coronary disease >20% (cvdrisk.nhlbi.nih.gov/)
- If increased cardiovascular or VTE risk, oral standard dosage estrogen-progestin should not be used.
- If increased cardiovascular risk (but not VTE risk), attempt to control symptoms with transdermal estrogen.

- If risk of VTE is increased and risk of CVD is usual and patient has no uterus, transdermal estrogen may be appropriate; if patient has an intact uterus, adding a progestin raises additional concerns.
- If neither VTE nor CVD risk is increased, estrogen (0.3–0.625 mg po daily for women who have had a hysterectomy) or estrogen-progestin (0.45/1.5 mg or 0.625/2.5 mg po daily, for those with an intact uterus) or transdermally at lowest dosage to control symptoms may be appropriate.
- Reassess risks and benefits every 2 y.
- If estrogen cannot be taken or if risks exceed benefits, try one of these alternatives. Expert opinion based on double-blind randomized trials and demonstrated safety and effectiveness suggests considering agents in the following sequence:
  ○ First, antidepressants: SSRIs[BC]: citalopram 10–20 mg/d; paroxetine 7.5–25 mg/d. Avoid SSRIs if patients are receiving tamoxifen; tamoxifen levels will be subtherapeutic. SNRIs[BC]: venlafaxine 75 mg/d; desvenlafaxine 50–200 mg/d
  ○ Second, anticonvulsants: gabapentin[BC] 900–2700 mg/d; pregabalin[BC] 75–300 mg/d
  ○ Third, α_2-Adrenergic agonists: clonidine 0.5–1.5 mg/d (Avoid in HTN[BC]); watch for orthostatic hypotension and rebound increase in BP if used intermittently. Common drug-related AEs: dry mouth, constipation, sedation.

Peter Hollmann, MD AGSF, 3/1/2019

Geriatricians focus on Medicare, but private payers—including Medicare Advantage plans—may use other valid CPT and HCPCS codes. Every procedure code (CPT or HCPCS) must be accompanied with a diagnosis code (ICD-10). The listed codes are particularly relevant for services performed by geriatrics healthcare professionals, but are not a complete list of all services geriatricians perform. CPT 2019 is an essential reference. A good rules reference is the Medicare Internet Only Manual for Claims Processing of Physician and Professional Services. Manual 100-04 (Claims Processing) Chapter 12. https://www.cms.gov/Regulations-and-Guidance/Guidance/Manuals/Internet-Only-Manuals-IOMs.html. **Codes that are new in 2019 are starred (*).** (New services may lack educational Medicare publications initially). Details are in the Final Rule, and you may search on the code number. https://www.govinfo.gov/content/pkg/FR-2018-11-23/pdf/2018-24170.pdf

Common Procedure Codes		
Procedure Code	**Description**	**Reference/Notes**
Evaluation and Management		
Documentation Guidelines available at: http://www.cms.gov/Outreach-and-Education/Medicare-Learning-Network-MLN/MLNEdWebGuide/EMDOC.html		
99201–99215	Office/Outpatient Visits	Also used for Office/Outpatient Consultations when reporting to Medicare
99217–99220 99224–99226 99234–99236	Observation Services	For Medicare, only the attending of record may use these observation codes. Others use the 99201–99215 series. 100-04; 12; 30.6.8
99241–99245 99251–99255	Consultations	Invalid for Medicare, but may be used by other payers. For Medicare use 99201–99215 for outpatient, 99221–99223 and 99231–99233 for inpatient, and 99304–99310 for nursing facility. 100-04; 12; 30.6.10
99291–99292	Critical Care	Used in all settings of care, geriatrician relevant.
99304–99318	Nursing Facility Services	
99324–99327	Domiciliary Care (eg, assisted living facility)	
99341–99350	Home Services	
99354–99359	Prolonged Services	Time-based codes; track exact time because it is needed for coding.
99387, 99397	Comprehensive Preventive Medicine	Noncovered Medicare (see Medicare Preventive Services), may be used by other payers (eg, Medicare Advantage plans).
99446–99449, 99451*, 99452*	Interprofessional Telephone/Internet/EHR Consultations	New codes in 2019 and newly recognized for payment existing codes. Includes "eConsult" and "eReferral".

(cont.)

99483	Cognition Assessment and Care Plan	An assessment for cognition and must include the creation of a care plan that is shared with patient and/or caregiver.
		May not report with other E/M.
99497, 99498	Advance Care Planning	If done with initial preventative physical exam or annual wellness visit (IPPE/AWV), use -33 modifier so no patient cost share.
		https://www.cms.gov/Outreach-and-Education/Medicare-Learning-Network-MLN/MLNProducts/Downloads/AdvanceCarePlanning.pdf
		https://www.cms.gov/Medicare/Medicare-Fee-for-Service-Payment/PhysicianFeeSched/Downloads/FAQ-Advance-Care-Planning.pdf

Care Management

https://www.cms.gov/Medicare/Medicare-Fee-for-Service-Payment/PhysicianFeeSched/Care-Management.html

99457*	Remote physiologic monitoring treatment management	This is similar to chronic care management (see next) but does not require a care plan, advanced practice, and 2 or more conditions. An example is monitoring management for congestive heart failure.
99487 99489 99490 99491*	Chronic Care Management	In 2019 CPT added Care Management by the physician, 99491.
		Monthly time-based codes with required services and practice structures (eg, EMR).
99495, 99496	Transitional Care Management Services	For 30 days post discharge hospital or skilled nursing facility.
99484	Care management for behavioral health conditions	This is the behavioral health equivalent of 99490, except that there does not need to be a comprehensive care plan or practice requirements (eg, EMR).
G0506	Comprehensive assessment of and care planning for patients requiring chronic care management services (list separately in addition to primary monthly care management service) (Add-on)	This is for assessment and care management initiation that is beyond the reported evaluation and management (E/M) initiating visit. It is added to the E/M or Medicare IPPE/AWV code.

Digital Services

99091	Collection and interpretation of physiologic data, 30 mins, each 30 days	May use for 30 min of physician time in 30 days, when no more specific code exists. Can use with 99487–99490
G2010*	Image evaluation	New HCPCS code for the interpretation of an image sent by a patient with report back to the patient
G2012*	Remote check-in	A check-in with patient to avoid a face-to-face visit

(cont.)

http://www.cms.gov/Outreach-and-Education/Medicare-Learning-Network-MLN/MLNProducts/PreventiveServices.html

https://www.cms.gov/Medicare/Prevention/PrevntionGenInfo/medicare-preventive-services/MPS-QuickReferenceChart-1.html

https://www.cms.gov/Outreach-and-Education/Medicare-Learning-Network-MLN/MLNProducts/Downloads/MedicarePreventiveServicesNationalEducationProducts.pdf

https://www.cms.gov/Outreach-and-Education/Medicare-Learning-Network-MLN/MLNProducts/Downloads/MLNPrevArticles.pdf

G0008, G0009	Flu and Pneumonia Vaccination	Use CPT and Q codes for vaccine supply
G0402	Initial Preventative Physical Exam; "Welcome to Medicare" Preventive Exam	http://www.cms.gov/Outreach-and-Education/Medicare-Learning-Network-MLN/MLNProducts/downloads/MPS_QRI_IPPE001a.pdf If necessary and performed, E/M may be reported same date with modifier -25.
G0438, G0439	Annual Wellness Visits	http://www.cms.gov/Outreach-and-Education/Medicare-Learning-Network-MLN/MLNProducts/Downloads/AWV_Chart_ICN905706.pdf If necessary and performed, E/M may be reported same date with modifier -25.
G0442, G0443	Alcohol Screening/Counseling	https://www.cms.gov/Outreach-and-Education/Medicare-Learning-Network-MLN/MLNMattersArticles/downloads/MM7791.pdf
G0444	Depression Screen	https://www.cms.gov/Outreach-and-Education/Medicare-Learning-Network-MLN/MLNMattersArticles/downloads/MM7637.pdf
G0446	Intensive Behavioral Therapy for CVD	https://www.cms.gov/Outreach-and-Education/Medicare-Learning-Network-MLN/MLNMattersArticles/downloads/MM7636.pdf
G0447	Intensive Behavioral Therapy for Obesity	http://www.cms.gov/Outreach-and-Education/Medicare-Learning-Network-MLN/MLNMattersArticles/downloads/MM7641.pdf

Other Important Procedure Codes

93793	Warfarin Management	Use for each INR reviewed with follow-up instructions to patient
G0179, G0180 G0181, G0182	Home Care Certification Home/Hospice Care Plan Oversight	These services are for time spent with professionals on patients who are receiving covered home care or hospice. https://www.cms.gov/Outreach-and-Education/Medicare-Learning-Network-MLN/MLNMattersArticles/Downloads/SE1436.pdf An educational item provided by one of the regional Medicare contractors is linked. There is limited official CMS information except on certification. https://med.noridianmedicare.com/web/jfb/specialties/em/care-plan-oversight-cpo
HCPCS "J" codes	Codes for drugs administered (eg, steroids)	

Many other codes are relevant to practice (eg, EKG), but not listed for brevity. Geriatric Mental Health and Neuropsychological Testing codes not listed—see CPT.

Index

Page references followed by *t* and *f* indicate tables and figures, respectively.
Trade names are in *italics*.

Hypotonic sodium loss, 199
Hypovolemic hyponatremia, 200
Hypoxemia, 64, 276*t*
Hypoxia, 74*t*

I

Pneumatic compression
    for DVT/PE prophylaxis, 31*t*
    for hip fracture surgery, 217
    for RLS, 347
    for venous insufficiency, 52
    for venous ulcers, 339
Pneumococcal vaccination, 105, 157, 158,
        160, 197, 289*t*, 290*t*
Pneumonia, 172–175
    treatment of, 174*t*, 179, 187*t*
    vaccination against, 289*t*, 290*t*
Pneumovax (PPSV23 pneumococcal
        polysaccharide vaccine), 197, 289*t*
POA (power of attorney) for healthcare, 273
Pocketalker, 149, 150
Podiatrists, 129*t*
Polacrilex gum *(Nicorette),* 353*t*
POLST (Physician Orders for Life-Sustaining
        Treatment), 11, 274
Polycarbophil, 137, 138*t*, 145
Polycythemia vera, 157
Polydipsia, 199, 200
Polyethylene glycol (PEG, *MiraLAX*)
    for constipation, 137, 138, 139*t*
    for FI, 170
Polyhexamethylene biguanide (PHMB), 334
Polymeric membrane dressings, 334*t*
Polymyalgia rheumatica, 232–233
Polymyxin B, 333
Polymyxin/trimethoprim, 120, 120*t*
Polypharmacy, 8
Polysomnography, 344
Polythiazide *(Renese),* 59*t*
Polyunsaturated fatty acids, 48, 51, 115
Polyuria, nocturnal, 168
Posaconazole *(Noxafil),* 191*t*–192*t*
Positioning devices, 338
Positive airway pressure (PAP), 345
Positron emission tomography (PET), 291
POST (Physician Orders for Scope of
        Treatment), 274
Post-herpetic neuralgia
    pain management, 253*t*, 261*t*, 270*t*
    pharmacologic management, 180, 246
Postmenopausal bleeding, 361
Postmenopausal state, 361

Post-prandial glucose (PPG), 106*t*
Postprandial hypotension, 70
Post-traumatic stress disorder (PTSD), 42,
        43, 259
Postural hypotension. *See* Orthostatic
        hypotension
Postural impingement of vertebral artery, 235*t*
Postural instability, 240*t*
Postvoid residual (PVR), 162, 294
Potassium
    for dehydration, 198
    for HTN, 58
    low-potassium diet, 196, 202
    for refeeding syndrome prevention, 204
Potassium, sodium, and magnesium sulfate
        (*Suprep* bowel prep kit), 139*t*
Potassium disorders, 196, 197, 201–202, 302
Potassium iodide, 102
Potassium phosphate, 204
Potassium-sparing drugs, 23*t*, 59*t*
Potassium supplements, 58
Povidone iodine, 334
Power of attorney (POA) for healthcare, 11,
        273
PPG (post-prandial glucose), 106*t*
PPIs. *See* Proton-pump inhibitors
PPSV23 pneumococcal polysaccharide
        vaccine *(Pneumovax),* 197, 289*t*
Pradaxa, 37*t*. *See also* Dabigatran
Praluent (alirocumab), 56*t*
PrameGel (pramoxifen), 145
Pramipexole
    for depression, 90
    for Parkinson disease, 90, 241*t*
    for periodic limb movement disorder, 348
    for REM sleep behavior disorder, 348
    for RLS, 347
Pramipexole ER, 241*t*
Pramlintide *(Symlin),* 109*t*
Pramoxifen *(Proctofoam, PrameGel),* 145
Prandin (repaglinide), 108*t*
Prasugrel *(Effient)*
    for ACS, 46
    for antithrombotic therapy, 30*t*
    cessation before surgery, 286, 287
    for chronic angina, 47